AFRICAN TRADITIONAL MEDICINE

AFRICAN TRADITIONAL MEDICINE

Philemon Omerenma Amanze

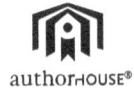

AuthorHouse™
1663 Liberty Drive
Bloomington, IN 47403
www.authorhouse.com
Phone: 1-800-839-8640

© 2011 by Philemon Omerenma Amanze. All rights reserved.

No part of this book may be reproduced, stored in a retrieval system, or transmitted by any means without the written permission of the author.

First published by AuthorHouse   11/10/2011

ISBN: 978-1-4670-0012-3 (sc)
ISBN: 978-1-4670-0013-0 (ebk)

Printed in the United States of America

Any people depicted in stock imagery provided by Thinkstock are models, and such images are being used for illustrative purposes only.
Certain stock imagery © Thinkstock.

This book is printed on acid-free paper.

Because of the dynamic nature of the Internet, any web addresses or links contained in this book may have changed since publication and may no longer be valid. The views expressed in this work are solely those of the author and do not necessarily reflect the views of the publisher, and the publisher hereby disclaims any responsibility for them.

TABLE OF CONTENTS

CHAPTER ONE

1.0	GENERAL INTRODUCTION	1
1.1	Statement of the Problem	4
1.2	Aims and Objectives	7
1.3	Theoretical Significance of the Study	8
1.4	Delimitations	8
1.5	Limitations	9
1.6	Definition of Terms	10
1.6.1	Traditional Medicine	10
1.6.2	Explicable form of Traditional Medicine	12
1.6.3	Inexplicable form of Traditional Medicine	12
1.6.4	Herbs	13
1.6.5	Herbal Medicine	13
1.6.6	Ellen Gould white	14
1.6.7	Seventh-day Adventist Church	14
1.6.8	Omnivorous Diet	15
1.6.9	Ovo-lacto Vegetarian Diet	15
1.6.10	Lacto Vegetarian Diet	15
1.6.11	Strict Vegetarian (Vegan) Diet	16
1.6.12	Diet Based on Meats	16
1.6.13	Bible	16
1.7	Review of Literature	17
1.8	Methodology/Instrumentation	52
1.8.1	Questionnaires	54
1.8.2	Interviews	55

1.9	Data Collection	56
1.10	Sampling Procedures	57
1.11	Validity of Instruments	57
1.12	Organization of the Thesis	58

CHAPTER TWO

2.0	IDENTIFICATION OF THE SEVENTH-DAY ADVENTIST CHURCH AND LOCATION OF REMOLAND	61
2.1	Identification of the Seventh-day Adventist Church	61
2.1.1	Word of God	63
2.1.2	The Godhead	63
2.1.3	God the Father	64
2.1.4	God the Son	64
2.1.5	God the Holy Spirit	65
2.1.6	Creation	65
2.1.7	The Nature of Man	65
2.1.8	The Great Controversy	66
2.1.9	The Life, Death and Resurrection of Christ	66
2.1.10	The Experience of Salvation	67
2.1.11	Growing in Christ	67
2.1.12	The Church	69
2.1.13	The Remnant and its Mission	70
2.1.14	Unity in the Body of Christ	70
2.1.15	Baptism	71
2.1.16	The Lord's Supper	71
2.1.17	The Spiritual Gift	72
2.1.18	The Gift of Prophecy	72
2.1.19	The Law of God	73
2.1.20	The Sabbath	73
2.1.21	Stewardship	74
2.1.22	Christian Behaviour	74

2.1.23	The Marriage and the Family	75
2.1.24	Christ's Ministry in the Heavenly Sanctuary	76
2.1.25	The Second Coming of Christ	77
2.1.26	Death and Resurrection	77
2.1.27	The Millennium and the End of Sin	78
2.1.28	The New Earth	78
2.2	Geographical Location of Remoland	79
2.3	Population	79
2.4	Origin of Remoland	81
2.5.	Culture and Social activities	82
2.6.	Economic Activities and Revenues	83
2.7	Religions in Remoland	85
2.8	African traditional Medicine and Remoland Worldview	85

CHAPTER THREE

3.0 THE HISTORY OF THE PRACTICE OF TRADITIONAL MEDICINE FROM BIBLICAL TIMES TO CONTEMPORARY PERIOD AND ITS RELEVANCE TO SEVENTH-DAY ADVENTISTS 90

3.1	The Background to the Practice of Traditional Medicine	90
3.2	China	94
3.3	India	94
3.4	Egypt	95
3.5	Middle East	100
3.6	Greece	100
3.7	The Romans	106
3.8	The Arabians	109
3.9	The Practice of Traditional Medicine in the Garden of Eden	110
3.10	The Practice of Traditional Medicine during the Old Testament	112

3.11	The Practice of Traditional Medicine during the New Testament	116
3.12	The Practice of Traditional Medicine in Contemporary Time	123
3.12.1	National Policy	126

CHAPTER FOUR

4.0	THE PRACTICE OF TRADITIONAL MEDICINE AMONG SEVENTH-DAY ADVENTISTS	128
4.1	Background of the Adventist Health Message	129
4.2	Adventist Lifestyle Highlighted	130
4.3	AH-NEWSTART	134
4.3.1	Attitude	135
4.3.2	Hygiene	137
4.3.3	Nutrition	143
4.3.3.1	Tea, coffee and Sudden death	144
4.3.3.2	Validation of Medical Science	147
4.3.3.3	Decaffeinated coffee and Tea	148
4.3.3.4	Alcohol, Brain Damage and Loss of Life	148
4.3.3.5	Confirmation by Medical Science	150
4.3.3.6	Fats Causing Heart and Blood-Vessel Diseases	152
4.3.3.7	The Witness of Medical Science	154
4.3.3.8	Sugar and Disease	163
4.3.3.9	Witness of Medical Science	164
4.3.3.10	Eating Right and Watching Calories	168
4.3.3.11	Height and Weight Guidelines	169
4.3.4	Exercise	173
4.3.4.1	Why is Exercise so Important	174
4.3.4.2	How Exercise Affects Glucose	175
4.3.5	Water	176
4.3.5.1	Water is Essential to Life	177
4.3.5.2	Water Aids Body Metabolism	178

4.3.5.3	Water is Necessary for Weight Loss	178
4.3.5.4	Water Helps the Digestive System Function Efficiently	179
4.3.5.5	Water Prevents Dehydration	179
4.3.5.6	Body Temperature	180
4.3.5.7	Water is needed for Breathing	180
4.3.5.8	The Brain Needs Water to Function Optimally	181
4.3.5.9	Water needed by the Kidneys	181
4.3.5.10	Body Joints need Water to work well	182
4.3.5.11	Adequate Water Intake Needed During Pregnancy	182
4.3.5.12	Drinking Water and other Beverages	183
4.3.5.13	How much Water should we drink?	184
4.3.5.14	Water is needed both internally and externally	184
4.3.6	Sunlight	188
4.3.6.1	Types of Light	189
4.3.6.2	Benefits of Sunlight	190
4.3.6.3	Sunshine Boots Immune System	190
4.3.6.4	Sunlight Aids Body Metabolism	191
4.3.6.5	Sunlight, Body and Cancer	192
4.3.7	Temperance	194
4.3.7.1	Conditions for Temperance	195
4.3.7.2	The Sense of Shame	195
4.3.7.3	The Sense of Honour	196
4.3.8	Air	198
4.3.8.1	Air Pollution and Health	199
4.3.8.2	Air Pollution adversely affects our Health	200
4.3.8.3	Relationship between Indoor and Outdoor Air	200
4.3.8.4	How to Improve Indoor Quality Air	201
4.3.8.5	Adverse Effects of Smoking	202
4.3.9	Rest	203
4.3.10	Trust in God	205

CHAPTER FIVE

5.0.	THE IMPACT OF THE PRACTICE AND USE OF AFRICAN TRADITIONAL MEDICINE AMONG SEVENTH-DAY ADVENTISTS	207
5.1	Herbal Medicine	207
5.2.	Bitter Leaf	209
5.3.	Pawpaw	212
5.4.	Coconut	217
5.4.1	History and Origin	217
5.4.2	Coconut Oil	218
5.5.	Aloe Vera	220
5.5.1	History of Aloe Vera	221
5.5.2	Maintenance of Skin Elasticity	222
5.5.3	Anti-viral Activity	223
5.5.4	Accelerated action of healing	223
5.5.5	Strong antioxidant and Immune-stimulant	223
5.5.6	Aloe Vera is also used for the treatment of burns	224
5.5.7	Raw or Processed Aloe Vera Gel	224
5.6.	Early Health and Medical Publications	225
5.7.	Endorsement of Adventist Lifestyle	227
5.8.	Relationship between Health and Gospel Messages	228
5.8.1	The Humanitarian Principle	229
5.8.2	The Evangelical Principle	230
5.8.3	The Stereological Principle	231
5.8.4	Health Care Institutions	232
5.9.	Churches and Health Relationships	233
5.10.	Seventh-day Adventist Hospital, Ile-Ife	238
5.11.	Seventh-day Adventist School of Nursing, Ile-Ife	241
5.12.	Seventh-day Adventist Postgraduate Medical Education	243
5.13.	Adventist Hospital, Aba	245

5.14. Seventh-day Adventist Hospital, Jengre, Plateau state 249

CHAPTER SIX

6.0 DATA ANALYSIS AND PRESENTATION OF FINDINGS ON THE PRACTICE AND USE OF AFRICAN TRADITIONAL MEDICINE AMONG SEVENTH DAY ADVENTISTS IN REMOLAND OGUN STATE 253

6.1 Introduction 253
6.2 Population 254
6.3 Sampling Procedures 255
6.4 Questionnaires Analysis 256
6.5 Frequency Tables on the Practice and Use of African Traditional Medicine among Seventh-day Adventists In Remoland of Ogun State 257
6.6 The Practice And Use of African Traditional Medicine Among Seventh-day Adventists in Remoland of Ogun State and Some Study Variables 341
6.7 Personal Interviews reports 350
6.7.1 Respondents' Understanding Of African Traditional Medicine 351
6.7.2 Materials Used In Traditional Medical Practice Responses 353
6.7.3 Who introduce you To African Traditional Medicine? .. 354
6.7.4 Benefits One Can Derive From The Use Of African Traditional Medicine? 355
6.7.5 Dangers That You Have Discovered In The Practice And Use Of This Medicine? 356
6.7.6 List Of Some Danger 356
6.7.7 Comparison of traditional with the Modern ways of Medication 358
6.7.8 Referral of Patients to a Traditional medical healer? (question for modern medical workers). 358

6.7.9	Referral of Patients by Other Medical Worker or Hospital? (question for traditional herbalist).	359
6.7.10	Nature Of The Sickness Referred To You?	359
6.7.11	Opinions on The Combination Of African Traditional Medicine And Modern Ways Of Healing	360

CHAPTER SEVEN

7.0	SUMMARY, RECOMMENDATION AND CONCLUSIONS	365
7.1	Summary of Findings	365
7.2	Suggestions	371

BIBLIOGRAPHY	375
PRIMARY/ORAL SOURCES	379
SECONDARY SOURCES	393
A. BOOKS	393
B. JOURNAL ARTICLES	404
C. ENCYCLOPEDIA	409
D. DICTIONAIRIES	409
E. COMMENTARIES	410
F. UNPUBLISHED MATERIALS	410
G. DAILIES	411
H. INTERNET - WORLD WIDE WEB	413
APPENDICES	417

LIST OF FIGURES

Figure I	Effect Of Alcohol On Different Parts Of The Human Body	152
Figure II	Products Derived From Soybeans	156
Figure III	Comparison Of Soyabeans With Meat Products	159
Figure IV	Different Types Of Diet Compared With Endurance During Physical Exercise	161
Figure V	Ten Generations Before The Flood (Ate Non-Flesh Food)	162
Figure VI	Ten Generations After The Flood (Ate Flesh Diet)	163
Figure VII	The Vegetarian Food Pyramid	167
Figure VIII	Daily Caloric Needs	169
Figure IX	Weight And Height Guidelines For Men And Women	171
Figure X	Daily Need Of Calories According To Profession	172
Figure XI	Physical Activities And Consumption Of Calories Per Hour Chart	176
Figure XII	Location Of Sda Health Institutions In Nigeria	236
Figure XIII	Medical Directors Of Sda Hospital, Ile-Ife (1940-2002)	240
Figure XIV	Seventh-Day Adventist Hospital, Le-Ife Statistics	241
Figure XV	Statistics Of Students Who Graduated 1994-2004	242

Figure XVI	Some Postgraduate Medical Education Students At Sda Hospital Ile-Ife, Osun State, Nigeria.	244
Figure XVII	Medical Directors Of The Seventh-Day Adventist Hospital And Motherless Babies' Home, Aba	246
Figure XIX	Seventh-Day Adventist Hospital And Motherless Babies' Home, Aba- Immunization Department— January-December, 2005	248
Figure XX	Seventh-Day Adventist Hospital And Motherless Babies' Home, Aba-Family Planning Department January-December, 2005	249
Figure XXI	Jengre Seventh-Day Adventist Hospital, Statistics 2001-October, 2004	251
Figure XXII	The Membership Of The 28 Different Seventh-Day Adventist Congregations In Remoland Of Ogun State	254
Figure XXIII	Summary Of Populations, Samples And Returns	256
Figure XXIV	Frequency Table On The Gender Of Respondents	257
Figure XXV	Frequency Table On The Ages Of Respondents	259
Figure XXVI	Frequency Table Of Tribes/Ethnic Groups Of Respondents	261
Figure XXVII	Frequency Table On The Nationalities Of Respondents	263
Figure XXVIII	Frequency Table On The Educational Status Of Respondents	265
Figure XXIX	Marital Status Of Respondents	267
Figure XXX	Frequency Table On Religious Affiliations Of Respondents Before Becoming Seventh-Day Adventists	269

Figure XXXI	Length Of Time Of Being Sda Church Member	271
Figure XXXII	Frequency Table Showing No. Of Sda Who Use Alternative Methods Of Healing	273
Figure XXXIII	Reasons For Traditional Medicine	277
Figure XXXIV	Motivation For Traditional Medicine	279
Figure XXXV	Parts Of The Body That Needed To Be Healed	281
Figure XXXVI	Forms Of Medicine Used	283
Figure XXXVII:	Length Of Time Medicine Was Used	285
Figure XXXVIII	The FreqUency Of Using Traditional Medicine	287
Figure XXXIX	Nature Of The Sickness	287
Figure XL	How Diseases That Defied Orthodox Medication Were Treated	289
Figure XLI	Support Of Traditional Medication By The Sda Church	291
Figure XLII	Ways Through Which The Sda Church Supports The Use Of Traditional Medicine	293
Figure XLIII	Why Do You Think The Sda Church Does Not Encourage Her Members To Embrace Traditional Medical Practice	296
Figure XLIV	Biblical Support For The Use Of Traditional Medicine	299
Figure XLV	Biblical Examples Where Traditional Medications Were Used	300
Figure XLVI	Who Introduced You To The Use Of Traditional Medicine	303
Figure XLVII	Is Traditional Medicine Better Than The Modern One?	305
Figure XLVIII	Nature Of Sickness That Led To The Use Of Traditional Medicine	307
Figure XLIX	Time For Traditional Medicine	308
Figure L	Reasons For Using Traditional Medicine	310

Figure LI	Are Members Aware You Are Using Traditional Medicine	313
Figure LII	Attitude Of The Church Towoards Traditional Medication	315
Figure LIII	Pastor's Attitude Towards The Use Of Traditional Medicine	317
Figure LIV	Any Education On The Importance Of Traditional Medication?	319
Figure LV	Has The Church Disciplined Any One Who Practiced Or Used Traditional Medicine?	321
Figure LVI	Has Traditional Medicine Made Any Observable Impact In Your Life?	323
Figure LVII	Has Traditioanl Medicine Made Any Impact In Your Life?	325
Figure LVIII	Has Traditional Medicine Made Any Impact On The Family?	327
Figure LVIX	Has Traditional Medicine Made Any Impact On The CHurch	330
Figure LX	What Is The Extent Of Using Traditional Medcine?	333
Figure LXI	Do You See Any Dangers In The Use Of Traditional Medicine?	335
Figure LXII	List Dangers Associated With Traditional Medicine	337
Figure LXIII	Why Some Sda Church Members Abhor Traditional Medicine?	339
Figure LXIV	Map Of Nigeria Showing Yoruba Speaking Area	435
Figure LXV	Map Of Nigeria Showing All The States Including Ogun Where The Study Was Made	436
Figure LXVI	Map Of Ogun State Showing Different Sections Of Remoland	437

DEDICATION

This book is dedicated to the Greatest Physician Who ever lived, Jesus Christ and to all medical missionaries who have contributed or would be contributing to the ministry of health and healing by using God's natural agencies.

ACKNOWLEDGMENTS

Many are the persons and organizations involved in this research. It is my pleasure, therefore to acknowledge these persons and groups who have contributed immensely to the successful completion of this work.

First of all, I am greatly indebted to my advisor, Dr. Elisha O. Babalola, who introduced me into African Traditional Religion with emphasis on African traditional medicine. It has been said that the closest academic relationship is that which exists between a doctoral student and his supervisor. This was proved true in my case. He afforded me the golden privilege of consulting him at any time for guidance, counsel, direction as well as throwing his personal collections and library open to my use. He finally saw me through my doctoral dissertation. It was both a pleasure and privilege to have been supervised by him.

I am grateful to the Babcock University Administrative Committee, BUADCOM, Ilishan Remo, Ogun State that gave both the approval and financial sponsorship that enabled me commence and complete this doctoral study. My thanks equally go to the Supervisory Committee of the Ellen G. White-SDA Research Centre, Babcock University, Ilishan Remo Ogun State and the Babcock University Board of Trustees, Ilishan Remo, Ogun State, Nigeria for granting me the rare opportunities of visiting both the Branch Office of the White Estate at Andrews University, Michigan as well as the White Estate at the General Conference headquarters, Maryland, both in USA for research materials.

Special thanks go to my doctoral committee members as well as the University Examiners who were both conversant in my area of study as well as versatile in research methodology, and this afforded me the opportunity of being objectively evaluated at every stage of the thesis writing. I thank Professors. M. A. Ojo, S. G. A. Onibere, E. O. Ogunbodede and Dr. S. A. Babalola for encouraging the consultation of qualified authorities to maintain high academic standards. The role of the University's External examiner, Professor M. Y. Nabofa in the accomplishment of this academic work is equally appreciated.

Other persons who were absolutely indispensable in many ways were Professor S. N. Chioma and Sal. Okwubunka, they encouraged me to go back to the university for a Doctorate Degree. That persuasion did not fall on deaf ears. Elder Emmanuel Egorugwu and Aunty 'Konye wrote constantly from Chicago and called my attention to the importance of a higher degree as far back as 1996 and Professor J. A. Kayode Makinde for reminding me severally that the time for that doctoral study has come. Thank you all for the confidence you had that I could do it by His grace.

My deep appreciation goes to Josiah A. Amanze, my father, whose 86th birthday marked the commencement of this research, yet he promised to attend my graduation after the completion of this study. I am grateful to Elder Samuel U. Amanze, my elderly brother, Shepherdess Christiana Ine, my mother in-law, Engineer James and Joy Amanze for providing the laptop computer which was used in typing this work and to the rest of our family for your supports and prayers. I am also grateful to Miss Abimbola O. Folorunso, the Research Assistant at the Ellen G. White-SDA Research Centre, Babcock University, Ilishan Remo, Ogun State, Nigeria for typing the original draft of this study and for taking care of the office during my numerous periods of absence. In the same way I express my thanks to Mr. Samuel Kehinde for interpreting for me during the interviews conducted in many communities within Remoland, Ogun State, Nigeria.

I remain very grateful to my beloved wife, Ruth, who for the five years it has taken to complete my Ph. D studies has constantly encouraged, prayed and provided a conducive home atmosphere that contributed to this success. This dissertation is as much your achievement as it is mine.

Finally, my praises, thanks, adoration and worship go to the Father of all mankind for His leadership in my life and for helping me complete this study. Indeed, *Ogechi ka Nma*—God's time is the best.

Philemon Omerenma Amanze,
Department of Religious studies,
Babcock University,
Nigeria.
May 2011

ABSTRACT

This study identified and assessed the patterns and the extent of the practice and use of traditional medicine among the Seventh-day Adventists in Remoland of Ogun State, Nigeria; it also examined the veracity of the claim that the practice and use of African traditional medicine amounted to idolatry; analyzed the social, economic and spiritual impacts of the practice and use of traditional medicine on Seventh-day Adventists in Remoland; and discussed the interplay between African traditional medical practices and Western medical practices in the health care delivery system of the Seventh-day Adventists.

A multi-dimensional methodology was adopted. Firstly, phenomenological method was used by applying the principle of epoche to observe and interpret Seventh-day Adventists' belief and practice on the use of African and Western medicine. Secondly, questionnaire and oral interview were used to gather information from Seventh-day Adventists and non Adventist. Fifty Seventh-day Adventists made up of ten pastors, fifteen men and women leaders respectively, ten medical personnel; and fifteen traditional birth attendants, two bone setters and thirty three traditional medical practitioners were interviewed to know the materials and forms of traditional medicine they used. The data generated through the questionnaire were analysized using descriptive and inferential statistics.

This study discovered that African traditional medicine played important roles among Seventh-day Adventists in particular and Christians in general. Among the Adventists, the use of herbal medicine had been confirmed through the Bible and the ministry of Ellen G. White, a pioneer Seventh-day Adventist. It was also discovered that African traditional medicine complemented the deficiencies in modern medicine in handling some birth related issues among others. It was also discovered that African traditional medicine was widely used by Seventh-day Adventists because it was affordable, available and effective to meet their health needs.

African traditional medicine was used in the explicable or inexplicable form. The inexplicable form involved the use of incantations, sacrifices, magic and mystic powers that were beyond human comprehension and empirical laboratory investigations. The explicable form on the other hand, used herbs, rhizomes, plants and other materials which could be pharmacologically and scientifically explained. It was further discovered that Seventh-day Adventists in Remoland of Ogun State, Nigeria used the explicable form of African traditional medicine to meet their health needs.

This study concluded that the Seventh-day Adventist Church in Remoland of Ogun State, Nigeria played an important role in the use of African traditional medicine to meet the health-care needs of the people in the area.

CHAPTER ONE

1.0 GENERAL INTRODUCTION

The present dissertation is written in the general context of the extensive tradition of academic inquiry dealing with the interfacing of medicine and religion among various religious groups in general and within the Seventh-day Adventists in particular. This study seeks to work within the academic evaluative and comparative traditions, which have been ably demonstrated in the works of P. A. Dopamu,[1] Abayomi Sofowora,[2] Anthony A. Elujoba,[3] Jethro Kloss,[4] Ellen G.

---

[1] P. Ade Dopamu. "Scientific Basis of African Magic and Medicine: The Yoruba Experience" in <u>African Culture, Modern Science and Religious Thought</u> (Ilorin: Decency Printers & Stationeries, 2003), pp. 442-461.

[2] Abayomi Sofowora: <u>Medicinal Plants and Traditional Medicine in Africa.</u> (Ibadan: Spectrum Books, 1993), pp. 68, 100-108.

[3] A. A. Elujoba. <u>Pharmacognosy for Health and Culture. The PHC Jungle Connection.</u> Inaugural Lectures series 134. (Ile-Ife: Obafemi Awolowo University Press, 1999), Pp. 4 - 50

[4] Jethro Kloss. <u>Back to Eden</u>. (California: Woodbridge Press Publishing Company, 1997), pp. 44-385; 666-667.

White,[5] Anselm Adodo,[6] J. Agbebahunsi,[7] Mervyn G. Hardinge,[8] A. O. Nkwoka,[9] M. O. Raimi,[10] Leo Van Dolson,[11] and Xiaorui Zhang.[12]

---

[5] Ellen G. White. Ministry of Healing. (Boise, Idaho: Pacific Press Publishing Association, 1942), pp. 271-337.

[6] Anselm Adodo. Nature Power. A Christian Approach to Herbal Medicine, (Akure: Don Bosco Training Center, 2002), pp. 9-175.

[7] J. M. Agbedahunsi. "Plant Utilization in Indigenous Medical System" Africana Marburgensia. Vol. XXVI, IX2, 1993, pp. 14-20

[8] Mervyn Hardinge. A Physician Explains Ellen White's Counsels on Drugs, Herbs, and Natural Remedies. (Hagerstown, MD: Review and Herald Publishing Association, 2001), pp. 28-205.

[9] A. O. Nkwoka. "Healing: The Biblical Perspective". Africana Marburgensia, vol. XXVI, IX2, 1993, pp. 59-69

[10] M. O. Raimi. "Religion, Fertility and Population Control - Iwo Yoruba Experience" Africana Marburgensia, Vol. XXVI, IX2, 1993, pp. 71-76

[11] Leo Van Dolson. Health, Happy, Holy. (Washington, DC: Review and Herald Publishing Association, nd), pp. 15-47

[12] Xiaorui Zhang. "Traditional Medicine and WHO" World Health Organization. The Magazine of the World Health Organization, 49th Year, No. 2, March to April, 1996, pp. 4-5

Others include Lateef A. Salako,[13] Markus Muller,[14] Isabel Carter,[15] Bolaji Idowu,[16] John S. Mbiti,[17] E. O. Babalola,[18] Elizabeth Kafaru,[19] Taryl Felhaber,[20] S. E. Ikenga-metuh,[21] L. Lagwuanya,[22]

---

[13] Lateef A. Salako. "An African Perspective" World Health. <u>The Magazine of the World Health Organization</u>, 51st Year No. 3, May-June, 1998, IX ISSN 0043-8502, pp. 24-25

[14] Markus Muller. <u>Footsteps</u>: A Quarterly Newsletter Linking Health and Development Workers Around the World, No. 48, September 2001, pp. 1-3
*Markus Muller is a medical doctor working with Innocent Balagizi who is a biologist with special emphasis on traditional medicinal plants.

[15] Isabel Carter. Footsteps. A Quarterly Newsletter Linking Health and Development Workers Around the World, No. 48, September, 2001, p. 3.

[16] Bolaji Idowu. <u>African Traditional Religion—A Definition</u>. (Ibadan: Fountain Publications, 1991), pp. 199-202.

[17] John S. Mbiti. <u>African Religions and Philosophy</u>. (Ibadan: Heinemann Education Books, 1985), pp. 166-171

[18] E. O. Babalola. "in <u>Africana Marburgensia</u>. Vol. XXVI, IX2, 1993, pp. 4-12.

[19] Elizabeth Kafaru has also done a lot of work on African Traditional Medicine.

[20] Taryl Felhaber. <u>South African Traditional Healers' Primary Health Care Handbook.</u> (Cape Town: Kagi So Publishers, 1997), pp. 1-93.

[21] E. Ikenga-Metuh. Article on "African Traditional Medicine and Healing". A Theological and Pastoral Reappraisal" contained in the proceeding of the August, 1982, Nigerian Zonal WAATI Conference and the August, 1983, West African Conference of WAATI, pp. 133-129.

[22] L. Lugwuanya. :Medicine, Spiritual Healing and African Response, 1857-1924: Concerns of Christianity in African Theological Journal, vol. 23, (2000) No. 1, pp. 17-32.

A. S. Oyalana,[23] Akinleye Omoyajowo[24] and several other scholars. Specifically, this dissertation is a contextual study of the practice and use of African traditional medicine among Seventh-day Adventists who are in Remoland of Ogun State, Nigeria.

1.1. Statement of the Problem

The problem of this dissertation grew out of interest, experience as well as out of a situation to investigate the impact of the practice and use of African traditional medicine among Seventh-day Adventists who are in Remoland of Ogun State. For over eight decades, the Seventh-day Adventist Church has been in existence in the Western part of Nigeria.

The Seventh-day Adventist Church has also gone ahead to establish various medical institutions based on her philosophy of health as portrayed in the Bible and the writings of Ellen G. White. Commenting on the principles which should govern the medical and health practices among Seventh-day Adventists, Ellen G. White said among other things that:

> God has caused to grow out of the ground, herbs for the use of man, and if we understand the nature of these roots and herbs, and make a right use of them, there would not be a necessity of running to the doctor so frequently,

---

[23] A. S. Oyalana. "Spiritual Healing: A Challenge to Mainline Churches in Contemporary Nigeria. "Religion and Spirituality. (Port Harcourt: Emhai Printing and Publishing Company, 2001), pp. 125-32.

[24] Akinleye Omoyajowo. Religion, Society and the Home. (Ijebu-Ode: Vicoo International Press, 2001), pp. 95-107

and people would be in much better health than they are today.[25]

She further gave this type of medicine practice many names such as "True Remedies", "Natural Remedies", "God's Remedies", "Heaven-sent Remedies", "God's Natural Remedies", "Simple Remedies", "God's appointed Remedies", and "God's Medicine"[26] among others. The problem is here presented under the following sections:

First the practice of African traditional medicine by Seventh-day Adventists in Remoland, as the custodians for over eight decades of the philosophy of health espoused by the Church, seems not to be in consonance with that portrayed in the Sacred Scriptures and Ellen G. White writings. According to the General Conference of the Seventh-day Adventist Church, Africa-Indian Ocean Division Committee,[27] the Seventh-day Adventist Church has since its organization promoted a philosophy of health and healing.[28]

While developing a system of health care institutions which are located around the globe, a health-promoting way of life both in practice and principle has been taught to the church membership. Teachings which are based on broad principles found in the Bible and more explicitly expressed in the writings given by Ellen G.

---

[25] Ellen G. White. Selected Messages, vol. 2. (California: Pacific Press Publishing Association, 19) pp. 297-298

[26] Mervyn Hardinge, p. 13

[27] General Conference of Seventh-day Adventist Church, African-Indian Ocean Division, Working Policy, (1998), p. 209.

[28] Ibid.

White, have in recent years been validated as well as substantiated by the findings of scientific research. These discoveries which have been made in different parts of the world, have clearly demonstrated the health superiority of Seventh-day Adventists, especially of those who more closely adhere to the health philosophy espoused by the Church[29]. The Adventist Church advocates positive steps to be taken to develop a healthful lifestyle, the Church also requires the members to refrain from the use of alcoholic beverages and tobacco. The Church equally advocates that the food Adam and Eve ate at the Garden of Eden was the best and members are strongly urged to refrain from the use of flesh foods, coffee, tea, other stimulants and harmful substances.[30]

We are living in a period of the world history when the sophistries of Satan and his agents one are rampant, both within and without the Church. The philosophy of the Health Ministries Department within the Seventh-day Adventist Church is to teach every member to bring his or her way of life to be in harmony with physical law, to enjoy the benefits of better health, to live longer, and be able to differentiate between right and wrong in all situations.[31] Although the argument that African traditional medical practices among Christians amount to idolatry is rather antiquated, some Christian fundamentalists still push it. This thesis attempts to negate the argument and determine the impact of the practice and use of African traditional medicine on the spirituality of Seventh-day Adventists in Remoland.

---

[29] General Conference of Seventh-day Adventist Church, Africa-Indian Ocean Division, Working Policy, (1998), p. 209.

[30] Ibid.

[31] Ibid, p. 210

1.2 Aims and Objectives

Traditionally, most Christians do not want to be associated with anything that could link them with magicians, native doctors, witchcraft or sorcery as many of them believe that these are what the traditional medicine man represents. Yet in times of great dangers and threats to life, the Christian breaks all bounds and restrictions posed by the Christian religion to get assistance even from the traditional healers.[32] Therefore, in view of the dual allegiance and hypocritical tendency of some Christians presented above, the specific objectives of this thesis are to achieve the following:

(a) identify and assess the patterns and the extent of the practice and use of traditional medicine among the Seventh-day Adventists in Remoland;

(b) examine the veracity of the claim that the practice and use of African traditional medicine by Christians amount to idolatry;

(c) analyze the social, economic and spiritual impact of the practice and use of traditional medicine on Seventh-day Adventists in Remoland; and

(d) discuss the interplay between African traditional medical practices and Western medical practices in the health care delivery system of the Seventh-day Adventists.

---

[32] E. O. Babalola. Interaction of Religions in Yorubaland: A Theological and Social analysis. (Ile Ife: Babs-Adedeji & Sons Press, pp. 34-39), 1994

1.3   Theoretical Significance of the Study

The topic of this study was selected in view of the centrality of the Christian's conception that man should be healthy, happy and holy as God intends him to be. However, the view of many Seventh-day Adventists as noted earlier, is that traditional medical practice should be left for the adherents of African Traditional Religion. Others are of the opinion that the use and practice of African traditional medical practice is tantamount to witchcraft and sorcery. An underlying assumption inherent in these arguments is that there is a basic misconception on what the people have understood to be the practice of African traditional medicine and what they actually need for their good health and well being. It is therefore proposed that the findings of this research will ultimately be a contribution to the educational, medical and health programmes of the Seventh-day Adventist Church in Remoland of Ogun State, Nigeria in particular and to the whole world in general.

1.4   Delimitations

According to Asika[33] delimitation enables the researcher to circumscribe his work within a manageable limit. Therefore, the data on the use and practice of African traditional medicine will be limited to that which would be provided by church members and ministers within the Seventh-day Adventist Church in Remoland of Ogun State, Nigeria in a random stratified manner. The information for this work was gathered from selected Seventh-day Adventists,

---

[33]   Nnamdi Asiak. Research Methodology in the Behavioural Sciences, (Ikeja: Longman Nigeria, PLC, 2002), p. 101.

traditional birth attendants, traditional bone setters, herbalists and other medical traditional practitioners.

1.5 <u>Limitations</u>

The responses from the participants in this study might reflect only their opinions at the time of the completion of the questionnaire or during the interview. In addition, the fact that more Seventh-day Adventist members and ministers would be involved in this study, may limit its generalizability. Another limiting factor is the fact that the researcher has to work through an interpreter to reach most of the traditional health personnel like herbalists, bone setters attendants, and other traditional healers.

In this study, it was assumed that the participants' perceptions of the use and practice of African traditional medicine among Seventh-day Adventists in Remoland of Ogun State could be objectively and effectively determined through the questions asked. It was also assumed that the respondents would accurately report and reflect their understanding of the practice and use of African traditional medicine through their responses in the questionnaire and interview.

1.6 Definition of Terms

Definition of terms has to do with the explanation of unfamiliar terms and concepts.[34] The following definitions are therefore used for the purpose of this study:

1.6.1 Traditional Medicine:

This term has evolved over many centuries of usage by mankind and according to Markus Muller and Innocent Balagizi, there is no one clear definition of traditional medicine. The World Health Organization, WHO, has however, defined traditional medicine as the sum total of the knowledge, skills, and practices based on the various theories, beliefs and experiences, indigenous to people of different cultures, which could be used in the maintenance of health, as well as on the prevention, diagnosis, improvement or treatment of physical and mental illnesses.[35]

Traditional medicine has also been described as:

> the total combination of knowledge and practices, which are used in the diagnosis, prevention, or elimination of a physical, mental, or social disease and which may depend solely on previous experience and observation that has

---

[34] T. I. Salau. Introduction to Research Methodology. (Ilaro: Limbs Press, 1998), p. 105.

[35] WHO. General Guidelines for Methodologies on Research and Evaluation of the Traditional Medicine: World Health Organization, (Geneva, 2000), p. 1

been handed down from one generation to another either verbally or in writing.[36]

On the other hand, traditional medicine is considered to be the sum total of the knowledge, skills, and practices of medicine based on the theory, beliefs and experiences indigenous to diverse cultures and in maintaining good health as well as in curing various diseases.[37]

Indeed, long historical usage of numerous practices of traditional medicine, with the established experiences passed from one generation to another, has ably demonstrated the efficacy, safety, availability and usefulness of traditional medicine. This, however, does not obliterate the need for further scientific research, which is needed to provide additional evidence of its efficacy and safety among various groups of people in Africa and the world in general.

In some parts of the world, terms such as complimentary, alternatives or non-conventional medicine are also used interchangeably with traditional medicine. Other terms, which have been used to describe the same term above, include simple remedies, natural remedies, true remedies, God's remedies, heaven-sent remedies, God's appointed remedies and God's medicine among others.[38] Traditional medication on the other hand involves the use of three outstanding components. These are herbal materials,

---

[36] Abayomi Sofowora, p. 2

[37] WHO. <u>Report on Interregional Workshop Intellectual Property Rights in the Context of Traditional Medicine</u>, (Bangkok, Thailand 6-8, 2000), p. 35.

[38] Mervyn Hardinge, p. 113.

animal parts and various minerals. In traditional medicine, however, herbal materials are the most widely used of all the three mentioned above.[39] Based on the above definitions, it is evident that there are two forms of traditional medicine. These are the explicable and the inexplicable forms of traditional medicine.

1.6.2   Explicable Form of Traditional Medicine:

The explicable form of traditional medical healing method uses different types of traditional medicine whose actions and potencies can be scientifically investigated and pharmacologically explained through experimental animal models. This form of traditional medicine uses herbs or other materials for healing and treating diseases just as Panadol is used for analgesic purposes.[40]

1.6.3   Inexplicable Form of Traditional Medicine:

The inexplicable form of traditional medicine involves the use of mystical, magical, psychic, supernatural, occultic and metaphysical practices in the healing process. This type of traditional medical practice cannot be probed scientifically in this era of modern science and technology. There is no physical law or theory, which can be used to explain this form of practice. This is the most dreaded and controversial form of traditional medical practice as it is shrouded in

---

[39]   WHO. General Guidelines for Methodologies on Research and Evaluation of the Traditional Medicine: World Health Organization, (Geneva, 2000), p. 3

[40]   A. A. Elujoba. "Pharmacognosy for Health and Culture". The PHC Jungle Connection. Inaugural Lectures series 134. Ile-Ife, Obafemi Awolowo University Press, p. 6

secrecy. It is beyond mere human intelligence. The unabated use of oracular diagnosis, cultic consultation, incantations, mystic activities and ritual sacrifices are part of this form of traditional medicine.[41]

1.6.4 Herbs:

These are the crude plant materials which include leaves, flowers, fruits, seeds, stems, wood, bark, roots, rhizomes or other parts of the plant which may be whole, fragmented or powdered. The herb is the source of all herbal materials which include fresh juices and fruits, gums, fixed oils, essential oils, resins, dried plant parts and powders so essential to life. These herbal materials are usually procured by indigenous procedures, which include but not limited to steaming, roasting, frying, stir baking with honey, alcohol or other beverages.[42]

1.6.5 Herbal Medicine:

Herbal medicine is a preparation derived from plant materials that have therapeutic benefits and it contains either raw or processed ingredients from one or more plants. Herbal medicine in some traditions may also contain inorganic or animal materials.[43]

---

[41] Ibid.
[42] WHO. General Guidelines for Methodologies on Research and Evaluation of the Traditional Medicine, p. 3
[43] Ibid, p. 27

1.6.6 Ellen Gould White:

This name would be used mostly as Ellen G. White or E. G. White throughout this research. She was one of the pioneer leaders of the Seventh-day Adventist Church. It was through her public ministry, which spanned over 70 years that God gave to the Seventh-day Adventist Church the divine principles, which should guide the establishment and operation of the church's health and medical institutions. She wrote over 100 books on a wide range of subjects including agriculture, marriage and family life, finance, health and medicine, education, youth development, administration, prophecy, and among others. [44]

1.6.7 Seventh-day Adventist Church:

This name would be used as SDA Church in most instances within this work. This is a World-wide Christian church organization that is established in 203 countries of the world with a membership of 16,049,101 baptized people. This church operates 7,597 educational institutions and 600 health and medical establishments around the world. [45]

---

[44] Herbert E. Douglas. Messenger of the Lord. (Ontario: Pacific Press Publishing Association 1998), pp. 40-60

[45] Seventh-day Adventist Church - Yearbook 2010 Proclaiming God's Grace. (Washington DC: Review and Herald Publishing Association, 2010), p. 4

1.6.8   Omnivorous Diet:

This is the diet followed by the greater number of people, who eat a great assortment of foods including an ample amount of animal and vegetable products.[46]

1.6.9   Ovolacto Vegetarian Diet:

An ovolacto vegetarian diet excludes meat, fish and fowl. It includes eggs and milk product in small or moderate quantities, and above all, vegetables, cereals, fruits, and garden products (vegetables, legumes and tubers). It is recognized that this provides a satisfactory diet from the nutritional point of view, and that it is easy to follow, is appropriate for children, and has great advantages over the omnivorous diet.[47]

1.6.10   Lacto Vegetarian Diet:

It includes only milk and dairy products as sources of food originating from animals. It is equally satisfactory in nutritional value. The proteins in the milk complement and enrich vegetable proteins, so that it is not difficult to obtain the essential amino acids. It is preferable that especially adults should use low or non-milk products.[48]

---

[46] George D. Pamplona. Enjoy It-Foods for Healing and Prevention. (Madrid: Editorial Safeliz, 1999), p. 61
[47] Ibid, p. 20
[48] George D. Pamplona, pp. 61, 62.

1.6.11   Strict Vegetarian (Vegan) Diet:

It includes only vegetable foods, omitting animal products. It provides all the necessary nutrients, including proteins, providing that precautions are taken at the time that selection and combination of foods are made. The strict vegetarian may need vitamin B12 supplement.[49] This kind of diet presents interesting advantages when compared to the omnivorous diet and provides the best results in the prevention and treatment of chronic degenerative diseases, such as arteriosclerosis (circulatory problems, angina pectoris, myocardial attacks), rheumatic diseases and cancer, among others.[50]

1.6.12   Diet Based on Meats:

Meat and fish are its basic components. This type of diets results in an excess of proteins and fats and a lack of carbohydrates and fiber, with negative repercussions upon health, for example, an excess of uric acid and cholesterol, intestinal putrefaction, and a greater possibility of cardiac problems (such as heart attacks, angina pectoris and cancer).[51]

1.6.13   Bible:

This is the book made up of sacred writings which are accepted by Christians as having divine authority because God inspired its writers. For the Jews, the Bible was made up of 24 separate

---

[49]   Ibid.
[50]   Ibid.
[51]   Ibid, p. 20

books. For Christians, the Bible is made up of 39 books of the Old Testament in addition to 27 other books which make up the New Testament. The Roman Catholic Bible has 12 additional writings which Protestants classify as Apocrypha. For the purpose of this work, the Christian Bible made up of 66 books has been used. All quotations in this thesis has been taken from the Authorized King James Version (KJV)

1.7 Review of Literature

This review focuses on various research studies which are related to the practice of traditional medicine in all its ramifications. The intent is to ascertain the numerous works that have been carried out by researchers and scholars to determine the efficacy and effectiveness of the use and practice of African traditional medicine. Indeed, major ideas highlighted in this section are used in the development of this dissertation.

Numerous studies provide helpful background material in terms of general information concerning the relationship between religion and medical science and other sciences on one hand, and the practice of traditional medicine among religious groups on the other hand.[52] It is also a fact that many works have been done on this subject of the use and practice of African traditional medicine but none has been specifically carried out among Seventh-day Adventists in Remoland of Ogun State. The present work will therefore fill that lacuna.

---

[52] Marco T. Terreros. <u>Theistic Evolution and Its Theological Implications</u>. (Columbia: Morter Editions, 1994), p. 18.

The first literature to be reviewed is the "Scientific Basis of African Magic and Medicine: The Yoruba Experience"[53] by Professor P. Ade Dopamu. According to Prof. Dopamu, magic, medicine, religion and science had played, and would continue to play important roles among the Yoruba of Western Nigeria. He went further to assert that although the concepts of medicine and magic are intermingled and usually related, their goals and intentions are always different. Both magic and medicine came into play as a result of finding solutions to the multiple needs and problems confronting humanity. In line with this, Yoruba medicine has been defined as:

> The traditional art and science of the prevention and cure of diseases. It is the use of natural substances to prevent, treat or cure diseases. It can also mean medication used internally or externally.[54]

---

[53] P. Ade Dopamu, et all. "Scientific Basis of African Magic and Medicine: The Yoruba Experience" in African Culture, Modern Science and Religious Thought. (Ilorin: Decency Printers & Stationeries, 2003), pp. 442-461.

[54] _____ "Yoruba Magic and Medicine and Their Relevance for Today" in RELIGIONS: Journal of the Nigerian Association for the Study of Religions, vol, 4, 1979, pp. 5-6.

.Magic on the other hand is:

The art of using available resources of nature to procure non-therapeutic needs of man. It is the art of influencing course of events by means of supernatural control of nature and invocation of particular spirit aids.[55]

Having defined magic and Yoruba medicine, we still observe that their interaction for the benefit of humanity represents an integral part of African science. The similarities in the practice of magic and medicine are evident in their names as both are "oogun", "egbogi" or "isegun". Next to that is that similar materials are also used in their preparations and these include herbs, leaves, roots, barks, stems, flowers, feathers, bones, water, honey and many other substances which might be gaseous, solid or liquid. After the preparation, both the magic and medicine are almost always used in the same way by drinking, eating, wearing, burying, among many other methods.

Some basic differences are, however, observable between medicines and magic. For instance, Yoruba medicine called "Oogun Iwosan" is used for both therapeutic and prophylactic purposes. Magic on the other hand is non-therapeutic but it is used for good harvest, protection from danger, success in education and business, protection against accident plus a host of other purposes. There are instances when both magic and medicine are used in the treatment of diseases of extraordinary nature. In such a complementary situation,

---

[55] _____ "Yoruba Magic and Medicine and Their Relevance for Today" in RELIGIONS: Journal of the Nigerian Association for the Study of Religions, vol, 4, 1979, p.5

it is understood that healing would be achieved through a process known as magical-medicine.[56] It is therefore significant to note that the interplay of magic and medicine for the benefit of man in some cases represent an integral aspect of African Science.

Prof. Dopamu further opined that medicine is an object used in restoring health or preventing disease, and as such it is always used to achieve good purposes. On the other hand, magic, when it is used to achieve evil purposes, is called sorcery. In the minds of foreigners, there are always confusion in the appropriate usages of medicine, magic and sorcery. With Yoruba practitioners, there is no contradiction at all. This is because when the Yoruba practitioner heals a stomach ache, he uses medicine, when he protects someone from accident, he uses magic, and when he invokes for the purpose of harming or killing a person, he uses sorcery.

It must however, be noted that in the practice of Yoruba Medicine, there is a big difference between disease <u>arun</u> and illness <u>aisan</u>. Disease <u>arun</u> is normally referred to as an unhealthy condition caused by germs, worms, infection and other conditions which could be proved scientifically and investigated in the laboratory. Illness is caused by hostile activities of witches, sorcery and other spiritual forces which cannot be detected pathologically in the laboratory. The former "arun" could be detected and cured while the later always leads to death.[57]

---

[56] Ibid, pp. 5-6.

[57] _____ Scientific Basis of African Medicine and Magic, pp. 448, 449

Finally, he made it clear that magic and medicine are based on scientific discovery. For instance, a sick individual who comes to a traditional healer would be interested in getting healing. The traditional healer will examine, diagnose, prescribe and also provide appropriate medicine. This is indeed a rational way of handling the sick and as such it is scientific. If magic and medicine had not been useful to Africans and especially to the Yoruba of Western Nigeria, it could have fizzled out of operation a long time ago. Its constant usages coupled with its current numerous demands as attested by the many beneficiaries have proved their practical useful services to mankind.[58]

If for any reason magic, medicine or a combination of both did not achieve desired purpose, it is not because it has failed completely but may be due to the fact that we are living in an imperfect world where even modern science and technology had failed to achieve its desired results in so many areas. The inability of African science in the form of magic and medicine to achieve its desired result may, apart from the imperfections of the world, be traced to incomplete ingredients, wrong usage, evil machination or differences in the physiological make-up of the people. This is similar to an engineer or scientist proffering reasons for the little or no services received from the National Electric Power Authority(NEPA), telephone and other communication organizations, e-mail failures, aeroplane and vehicle service failures.

---

[58] _____ Scientific Basis of African Medicine and Magic, p. 447

The second literature to be reviewed is "Medicinal Plants and Traditional Medicine in Africa [59] written by Professor Abayomi Sofowora. This work began by providing a comprehensive definition of traditional medicine. He went further to reveal that traditional medicine is practiced throughout the world. Other phases of traditional medicine which include Juju, Folk medicine, ritual rites, incantation, bone setting, vegetable drug, concoction, decoction, infusion among others were equally emphasized.

This section on the Historical Review of traditional medicine actually made clear its World-wide application. Beginning with the work of Emperor Shem Nung of China between 2730 and 3000 B.C. to the materia medica of Hippocrates, the father of medicine; through the writings of Galen of Pergamas who was born about A.D. 31 and who essentially treated diseases with herbs down to current century are examples of the usage of traditional medicine for the good of humanity.

The Ayurveda, which considers the human being as small universe is an outstanding example of an indigenous system of medicine in India while acupuncture is a traditional form of therapy, which has been popularly accepted in China. The various major region of the world such as Africa, America, South-East Africa, Western Pacific-European, and the Eastern Mediterranean region have imbibed the use of traditional medicine in one way of the other.

---

[59] Abayomi Sofowora, pp. 1-23.

Finally, according to Professor Sofowora, the World Health Organization (WHO) has established a programme to coordinate the practice of traditional medicine with the objectives of fostering a more realistic approach to enable it contribute more effectively to the health care of our people; to examine its merits and maximize its useful aspects while discouraging its harmful ones and promoting the use of tested and proven knowledge and practices in traditional medicine.[60]

Dr. E. O. Babalola did another important work under the title "The Persistence of African Traditional Medicine in the Contemporary Nigeria Society—The Yoruba Case Study"[61] In this paper Dr. E. O. Babalola posits that the inability of Western Medicine to fully address and fulfill the health needs of the Africans has lead to the continuity of African traditional medicine. This has also led to the use and practice of oogun among the Yoruba of South Western Nigeria.

Traditional medicine is used to cure mystical diseases, which are not within the scope of the scientific medicine. From another direction, he submits that ailments that belong to the natural category are cured with roots and herbs. However, when the ailments are in the corridor of the supernatural, divination, which will involve offerings and sacrifices, will definitely be involved. Apart from this, healing is also holistic, and this involves soundness of the body, mind and soul. He maintained that healing also has a religious dimension.[62]

---

[60] Abayomi, Sofowora, p. 22
[61] E. O. Babalola. Africana Marbugensia, Vol. XXVI, IX2, 1993, pp. 4-12.
[62] E. O. Babalola. Africana Marbugensia, p. 9

"Plant Utilization in Indigenous Medical System"[63] was another important work done by Dr. J. M. Agbedahunsi. He traced the origin of herbal remedies to the Bible. Relevant scriptural texts were also cited to support the fact that man who was created by God was to eat the fruits of the tree and use the leaves for medicine. From the above it is discovered that plants are selected and utilized for either their medicinal purposes or dietary needs. That is not all; some other plants are equally selected due to the belief attached to them. For example, a plant with heart-shaped leaves is believed to be good for the treatment of heart diseases. Dr. J. M. Agbedahunsi further explained that the collection of the medicinal plant would influence its effectiveness and the quality of drug that could be produced from it. The season of the year and the time of the day or night are also to be noted. The age of the plant to be collected should also be taken into consideration as this might eventually affect its active pharmacological constituents.

Finally, he asserts that there should be a closer cooperation between medical scientists and traditional healers in order to achieve better results in the utilization of medicinal plants. Indeed, the training of traditional medicine practitioners will bring marked improvement in plant collection, processing formulation, standardization, packaging and preservation.[64] So I quite agree with him that there should be a coming together of the orthodox and traditional practitioner for greater efficiency and effectiveness in the practice of medicine.

---

[63] J. M. Agbedahunsi., In E. O. Babalola, <u>Africana Marbugensia</u>, pp. 14-20.

[64] J. M. Agbedahunsi., In E. O. Babalola, <u>Africana Marbugensia</u>, pp. 19 - 20

Next in the series is <u>South African Traditional Healers' Primary Health Care Handbook</u>,[65] which Taryl Felhaber edited. Commenting on traditional diagnosis, he opined that observation, Patient Self-Diagnosis and Divination are involved.

Observation: This involves taking note of symptoms, which can be seen, for instance, weak and watery eyes, restlessness, swelling or lack of concentration.

Patient Self-diagnosis: Patient Self-Diagnosis involves giving the patient the opportunity to state his or her symptoms of disease. The individual tells how the sickness develops and any possible step, which have been taken to cure it. The ability to take note of the medical history, and to ask patients questions when necessary and also to pay particular attention to the sick is important.

Divination: Three materials are used to carry out divination. These include bone throwing, psychic (Clairvoyance or telepathy) and visions or dreams. These methods are to help one get the root causes of the diseases and the method of curing them. He went further to discuss traditional treatment as being both comprehensive and holistic. It also has elements of being curative, protective, and preventive and could be natural, ritual or both. He further commented that in preparing traditional medicine, the sex of the patient is taken into consideration. This is because certain preparations are used exclusively for either a man or a woman in accordance with the individual's health need. And once medicine is prepared, it could be administered in any of these five ways: Orally (by mouth); dermally

---

[65] Taryl Felhaber. ed., pp. 28-38

(through the skin); nasally (in the nose); vaginally (through the virginal or auricularly (through the ear).

According to Felhaber, 17 other ways of administering Traditional medicine are mentioned below:

1. <u>Bathing</u>: Bathing is used as a topical application of medicine through the skin to reach the whole body. This process heals, stimulates and invigorates the body. Bathing is also used to wash off bad luck to ward off evil spirits.
2. <u>Behaving</u> This involves the role of counseling and encouragement in getting the desired compliance from the sick person. It is also used to encourage the traditional medicine leader to respect the order of this type of medication.
3. <u>Blood Cleansing:</u> This is done when the need arises to detoxify the body if possible blood-borne toxins that might have gained entrance into the body.
4. <u>Charm:</u> It is prepared for good luck, protection and for driving away bad spirits.
5. <u>Cuts (Incisions):</u> These are made in order to introduce medicine directly into the blood streams. It is also the African mode of injection and inoculation.
6. <u>Dancing:</u> Dancing is used to relieve stress while giving the body the required exercise that it needs. It is also used to communicate with the ancestors during initiation and other special occasions.

7. Diet: During the application of a particular drug, or when a patient is recuperating, instructions are given on what to eat and drink.
8. Drumming: Drumming is essential in reinforcing treatments that involves ritual activities. It serves as a relief to ancestral stress. It is also used to facilitate communication with the ancestors during healings and other activities.
9. Emetics: Emetics are used for expectoration purposes. They are used to cleanse the chest of wheezing and congestion. They are also used to cleanse the upper gastrointestinal tract of poisons, dirt, excess mucus or bile.
10. Enemas: This is also a cleansing method which is employed to clear foreign bodies from the lower section of the gastrointestinal tracts. It handles such health problems as constipation, backaches, womb complications, certain types of sexually transmitted diseases and for aphrodisiac purposes in men and women.
11. Prayer/Sacrifice to Ancestors: This type of prayer works at the psychological level as reinforcement to cultural rituals and sacrifices. The occasion is also used to seek favour from the ancestors in curing ancestor related diseases or illness. It is equally used during initiatory ceremony.
12. Reassurances: This is a Counseling skill, which is used to instill confidence in a patient about the competence of a healer. Reassurance is also used to encourage the patient to take his/her drugs according to the given instructions in order to speed up recovery.

13. Rest: Rest is encouraged during the period of medication to relieve the body of stress. Rest gives the body a better condition for drug assimilation into the system.
14. Smoke Inhalation: Smoke inhalation is applied when medicine is to be introduced into the body very quickly.
15. Snuff: Snuff is an example of traditional medicine which is used in its powered form. It is usually made with a mixture of two or more herbs.
16. Steaming: Steaming is used as a topical application of a particular medicine through the pores of the skin to penetrate, stimulate, invigorate and to heal the body.
17. Piercing (African Acupuncture): African Acupuncture is a method used to treat pain or bodily discomfort in areas with no wound or open sore. A porcupine's quill is commonly used in this case as a needle to pierce the affected area. This piercing is then followed with the application of powered medicine or poultice as needed.

Back to Eden[66] written by Jethro Kloss is the next book to be reviewed. He sees and recommends water in all its forms as the most abundant element of nature for remedial use. Water makes up about four-fifth of the composition of the human brain and blood. The chemical formula for this important liquid is H_2O. It is made up of two volumes of hydrogen and a volume of oxygen. Both of these gases are odourless.[67]

---

[66] Jethro Kloss, p. 44-53, 108, 166, 338-339
[67] Ibid, p. 108

In spite of the availability of many different kinds of liquids for drinking, water is still the only substance, which really quenches thirst. However, exclusive breastfeeding without any additional food or water is recommended for new born babies. This is because the breast milk contains all the energy and nutrients that the infant needs for the first six months of life[68]. On the other hand, every average person must take at least six glasses of water daily. Among the many reasons for enough water intake are:-

1. Water dissolves nutrient materials in the cause of food digestion to absorption.
2. Water keeps all the mucous membranes of the body soft and free from friction as they function day after day.
3. Water helps in regulating the body temperature and all other body processes. It aids fluid circulation in the body.
4. Water is a laxative. It corrects constipation and it is not violent or purgative.
5. Water is also an astringent. Its use arrests hemorrhages.
6. Water is a perfect eliminator. It dissolves all poisonous waste materials thereby helping their elimination. Here we note that water is diaphoretic-it helps in producing profuse perspiration—which is another way of eliminating wastes through the pores of the skin.
7. One of the most important properties of water is its powerful cleansing effect. Water works wonders both in the body and out of the body to keep it clean. Dr. Kloss still went further

---

[68] http://www.who.int/child-adolescent-health/NUTRITION/infant_exclusive.htm

to discuss some basic rules, which should be applied when using water for bathing.

Rules for Bathing

1. Always use the thermometer when possible in preparing bathing water for the sick. Test the water by placing the elbow on it when thermometer is not available.
2. Room temperature where bath is taken should be between 70 and 85^0F. Patients and invalids require warmer temperature.
3. Extremely hot or cold baths should not be used for old or nervous patients.
4. Never take a cold bath when you are extremely fatigued. It is always better to begin with tepid water and later increase to the cold water.
5. Cold bath should not be taken during menstruations.
6. Pure and soft water should be used for baths.
7. Patients should exercise before and after bathing.
8. Hydrotherapy treatments are best given to patients about three hours after their breakfast.
9. Cleansing baths should be taken once every three or four days.

All the above-mentioned rules for bathing should be applied appropriately for optimum well-being. Appropriate care and measures should equally be taken for footbath, leg bath, eye bath, ear bath and nose bath.

Finally, Kloss divided baths into seven different classes depending on the temperature of the water. The condition of the patient will ultimately influence the temperature of the bath.[69]

1. Very Cold Bath   32-55°F.
2. Cold Bath   55-65°F.
3. Cool Bath   65-80°F.
4. Tepid Bath   80-92°F.
5. Warm Bath   92-98°F
6. Hot Bath   98-104°F.
7. Very Hot Bath   104°F and above.

Anselm Adodo in <u>Nature Power- A Christian Approach to Herbal Medicine</u>[70] presents God's gift from nature as leaf, paw-paw, coconut, aloe Vera, lemon and garlic among others. He also went ahead to point out the various health benefits of these gifts from nature.

<u>Bitter Leaf</u>: As its name suggests, it is bitter and when the tender stem and leaves are chewed and swallowed, it is a wonderful remedy for stomachaches. Pure undiluted extract of bitter leaf is also used to cure skin infections like ringworm, eczema and itching rashes. This leaf is also used in treating diabetic patient. That is not all, according to Adodo, bitter leaf is also an antidote to prostate cancer. Prostate cancer seems to be common among men who are over forty years old. Some of its symptoms include difficult and painful urination. In all the above cases, the bitter leaf fresh leaves are squeezed in water and the dosage taken as specified. It is also useful in counteracting the

---

[69] Jethro Kloss, p. 124

[70] Anselm Adodo, pp. 9-124

following general body weaknesses: stroke, pneumonia, insomnia and arthritis.[71]

Paw Paw: The Paw-paw is also noted as one of God's gifts to man and the leaves of the paw-paw could be used as soap for bathing. The unripe paw-paw fruit could be used to treat wound or sore. The ripe one is rich in vitamins A, B, and C. Paw-paw helps the digestion of protein and equally expels worm from the body.[72] Specific parts of the paw-paw tree have specific healing properties. This makes all the parts of the paw-paw very valuable. Some examples include:[73]

1. The yellow leaves are used in curing malaria fever.
2. The green leaves are used in curing diabetes and diabetes-induced hypertension.
3. The unripe paw paw is used in curing stomach ulcer.
4. The white milky sap of the unripe paw paw is used in curing external bodily ulcers.
5. The dried brown paw paw leaves are good remedies for convulsion in little children.
6. The inhalation of the burnt dried leaves of the paw paw brings quick relief to attacks of asthma.
7. The roots of paw paw on their own parts are effective remedies for bronchitis, piles, and impotence. The use of different parts of coconut, Aloe Vera and other plants will result in the total good health of humanity.

---

[71] Ibid, pp. 36-37
[72] Ibid, p. 39
[73] Ibid, pp. 40-41

Coconut: Coconut is another tree that has so many useful parts. The bark of it is boiled and served as soap for bathing. The roots could be used to cure bronchitis, fibroid as well as hepatitis. The water of coconut is an excellent cleanser while the white pulp of the immature coconut is very useful for the memory.[74]

Aloe Vera: This has been called natures wonder plant with high nutritive values. It is used in curing a lot of diseases such as cancer, constipation, intestinal disorder, impotence and suppressed menstruation.[75]

Garlic: Garlic is a strong antibiotic which could be eaten in cloves or in mashed form. Scientifically, it has been proved that garlic works against intestinal and urinary infections, typhoid fever, bacillus dysentery and infections of the genital organs. Its constant usage lowers both blood and cholesterol levels. It is also an anti-tumor and anti-hypertensive.[76]

Lemon: Some people have called lemon the tree of life because of its many medicinal properties. The leaf is sedative and antispasmodic. The fruit is good remedy for lack of appetite, indigestion, constipation and typhoid fever. The juice is an excellent remedy for scurvy, a disease caused by lack of vitamin C. It is also used in treating sore throat, kidney stones, arthritis and other human ailments.[77]

---

[74] Anselm Adodo, pp. 42-44
[75] Ibid, p. 45-49
[76] Ibid, pp. 68-73
[77] Ibid, pp. 64-67

<u>Counsels on Diet and Foods</u>[78] authored by Ellen G. White contains timeless admonitions on how to be healthy by eating the right kind of natural food. She is advising people who live in places where it is possible to secure fruits, vegetables, nuts, herbs and plant foods to subsist on these. This is because flesh foods are injurious to the physical well-being of man. People should not just eat and drink as they please. Sound reason should guide in the selection of food for man's consumption.

This counsel is for all members of the family. Even children should be involved in this self-denial. Students in our schools are not to be served with flesh food or anything that is known to be unhealthful. These actions, if properly applied, will lead to healthier and longer lives. [79]

The use of water externally can also accomplish a lot in restoring the health of those who are sick. Bathing at night just before retiring to bed or upon rising in the morning is very beneficial. Still on the good effects of bath, Ellen G. White said;

> Bathing helps the bowels, stomach, and liver, giving energy and new life to each. It also promotes digestion. Instead of increasing the liability to cold, the circulation is improved, and the uterine organs which are more or less congested, are relieved. [80]

---

[78] Ellen G. White. <u>Counsels on Diet and Foods</u>. (Washington, DC: Review and Herald Publishing Association, 1976), pp. 380-404.

[79] Ibid,

[80] <u>Ibid</u>.p. 228

Furthermore, in the Ministry of Healing[81] Ellen White noted that we are to study God's original plan for man's diet. God, the Omniscient One appointed the food for Adam and Eve after creating them. God told them that He had given to them every herb yielding seed, every tree, in which is the fruit if a tree yield seed, to be food for them.[82] Even when they left the Garden of Eden under the curse of sin, God still gave man the permission to eat the herbs of the field.[83] Therefore, grains, fruits, nuts, and vegetables still remain and constitute our best diet from God, the Creator. It is true natural foods are the best, care must be exercised in the selection and mixture of the food that we eat. The foods we eat should suit the season, the climate and our various chosen occupations.[84]

Another physician, Mervyn G. Hardinge, in his book, A Physician Explains Ellen White's Counsels on Drugs, Herbs & Natural Remedies[85] gave a candid explanation on herbal remedies. He first of all grouped plants into four categories: food plants, plants that are not edible due to their taste and odor, medicinal plants and poisonous plants. A lot of wisdom is needed to distinguish between the last two categories. As a matter of fact, God, the Creator had made plants wonderful chemists. And when they are examined very well, every plant might prove to be a blessing when used properly or a curse when misused. Dr. Hardinge still went ahead to give the background of herbal medicine. This according to him started in

---

[81] Ellen G. White. Ministry of Healing. (Ontario: Pacific Press Publishing Association), pp. 271-325

[82] Genesis 1:29

[83] Genesis 3:18

[84] Ellen G. White: Ministry of Healing, p. 297

[85] Mervyn Hardinge, pp. 113-170

India with the Ayurvedic (knowledge of life) medicine as contained in the four books. Vedas. This knowledge continued in China where the yin and yang system of medicine was developed. The Chinese on their part believed that two forces existed in life, and any imbalance in any of these forces of yin and yang will result in sickness. Even from Africa, archaeological findings reveal that Egypt was advanced in the knowledge and practice of medicine with herbal plants. [86]

German Egyptologist, found out that the Ebers papyrus contained full information on medicinal plants and their preparations. Even during the early and middle nineteenth century, there was revulsion on the practice of orthodox medicine among medical experts and the laity. This was due to the bloodletting, blistering and other harsh methods of treating patients. This attitude once again gave rise to the practice of herbal medication. [87]

The work of A. O. Nkwoka titled "Healing: The Biblical Perspective" was also reviewed. This work was a contribution to the 1993 edition of African Marburgensia.[88] He has defined healing as restoration to sound health. Health on its own part has been defined by WHO as a "state of complete physical, mental and social well being, and not merely the absence of disease or infirmity."[89] From the above definition, we see that the moral, religious or spiritual aspect of health is not mentioned. But the Hebrew word for Health,

---

[86] Ibid.

[87] Ibid

[88] A. O. Nkwoka, "Healing: The Biblical Perspective" in African Marbugensia, pp. 59-60

[89] Preamble to the Charter of WHO as cited in Encyclopedia Britannica, vol. 8 p. 68.

Marpeh which is derived from rapha embraces the full meaning to include healing[90] and general well-being.[91] We therefore note that there is a very close relationship between religion and health.

The traditional African believes that if one is sick when that individual is at peace with the "gods", then some evil or spiritual forces are at work. In such an instance, a mystico-religious healing is needed.[92] This seems to be the case with the biblical Job who was inflicted with all kinds of misfortune and sickness by the devil with God's permission.[93] There have been other diseases, which Orthodox medicine cannot help, or cure. Such cases which haven been termed helpless by the orthodox medical practitioners have found help and restoration from religious experiences. In this situation, closer interactions should be developed between orthodox and African religious healers to achieve better results.

Dr. Nkwoka went further to draw other healing instances from the Old and New Testaments. He made it clear that the Lord Himself is responsible for healing His people. That was why the Lord normally frowned at His people when they go to other people for their healing needs. While Jesus Christ was here, He healed, drove out evil spirits and even raised the dead. These equally demonstrate Christ's holistic and complete healing ministry.[94]

---

[90] Proverbs 12:18; Jeremiah 8:15.
[91] Acts 3:16; 2 John 2
[92] A. O. Nkwoka, p. 61
[93] Job 1:6-2:10
[94] A. O. Nkwoka, p. 68.

In the same way, Leo Van Dolson in his book Healthy, Happy, Holy[95] is strongly convinced that religion and medicine should collaborate as equals in dealing with the health problems of mankind. He further pointed out that recent medical research findings confirm that religion has a correlation to personal health. For example, he pointed out that the Israel Ischemic Heart Diseases Project reports that Orthodox Jews, who prayed to Yahweh daily, had a fewer heart attacks than people who rarely went to worship in the synagogue.[96]

Xiaorui Zhang, writing under the title "Traditional Medicine and WHO"[97] mentioned that traditional medicine is playing a very important role in the primary health care of many African Countries. The World Health Organization, WHO, in order to enhance the effectiveness and safety of traditional medicine is supporting training and retraining programme among member states. WHO is also currently encouraging and supporting countries in their efforts to find remedies through traditional medicine. Tremendous progress is being made in incorporating traditional medicine in national policies.[98]

---

[95] Leo Von Dolson and Robert Spangler. Healthy, Happy, Holy, (Washington, DC: Review and Herald Publishing Association, 1975), pp. 16-19

[96] Ibid, p.17

[97] Xiaorui Zhang, World Health Organization, 49th year. No. 2, March-April, 1996. IX ISSN 0043-8502, pp. 4-5, Dr. Ziaorui Zhang is the Chief of the Traditional Medicine Unit, World Health Organization, 1211, Geneva 27, Switzerland.

[98] Ibid, p. 4

It is a known fact that there is acute shortage of medical doctors and pharmaceutical products in all developing countries. As a result of this, most of the population in the developing nations like Nigeria and Ghana still depend on the traditional practitioners for medications. Traditional birth attendants, bonesetters, herbalists and others still abound. For example, in the federal republic of Ghana, the ratio of orthodox medical doctors to the general population is 1:20,000, whereas, the same ratio for traditional practitioners is 1:200. In Swaziland, the ratio of medical doctors to the total population is 1:10,000 while it is 1:100 for traditional practitioners.[99] In view of this acute shortage of orthodox medical personnel and products to adequately meet the health needs of the people and considering the fact that traditional medicine is playing important roles in the primary health delivery system in many developing countries, the need for a national policy on traditional medicine cannot be overlooked any longer.[100]

The work of Lateef A. Salako titled "An African Perspective" has also been reviewed.[101] This work is indeed a contribution to the 1998 World-Health—The Magazine of the World Health Organization. In this paper, Professor Salako submits that in many African countries today, unofficial health care system work side by side with the official ones. This unofficial one includes traditional healers, medicine vendors, spiritual healers and others. The interesting aspect is that the unofficial-alternative medicine is more readily available, more accessible and even cheaper than the official one. As a result, more

---

[99] Ibid., P. 5
[100] Ibid.
[101] Lateef A. Salako. World Health Organization, pp. 24-25

patients seek treatment from the cheaper and more readily available alternative traditional healer than the orthodox ones.[102] This has supported what Dr. Xiaorui Zhang, Chief of the traditional medicine units of the World Health Organization has emphasized earlier on.

Professor Salako went further to point out a salient fact that since greater majority of Africans surge to traditional healer for their medical welfare, there is the urgent need for these alternative traditional healers to be recognized and empowered. Not only that, they should be empowered through adequate training and orientation to be verse in proper health care delivery methodologies. If this is done the traditional healers can then diagnose and treat a disease such as malaria correctly.[103]

Malaria, Professor Salako submits is not a homogenous disease but its incidence varies from place to place. The over 300 million cases of malaria around the world result in about two million deaths every year. Malaria is also responsible for 9% of the disease burden in Africa. Complicated, severe malaria on the other hand is the cause of over 85% of all deaths caused by this disease. In view of the endemic nature of malaria in Africa, it is important to enlighten and have competent traditional healers who would give correct diagnosis and treatment of malaria.[104]

---

[102] Lateef A. Salako. p.24
[103] Ibid, p. 25
[104] Ibid.

Marcus Muller[105] wrote on the urgent need for traditional and modern medicine to cooperate with each other in handling the ills of humanity while Isabel Carter[106] posits that up till now more than an estimated 80% of the world's population still depends on traditional medicines for their health security. That is why enough and adequate information must be provided for more wisdom and caution in handling traditional medicine.[107]

Another outstanding scholar who has contributed immensely to our wealth of knowledge is E. Bolaji Idowu through his work, "African Traditional Religion: A Definition"[108] Bolaji Idowu posits that some forms of rituals accompany the dispensing and application of African Traditional Medicine. He further stated that apart from God, the ancestors who first practiced the medicine must be given due honour. For example, in Yorubaland, the first traditional doctor was Elesiji and he must be invoked before the medicine can be effective.

According to John S. Mbiti,[109] the medicine men are the greatest gifts to any African society. They are also called herbalists or traditional doctors. They are not witch doctors. This is an inappropriate term which American and European writers have wrongly applied to them. Medicine men are expected to be trustworthy, upright

---

[105] Markus Muller. "Traditional and Modern Medicine, The Need for Co-operation", Footsteps, No. 48, September, 2001, p. 125.
[106] Isabel Carter. Footsteps, No. 48, September, 2001, p. 3
[107] Marcus Muller, p. 2
[108] Bolaji Idowu, African Traditional Religion. A Definition. (London: Fountain Publication, 1991), p. 202
[109] Ibid, p. 200.

morally, friendly and willing to serve any time.[110] People are trained before they can do this work. The training also involves some apprenticeship whereby the candidate is taught the medicinal value, quantity and use of various herbs, leaves, roots, fruits, barks, grains, dead insects, bones, feathers, powders, smoke of different objects, excreta of animals, and insects, shells, eggs, etc. They also learn the causes, prevention and cure of diseases and suffering.[111]

Elizabeth Kafaru[112] gave some outstanding reasons for the present interest in traditional healing methods. The first is that many ailments, which are said to be incurable, respond to traditional medicine. The high cost of sustaining orthodox medicine for some of the common health problems is beyond the reach of even the wealthy among us. Finally, the availability and proximity of the forest which are full of medicinal plants, which can be used and have always been used for the treatment of various diseases is here with us.[113]

The dosage of traditional medication which has raised a lot of criticism should not be so. She posits that the effectiveness of the medicine and its dosage could be seen in the over 70% of the inhabitants of our continent who are currently being cared for by this same method. However, for the sake of development, the dosage

---

[110] John S. Mbiti. African Religions and Philosophy, (London: Heinemann Educational Books, 1975), pp. 166-167.
[111] John S. Mbiti. African Religions and Philosophy. pp. 167-168
[112] Elizabeth Kafaru. "Application of Dosages and Norms in the Nigerian Traditional Healing Methods" in Traditional Medicine in Nigeria, (Ibadan: Toyin Okebunmi Printers, 1997), pp. 7-16.
[113] Ibid. p. 10

may be converted for the benefits of those who find it difficult to accept simple things.[114]

Professor A. A. Elujoba[115] in his inaugural lecture dated the use of medicinal plants to the beginning of creation starting from Adam and Eve who lived in the Garden of Eden. Housewives made further usage of these plants and hunters have observed various animals using different plants for different purposes.[116] Furthermore, he said that traditional medicines are in two forms namely, the explicable and inexplicable forms.[117]

The explicable form has to do with the case of medicinal substances, which could be probed scientifically. The inexplicable one has to do with mystical, magical, psychic, supernatural, metaphysical and occultic practices to effect healing and this cannot be probed scientifically.[118]

In his article, "African Traditional Medicine and Healing: A Theological and Pastoral Reappraisal,"[119] Dr. Ikenga-Metuh made it clear that in traditional African societies, the medicine-man is

---

[114] Elizabeth Kafaru. "Application of Dosages and Norms in the Nigerian Traditional Healing Methods" in <u>Traditional Medicine in Nigeria</u>, p. 16

[115] A. A. Elujoba, "<u>Pharmacognosy for Health and Culture</u>" The PHC <u>Jungle Connection</u> (Ile-Ife: Obafemi Awolowo University Press, 1999), p. 4.

[116] <u>Ibid</u>. pp. 4-52

[117] <u>Ibid</u>, p. 5

[118] <u>Ibid</u>, p. 6

[119] <u>Ibid</u>

erroneously and unjustly called the witch doctor. He pointed out still that the main concern of the medicine man is to handle diseases, sickness and misfortune generally. And in order to meet the multiple needs of restoring the people's health, the medicine man acts as a physician, psychiatrist and a wonder worker at other times.[120]

L. Lugwuanya[121] contends that all over the African continent, medicine is conceived to have physical, metaphysical and spiritual dimensions. Among the Igbo and Yoruba people and in their practices of religions, "*Ogwu*" Igbo, and "*Ogun*" Yoruba cover herbal or similar remedies, charms, poison, or spell. So the concept of medicine carries the idea of physical cure and spiritual healing.[122]

Dr. A. S. Oyalana in writing the article "Spiritual Healing: A Challenge to Mainline Churches in Contemporary Nigeria"[123] emphasized the fact that healing constitutes the removal of factors which cause disease and infirmity.[124] In the African conception, these factors could be physical, environmental and spiritual through

---

[120] E. Ikenga-Metuh. "African Traditional Medicine and Healing. A Theological and Pastoral" Reappraisal" contained in August 1982 Nigerian Zonal WAATI Conference and the August 1983, West African Conference of WAATI, pp. 113-127.

[121] L. Lugwuanya. "Medicine, Spiritual Healing and African Response 1857-1924: Concerns of Christianity in Africa in the 21st Century" African Theological Journal, vol. 23, (2000), No. 1, pp. 17-31.

[122] Ibid, p. 20

[123] A. S. Oyalana. "Spiritual Healing: A Challenge to Mainline Churches in Contemporary Nigeria" in Religion and Spirituality, Port Harcourt: Emhai Books, 2001, pp. 125-132

[124] Ibid, p.125

the actions of Witches and Sorcerers. Divine healing on the other hand had led to the growth and popularity of the Aladura Churches[125] Other mainline churches because of the absence of this healing are not experiencing this geometric growth.[126]

Writing under the topic: "The Church's Healing Ministry" Akinyele Omoyajowo[127] maintained that a healthy person is one who is in the right relationship with God and others. More so, a healthy society is one in which the racial, political, economic, religious and sexual activities are not torn apart. Christ during His earthly ministry healed people physically, spiritually, emotionally and mentally because of His unique relation with God.[128]

Six other valuable manuscripts prepared by Dr. E. O. Babalola have equally been devoted to different aspects of traditional medicine. The first one is titled: "The Concepts of (Ofo) Incantation as an Aspect of Traditional Medicine in Yorubaland."[129] In this article he submitted that the phenomena of magic, medicine, prayers, and incantations are so related that they cannot be separated when it comes to healing.[130]

---

[125] Ibid, p. 131
[126] Ibid, p. 132
[127] Akinleye Omoyajowo, Religion, Society and the Home (Ijebu-Ode: Vicoo International Press, 2001), pp. 95-104.
[128] Ibid, p. 96
[129] E. O. Babalola. "The Concept of (Ofo) Incantation as an Aspect of Traditional Medicine in Yorubaland", Department of Religious Studies. Obafemi Awolowo University, Ile-Ife, 2002, pp. 1-13
[130] Ibid, p. 6

A vivid example is in the use of Ficus degans leaves to cure piles, stomachache, constipation and diarrhea. The incantation for the cure of diarrhea goes thus:

Ejiogbe very early in the morning I call you!
Ejiogbe very early in the morning I call you!
Ejiogbe very early in the morning I call you!
When the Creator made man
He made body and blood together
He did not create illness and disease with man
Because of this
Whoever uses this drug
Shall be relieved of any kind of disease
Therefore, the disease shall abandon the patient.[131]

Another example of the close relationship between medicines, magic, prayers and incantations is in the treatment of mental derangement and insanity. Effective treatment for this case will involve taking the patient to Ogun Shrine (the god of iron) with a live dog, oil, medicinal soap and other related materials. The healing ritual involves killing the dog and using its blood and the medicinal soap to bath the patient. And before that medicine can be efficacious, the following incantations will be used:

Asagijan! Asagijan!! Asagijan!!!
Oku aja kii gbo
Oku aja kii gbo
B'opa ba pejo, a poro moo ninu
Asagijan! Asagijan!! Asagijan!!!

---

[131] Ibid. p. 8

A dead dog never barks
A dead goat never fights
A trap normally kills the snake with its poison
Surrender your sword!!! [132]

The second article is titled "African Traditional Medicine as an important Factor of social Integration in Yorubaland."[133] This article highlights the facts and the important roles of African Traditional Medicine in the selection process and also in the installation of Chiefs, Obas, and other political heads. In this aspect, the Yoruba people believe that there is equally no harm in using magic to get whatever one needs. In the larger society, African magic is used to solve problems of laziness on the part of a man who could not care for his family needs, it is applied when seeking for a future spouse, and it is equally used in solving other community problems such as untimely deaths, accidents and famine.

"The Scientific Basis of African Traditional Medicine: The Yoruba Example"[134] is the third work by Dr. E. O. Babalola to be reviewed. He argued that African Traditional Medicine has been known to be scientific; it is still scientific and will continue to be scientific. This has been found to be true due to the various usages of the biological and chemical contents of indigenous medicinal plants in the healing process. In addition to that, the selection of different plants for various medicinal processes and the period when the plants

---

[132] Ibid, p. 10
[133] Ibid.pp. 1-14
[134] Ibid, pp. 8-9

were collected attest to the scientific nature of African traditional medicine.[135] For instance, herbalist may advocate that certain plants be collected at night because they will be more effective in medicinal preparations than those collected in the day. Elipatorium Odorantum is a good example of a plant whose volatile oil loses its essential contents to evaporation in the bright sunlight.[136]

E. O. Babalola's article "Clinical Management of Coronary Heart Disease with the use of herbal Medicine and Food Therapy: A Comparative Analysis"[137] is the fourth article to be reviewed. Heart disease among human beings is a reality. Among its various causes are wrong feeding habits, faulty lifestyles, stress in all its forms, high level of cholesterol in the blood, elevated blood pressure, diabetes, obesity, smoking and lack of physical exercise. Heart disease, which may arise from the above mentioned factors or other causes, might be congenial or acquired. No matter the type of heart problem which one has, it is always very expensive to handle heart problems. It has, however, been discovered that many of the risk factors involved in heart problems are dietary in nature.[138]

---

[135] E. O. Babalola. "The Scientific Basis of African Traditional Medicine: The Yoruba Example", Department of Religious Studies, Obafemi Awolowo University, Ile-Ife, 2002. pp. 1-21

[136] Ibid, p. 11

[137] Ibid. p. 16

[138] E. O. Babalola. "Clinical Management of Coronary Disease with the use of Herbal Medicine and Food Therapy: A Comparative Analysis" Department of Religious Studies, Obafemi Awolowo University, Ile-Ife, Nigeria, pp. 1-16

In spite of the fact that it is advisable to see orthodox medical personnel concerning heart disease, the important role of natural remedies should not be overlooked. Fruits and vegetables, which are used to tone up the heart, should be used generously. Specifically:

A. Grapes, oranges, lemons, and other source of vitamin C should be taken to control heart palpitation
B. Onions and Garlic should be eaten first thing in the morning to normalize blood cholesterol.
C. Honey, which improves circulation, should be taken each morning to tone up the heart.
D. Mistletoe, which has a balancing effect on the blood pressure, repairs pancreases and is good for treatment of diabetes, should be used regularly
E. Whole meal products such as green vegetables, carrots, pears, lettuce, nuts that are rich in Vitamin E, which improves muscle strength, and circulation should equally be taken daily.[139]

Subsisting daily on the above mention fruits and herbs will go a long way in both preventing and curing heart problems. "Medical Dialogue Between Orthodox and Traditional Healers: The Complete Solution to Basic Medical Problems in the Nigerian Community"[140] is the next article to be reviewed. This article is a research proposal, which has been submitted to the National Universities Commission, Abuja for approval and funding. The proposal unveils certain factors that are militating against the work of traditional healers.

---

[139] Ibid. p. 4
[140] Ibid, p. 5

Some of them include religious fanaticism concerning the use of herbal medicine by Christians and Muslims; uncooperative attitudes of orthodox medical practitioners with herbal medical practitioners; unemployment of the wonderful benefits of traditional medicine. Since the Nigerian economy is very bad, not every one can embrace orthodox medicine, it is therefore necessary to go for alternatives in the form of Divine healing, natural medicine, herbal medicine and traditional medicine[141]

The last in this series is "The Relevance of Herbal Medicine to the Practice of African Traditional Religion—Islam and Christianity in Yorubaland.[142] Dr. E. O. Babalola in this article pointed out the fact that traditional medicine gave rise to orthodox medicine, and that traditional medicine has a divine origin and not satanic as some religious extremists have come to regard it. He went further by pointing out the relevance of Herbal Medicine to both Islam and Christianity. In the Qur'an, Sura 2:168 states:

> O ye people!
> Eat of what is on earth
> Lawful and good.

The above quotation and many others are used to buttress the fact that Islam endorses herbal medicine. On the other hand, the Christian religion embraces it too. In Ezekiel 47:12, is contained

---

[141] Ibid, pp.12-14

[142] E. O. Babalola. "Medical Dialogue Between Orthodox and Traditional Healers: The Complete Solution to Basic Medical Problems in the Nigeria Community" A Research proposal submitted to the National Universities Commission, Abuja-Nigeria, 2002, pp. 3-21

the injunctions to eat the fruit of trees as food and to use the leaves as man's medicine. Dr. Babalola finally made a call to all religious leaders to embrace herbal medicine and to teach their members to accept its practice in order to positively contribute to the health care delivery system of our land.[143]

George E. Simpson[144] further observed that the most common methods of treating patients involves the use of preparations made from mixing leaves, barks, roots, rhizomes, flowers of plants, honey and some specific parts of animals. These mixtures are also administered through drinking, bathing or scarification methods after the causes of the disease had been investigated. The causes of the disease may be natural, preternatural or supernatural. Commenting on the changes which have taken place in Yoruba traditional religion and medicine since 1964, Simpson opines that four major factors seem to be responsible for these and they include:

A. The conversion of the adherents of Yoruba religion to Christian and Muslim faiths
B. Observable decrease in full participation by the Yoruba people on annual ceremonies
C. Compromises, concessions and rationalization by many Yoruba families and individuals
D. Syncretism of traditional and non-traditional elements which are present in many religious organizations

---

[143] Ibid, pp. 6-8
[144] George E. Simpson, Yoruba Religion & Medicine in Ibadan. (Ibadan: Ibadan University Press, 1994), Pp. 97-113, 143-167

Finally, he maintained that despite all the conversions which other religious groups have made on traditional religion, the real test of the strength and impact of traditional beliefs comes in times of crisis or trouble to individuals or communities. It has been found out that at this critical moment, a larger percentage of Yoruba, educated, uneducated and irrespective of former religious inclination will come to the traditional leader or healer for guidance[145] From all the books which have so far been reviewed, it is evident that the practice of traditional medicine in all its phases started with the origin of man. The current use of traditional medicine in handling the health problems of man cannot be overemphasized. The fact also that about 70%-80%[146] of the people in Africa use traditional medicine to meet their health needs indicates its efficaciousness and effectiveness.

1.8   Methodology/Instrumentation

(a)   Field Work

The data for this dissertation was collected through two widely accepted descriptive and comparative research procedures, namely, the primary and secondary sources. The secondary sources included already existing records dealing with various aspects of the work being done. These were made up of both published and unpublished studies. The primary sources on the other hand, were through personal/group interviews and questionnaires. Questionnaires,

---

[145]   E. O. Babalola. "Medical Dialogue Between Orthodox and Traditional Healers: The Complete Solution to Basic Medical Problems in the Nigeria Community", pp. 6-8

[146]   Ebenezer, O. Olapade, ed. Traditional Medicine in Nigeria. (Ibadan: Toyin Okebunmi Printers, 1997), Pp. 1 - 10

however, were the main instruments to be used. Indeed, the study adopted a multi-dimensional methodology.

(b) Theoretical Frame Work

Firstly, the phenomenological method was used by applying the principle of epoché to observe and interpret Seventh-day Adventist's belief on healing, and the use of traditional and Western medicine. This was further accomplished by observing Seventh-day Adventist traditional healers as well as modern medical personnel carry out their work of providing preventive and prophylactic materials to their patients without passing any value judgment by me.

Secondly, using the sociological method, questionnaires were administered on one thousand members of the Seventh-day Adventist Church out of a total population of seven thousand in Remoland. The sampled members were made up of one hundred pastors, four hundred men, and four hundred women. The data was analyzed using simple frequency table.

Thirdly, one hundred people were also interviewed and it was on a ratio of 50 percent Seventh-day Adventists to 50 percent non-Seventh-day Adventists. The Seventh-day Adventists in this group were ten selected pastors, fifteen men leaders, fifteen women leaders, and ten medical personnel, while the non-Seventh-day Adventists were fifteen traditional birth attendants, two bone setters and thirty three herbal and other traditional medical practitioners. The most elderly interviewee was 95 years old while the youngest was 23 years old. Lastly, relevant journal articles and books on herbal medicine and Christian health care were also consulted.

1.8.1 Questionnaires

According to Van Dalon[147] the questionnaire is one instrument for the collection of information that allows for objectivity, integrity and standardization of the respondents' observation. Similarly, Salau[148] opines that the questionnaire forms a major instrument in eliciting information for the research work. Some understanding features, which are taken into consideration while using the questionnaires, are[149]

- The questions should be easy to elicit simple answers
- Instructions on what should be done must be supplied
- The wording and phrasing of the questions should be short and simple
- Offensive questions should be avoided as much as possible
- Typographical layout is equally considered
- The number of copies to be reproduced are determined

Two types of questionnaires were used for this dissertation. The first one was a structural questionnaire and it was used to get appropriate information from Seventh-day Adventist in Remoland. The questionnaire had two sections namely:

Section I: This section was designed to collect the demographic information of the respondents. Specifically, the information

---

[147] Van Dalon

[148] T. I. Salau, Introduction to Research Methodology (Ilaro: Limbs Press, 1998), p.73

[149] E. C. Osuala, Introduction to Research Methodology, (Ibadan: African-Fep Publishers, 1993), pp. 196 - 204.

requested for included the gender, the age of the respondents, levels of education, marital status, and religious affiliation among others.

Section II: In this section, the respondents provided information as it concerns the impact which the practice and use of traditional medicine had made on them as Seventh-day Adventists in Remoland. They also indicated how long they have been members of the Seventh-day Adventist Church, what motivated them to embrace traditional medicine in the first place, the length of time they have used traditional medicine, and who introduced them to the use of traditional medicine among others. The second questionnaire was an unstructured or open-ended one. This was used to collect information from selected individuals during the personal interviews According to T. I. Salau,[150] this type of unstructured or open-ended questionnaire is the most appropriate. This is because it does not give the researcher the opportunity of predicting what the respondents' responses would be like. This type of questionnaire leads to more objectivity from the responses of the respondents.

1.8.2   Interviews

Interviews, according to Oluikpe[151] are respectable sources of collecting material for research work. Borg and Gall[152] believe that the semi structural interview is the most appropriate since it has the

---

[150]   T. I. Salau, Introduction to Research Methodology. (Ilaro: Limbs Press, 1998), p. 10

[151]   Benson Oluikpe, Thesis Writing: Its Form and Style, (Onitsha: Africana Publishers, 1982), p. 93

[152]   W. R. Borg and M. D. Gall, Educational research: An Introduction, 4th ed. (New York: Longman, 1983), p. 447.

advantage of being reasonably objective. On the other hand, Salau[153] contends that the personal interview technique is very useful where great depth of study is needed. Mencher[154] is of the opinion that the key to any successful interview lies in knowing what to find out.

The interview guides for this study was semi-structured and it has two sections. The first section was designed with the intent of getting the demographic information of the respondents. The second section was to get the various reasons people have for embracing traditional medicine. The purpose was to obtain more in-depth information, which was not possible with the questionnaires. Furthermore, the interviews were also used to establish the validity of the questionnaires.

1.9   Data Collection

Data collection, according to Salau[155] involves the process of using the instrumentation to obtain materials for the research work. Permission to conduct this study among SDA members has been requested from the Executive Committee of the South-West Nigeria Conference of the Seventh-day Adventist Church with headquarters located at Akure, Ondo State of Nigeria. The researcher also visited all the Seventh-day Adventist Churches, which are located in Remoland for the purpose of distributing the questionnaires and conducting the interviews. The researcher distributed the questionnaires to all churches, all the members and to all the gospel ministers under

---

[153]   T. I. Salau, p. 10
[154]   Mencher, p.223.
[155]   Salau, p. 73

consideration with the instruction to complete and return them in three large different envelops. The first envelop was set aside for collecting all the questionnaires, which would be completed by the pastors. This was accomplished during one of the monthly meetings of the pastors. The second and third large envelops were used in collecting the completed questionnaires of the Adventist men and Adventist women members respectively in each local church within Remoland. Each large envelop was marked accordingly either for men or women for easy collection, collation and interpretation of the various data, which would be collected from the questionnaires.

1.10   Sampling Procedures

According to T. I. Salau[156] the sample is the proportion of the population that is being surveyed or interviewed. The population represented in this study is made up of all the men and women of the Seventh-day Adventist Church in Remoland of Ogun State. The church membership is seven thousand. This study comprised all the members and ministers of the Seventh-day Adventist Church in Remoland of Ogun State.

1.11   Validity of Instruments

Salau[157] opines that validation has to do with ensuring that the instrument used has measured what it was designed to measure. Asika[158] on the other hand had defined validity as the degree to

---

[156]   Salau, p.15

[157]   Ibid.

[158]   Nnamdi Asika, p. 69

which a measuring instrument has measured what it was designed to measure. And to help ensure the validity, clarity of statements, un-ambiguity and logical sequence of questions, the questionnaires were reviewed severally by selected faculty members of the Department of Religious Studies, Obafemi Awolowo University, Ile-Ife, Nigeria. The questionnaires were finally modified based on the recommendations of the above staff members.

1.12   Organization of the Thesis

The organization of this thesis is as follows:

Chapter one provides the basic introduction to the study which has been done on the impact of the practice of traditional medicine among Seventh-day Adventists in Remoland of Ogun State. This is further made up by the statement of the problem, purpose of the study, delimitations, limitations, assumptions, definition of terms, review of relevant literature and the research methodology and design being used.

The second chapter has to do with the identification and location of the Seventh-day Adventist Church and Remoland respectively. This section also considers the Church and Remoland in their historio-graphical setting. Furthermore, the sociogenic, economic and the culture of the people were considered. Finally, the interactions and the interfacing of the three major religions, notably African Religion, Christianity and Islam, which are prevalent within Remoland, were considered.

The third chapter deals with the history of the practice of traditional medicine from biblical times to the contemporary period. This section surveys the practice of traditional medicine from the Garden of Eden through the Old Testament time, the Inter-Testamental period, the New Testament era and the Hellenistic epoch to the contemporary time.

Chapter four is devoted to the practice of traditional medicine among the various established groups of Seventh-day Adventists in Remoland. These groups are made up of the youth, men, women and ministers as earlier expatiated in this research. Two major sections of this chapter include the prophetic background of the Seventh-day Adventist health message and a synopsis of the Adventist life style which has been simplified with the acronym AH-NEWSTART.

The fifth chapter examines the various ways in which Seventh-day Adventists use traditional medications. For instance, members of the SDA Church use bitter leaf for treating boils, stomach aches, diabetes and prostate cancer. Seventh-day Adventist health institutions in the East, West and Northern part of Nigeria also emphasize the use of natural products like Pawpaw, coconuts, Aloe Vera among others for health and healing

Chapter six is the data analysis on how Seventh-day Adventists in Remoland use African traditional medication in all its phases. Some study variables among some groups within the SDA Church in Remoland were presented. Lastly, this chapter contains the full record of the personal interviews.

Chapter seven is basically the summary, recommendation as well as the conclusion of this research. God has put the herbs and other natural products in place for the benefit of humanity. Herbal medication, which is an integral part of traditional medicine, should be restored to its rightful position in this era of science and technology for the benefit of all.

CHAPTER TWO

2.0 IDENTIFICATION OF THE SEVENTH-DAY ADVENTIST CHURCH AND LOCATION OF REMOLAND

2.1 <u>Identification of the Seventh-Day Adventist Church</u>

Identification according to the New English Dictionary and Thesaurus is that which identifies. Identity as defined by The New Collins Concise English Dictionary is the "individual characteristics by which a person or thing is recognized". This section will deal with those traits and characteristics which set the Seventh-day Adventist Church apart from others. These would include basically her peculiar orthopraxy and orthodoxy. What Seventh-day Adventists teach invariably affect what the church practices. These have been called 'LANDMARK' doctrines or 'PRESENT TRUTH' and they are non-negotiable in Seventh-day Adventist Theology. Each of these doctrines has been biblically and carefully studied and they have given the Seventh-day Adventists an identity.[159]

Specifically, the first segment of these "Landmarks" was developed during the early years of Adventism and they include:

---

[159] George R. Knight, <u>A Search for Identity: The Development of Seventh-day Adventist Beliefs.</u> (Hagerstown, MD: Review and Herald Publishing Association, 2000), p. 27.

1. The Seventh-day Sabbath,
2. The Second Advent, the two-phase
3. Ministry of Jesus Christ in the heavenly sanctuary,
4. Conditional Immortality and
5. The perpetuity of spiritual gifts (including the gift of prophecy) until the end of time.

The second group of "Landmarks" and Adventist Theology is made up of a number of beliefs which Adventist share with other Christians. Some of these "Landmarks" or distinctive doctrines or beliefs include the Godhead; the divine inspiration of the Bible; the problem of sin, the life, substitutionary death and resurrection of Jesus Christ and the plan of salvation.[160]

Interestingly, the uniqueness of the Seventh-day Adventist Church does not lie so much on these doctrines that make it distinctive or in those beliefs that it shares with other Christians. Rather, what makes it unique is a combination of these two sets of understanding within the framework of the Great Controversy Theme. This Great Controversy theme is found in the apocalyptic book of Revelation starting from Revelation 11:19 to the end of the Chapter 14. It is the prophetic understanding of the above periscope that distinguishes the Seventh-day Adventists from all other Christians. Indeed, Seventh-day Adventists identity is found in John the Revelator's vision that at the end of time, God will have a peculiar people on earth. The group of people will be patiently waiting for the Parousia. During the period of waiting for Christ's Second Advent they will also keep the commandments of God including the fourth which calls

---

[160] Ibid. p. 203

all to remember the Sabbath and keep it holy. These are to be obeyed in the context of a saving faith relationship with Jesus Christ.[161] This is where the Seventh-day Adventist derive their name.

Seventh-day Adventists uphold the Bible as their only creed and they hold specific teachings of the Holy Scriptures very dear to them. Twenty-eight of these Bible teachings known as the fundamental beliefs of the Seventh-day Adventists have been presented below as a mark of the church's identification in terms of teaching and practical Christian living.[162] They include:

2.1.1 Word of God:

The Holy Scriptures, Old and New Testaments, are the written word of God, given by divine inspiration through holy men of God who spoke and wrote as the Holy Spirit moved them. In this word, God had committed to man the knowledge necessary for salvation. The Holy Scriptures are the infallible revelation of His will. They are the standard of the character, the test of experience, the authoritative revealer of doctrines, and the trustworthy record of God's acts in history. (2 Peter 1:20, 21; 2 timothy 2:16, 17; Psalms 119:105).[163]

2.1.2 The Godhead:

There is one God: Father, Son and Holy Spirit, a unity of three co eternal persons. God is immortal, all-powerful, all-knowing,

---

[161] 2 Ibid. p. 205
[162] 3 Seventh-day Adventist Church-2005 Year Book. p.5
[163] Ibid. P.23

above all, and ever present. He is infinite and beyond human comprehension, yet known through His self-revelation. He is forever worthy of worship, adoration and service by the whole creation. (Deuteronomy 6:4, Matthew 28:19; 2 Corinthians 13:14).[164]

2.1.3 God The Father:

God the Father is the Creator, source, sustainer and sovereign of all creation. He is just and holy, merciful and gracious, slow to anger, and abounding in steadfast love and faithfulness. The qualities and powers exhibited in the Son and the Holy Spirit are also revelations of the Father. (Gen. 1:1; Rev. 4:11; 1 Cor. 15:28).[165]

2.1.4 God The Son:

God the eternal Son became incarnate in Jesus Christ. Through Him all things were created, the character of God is revealed. The salvation of humanity is accomplished, and the world is judged. Forever, truly God, He became also truly man, Jesus the Christ. He was conceived of the Holy Spirit and born of the Virgin Mary. He lived and experienced temptation as a human being but perfectly exemplified the righteousness and love of God by His miracles. He manifested God's power and was attested as God's promised Messiah. He suffered and died voluntarily on the cross for our sins and in our place, was raised from dead, and ascended to minister in the heavenly sanctuary in our behalf, He will come again in glory for

---

[164] Ibid.

[165] Ibid.

the final deliverance of His people and the restoration of all things. (John 1:1-3; 14:1-2; Col. 1:15-19; John 10:30). [166]

2.1.5 God the Holy Spirit:

God the eternal Spirit was active with the Father and the Son in the creation, incarnation and redemption. He inspired the writers of the scriptures. He filled Christ's life with power. He draws and convicts human beings; and those who respond He renews and transforms into the image of God. Sent by the Father and the Son to be always with His children, He extends spiritual gifts to the church, empowers it to bear witness to Christ and in harmony with the scriptures leads into all truth. (Gen. 1:1, 2; Luke 1:35; Acts 10:38).[167]

2.1.6 Creation:

God is creator of all things, and has revealed in Scripture the authentic account of His creative activity. In six days the Lord made "the heavens and the earth" and all living things upon the earth, and rested on the seventh day of the week. Thus, He established the Sabbath as a perpetual memorial of His completed creative work. The first man and woman were made in the image of God as the crowning work of creation, given dominion over the world, and charged with responsibility to care for it. When the world was finished it was "very good" declaring the glory of God. (Gen. 1:2; Ex. 20:8-11; Ps. 19:1-1) [168]

---

[166] Ibid. P.23
[167] Ibid. p.24
[168] Ibid.

2.1.7 The Nature of Man:

Man and woman were made in the image of God with individuality, the power and freedom to think and to do. Though created free beings, each is an indivisible unity of body, mind and soul, dependent upon God for life and breath and all else. When our first parents disobeyed God, they denied their dependence upon Him and fell from their high position under God. The image of God in them was marred and they became subject to death. Their descendants share this fallen nature and its consequences. They are born weak with weaknesses and tendencies to evil. But God in Christ reconciled the world to their maker. Created for the glory of God, they are called to love Him and one another, and to care for their environment. (Gen. 1:26-28; Ps. 51:10, 1 John 4:7) [169]

2.1.8 The Great Controversy:

All Humanity is now involved in a great controversy between Christ and Satan regarding the character of God, His law and His Sovereignty over the universe. This conflict originated in heaven when a created being, endowed with freedom of choice, in self exaltation became Satan, God's adversary, and a portion of the angels led into rebellion. He introduced the spirit of rebellion into this world when he led Adam and Even into sin. This human sin resulted in the distortion of the image of God in humanity, the disordering of the created world, and its eventual devastation at the time of the worldwide flood. Observed by the whole creation, this world became the arena of the universal conflict, out of which the

---

[169] Ibid. P.24

God of love will ultimately be vindicated. To assist His people in this great controversy, Christ sends the Holy Spirit and the loyal angel to guide, protect and sustain them in the way of salvation. (Rev. 12:4-9; Isa. 14:12-14; Ezekiel 28:12-18).[170]

2.1.9 The Life, Death and Resurrection of Christ:

In Christ's life of perfect obedience to God's will. His suffering, death and resurrection, God provided the only means of atonement for human sin, so that those who by faith accept this atonement for human sin, and whole creation may better understand the infinite and holy love of the creator. This perfect atonement vindicated the righteousness of His character; for it both condemns our sins and provided for our forgiveness. The death of Christ is substitutionary and expiatory, reconciling and transforming. The resurrection of Christ proclaims God's triumph over the forces of evil, and for those who accept the atonement assures their final victory over sin and death. It declares the Lordship of Jesus Christ, before whom every knee in heaven and on earth will bow. (John 3:16; Isa. 53: 1 Peter 2:21, 22).[171]

2.1.10 The Experience of Salvation:

In infinite love and mercy God made Christ, who knew no sin to be sin for us, so that in Him we might be made the righteousness of God. Led by the Holy Spirit we sense our need, acknowledge our sinfulness, repent of our transgressions and exercise faith in Jesus

---

[170] Ibid. p. 25

[171] Ibid.

as Lord and Christ, as Substitute and Example. This faith, which receives salvation, comes through the divine power of the word and is the gift of God's grace. Through Christ we are justified, adopted as God's sons and daughters, and delivered from the lordship of sin. Through Holy Spirit we are both born again and sanctified,. The spirit renews our minds, writes God's law of love in our hearts and we are given the power to live a holy life. Abiding in Him we become partakers of the divine nature and have the assurance of salvation now and in the judgment. (2 Cor. 5:17-21; John 3:16; Gal. 1:4) [172]

2.1.11   Growing In Christ:

By His death on the cross Jesus triumphed over the forces of evil. He who subjugated the demonic spirits during His earthly ministry has broken their power and made certain their ultimate doom. Jesus' victory gives us victory over the evil forces that still seek to control us, as we walk with Him in peace, joy and assurance of His love. Now the Holy Spirit dwells within us and empowers us. Continually, committed to Jesus as our Saviour and Lord, we are set free from the burden of our past deeds, No longer do we live in the darkness, fear of evil powers, ignorance, and meaninglessness of our former way of life. In this new freedom in Jesus, we are called to grow into the likeness of His character, communing with Him daily in prayer, feeding on His word, meditating on it and on His providence, singing His praises, gathering together for worship and participating in the mission of the church. As we give ourselves in loving service to those around us and in witnessing to His salvation,

---

[172] Ibid p.26

His constant presence with us through the Spirit transforms every moment and every task into a spiritual experience (Psalms 1:1-23; 23:4; Colossians 1:13-14; Luke 10:17-20; Matthew 20:25:28; Hebrews 10:25) [173]

2.1.12 The Church:

The church is the community of believers who confesses Jesus Christ as Lord and savior. In continuity with the people of God in Old Testament times, we are called out from the world; and we join together for worship, for fellowship, for instruction in the word, for the celebration of the Lord's Supper, for services to all mankind and for the worldwide proclamation of the gospel. The church derives its authority from Christ, who is the incarnate word and from the Scriptures, which are the written word. The church is God's family; adopted by Him as children, its members live on the basis of the new covenant. The church is the body of Christ, a community of faith of which Christ Himself is the head. The church is the bride for whom Christ died, sanctified and cleansed. At His return in triumph, He will present her to Himself a glorious church, the faithful of all the ages, the purchase of His blood, not having spot or wrinkle, but holy and without blemish. (Gen. 12:3; Acts 7:38; Ephesians 4: 11-15) [174]

---

[173] Ibid.

[174] Ministerial Association- General Conference of Seventh-day Adventist. Seventh-day Adventist Believe…A Biblical Exposition of Fundamental Doctrines, (Boise ID: Pacific Press Publishing Association, 2005), Pp. 149-150

2.1.13 The Remnant And Its Mission:

The universal church is composed of all who truly believe in Christ, but in the last days, a time of widespread apostasy, a remnant has been called out to keep the commandments of God and the faith of Jesus. These remnants announce the arrival of the judgment hour, proclaim salvation through Christ and herald the approach of His second advent. The three angels of Revelation 14 symbolize this proclamation; it coincides with the work of judgment in heaven and results in a work of repentance and reform on earth. Every believer is called to have personal part in this worldwide witness. (Rev. 12:17; 2 Peter 3:10-14; 2 Corinthians 5:10)[175]

2.1.14 Unity In The Body Of Christ:

The church is one body with many members, called from every nation, kindred, tongue and people. In Christ we are new creation; distinctions of race, culture, learning; and nationality, and differences between high and low, rich and poor, male and female, must not be divisive among us. We are all equal in Christ, who by one spirit has bonded us into one fellowship with Him and with one another; we are to serve without partiality or reservation. Through the revelation of Jesus Christ in the scriptures we share the same faith and hope, and reach out to witness to all. This unity has its sources in the oneness of the triune God, who has adopted us as His children. (Rom. 12: 4, 5 1 Cor. 12:12-14; Matt. 28:19, 20)[176]

---

[175] Ibid. Pp. 163-169
[176] Ibid. p. 181

2.1.15 Baptism:

By baptism we confess our faith in the death and resurrection of Jesus Christ, and testify of our death to sin and our purpose to walk in the newness of life. Thus, we acknowledge Christ as Lord and Saviour, become His people, and are received as members by His church. Baptism is a symbol of our union with Christ, the forgiveness of our sins and our reception of the Holy Spirit. It is by immersion in water and is contingent on an affirmation of faith in Jesus and evidence of repentance of sin. It follows instructions in the Holy Scriptures and acceptance of their teachings. (Rom. 6:1-6; Col. 2:12-14; Matt. 28:19, 20)[177]

2.1.16 The Lord's Supper:

The Lord's Supper is a participation in the emblems of the body and the blood of Jesus as an expression of faith in Him, our Lord and Saviour. In this expression of communion Christ is present to meet and strengthen His people. As we partake, we joyfully proclaim the Lord's death until He comes again. Preparation for the supper includes self-examination, repentance and confession. The master ordained the service of foot washing to signify renewed cleansing, to express a willingness to serve one another in Christ like humility, and to unite our hearts in love. The communion service is open to all believing Christians. (1 Cor. 10:16; 17; Matt. 26:17-30; Rev. 3:20)[178]

---

[177] Ibid. Pp. 201-210
[178] Ibid., Pp. 211-220

2.1.17 The Spiritual Gifts And Ministries:

God bestows upon all members of his church in every age spiritual gifts, which each member is to employ in loving ministry for the common good of the church and of humanity. Given by the agency of the Holy Spirit, who apportions to each member as he wills, the gifts provide all abilities and ministries needed by the church to fulfill its divinely ordained functions. According to the scriptures, these gifts include such ministries as faith, healing, prophecy, proclamation, teaching administration, reconciliation, compassion, self-sacrifice service, charity for the help and encouragement of people. Some members are called of God and endowed by the spirit for functions recognized by the church in pastoral, evangelistic, apostolic and teaching ministries particularly needed to equip the members employ these spiritual gifts as faithful stewards of God's varied grace. The church is protected from the destructive influence of false doctrine, grows with a growth that is from God, and is built up in faith and love (Rom. 12:4-8; 1Cor. 12:9-11, 27, 28; Ephesians 4:8)[179]

2.1.18 The Gift of Prophecy:

One of the gifts of the Holy Spirit is prophecy. This is an identifying mark of the remnant church and was manifested in the ministry of Ellen G. White. As the Lord's messenger, her writings are a continuing and authoritative source of truth, which provide for the church, comfort, guidance, instruction and correction. They also make clear that the Bible is the standard by which all teachings

---

[179] Ibid. Pp. 225-233

and experience must be tested. (Joel 2:28, 29; Acts 2:14-21; Heb. 1:1-3).[180]

2.1.19 The Law of God:

The great principles of God's law are embodied in the life of Christ. They express God's love, will and purposes in every age. These precepts are the basis of God's covenant with all people and the standard in God's judgment. Through the agency of the Holy Spirit they point out sin and awaken a sense of the need for a saviour. Salvation is all of grace and not works. Fruitage is obedience to the commandments. This obedience develops Christian character and results in a sense of well-being. It is an evidence of our love for the Lord and our concern for our fellow men. The obedience of faith demonstrates the power of Christ to transform lives and therefore strengthens Christian witness. (Exodus 20:1-17; Psalms 40:7, 8; Matt. 5:17-20).[181]

2.1.20 The Sabbath:

The beneficent creator, after six days of creation, rested on the Seventh day and instituted the Sabbath for all people as a memorial of Creation. The fourth commandment of God's unchangeable law requires the observance of this seventh-day Sabbath as the day of rest, worship and ministry in harmony with the teachings and practice of Jesus, the Lord of the Sabbath. The Sabbath is a day of delightful communion with God and one another. It is a symbol of

---

[180] Ibid. Pp. 237-244
[181] Ibid. Pp. 247-259

our redemption in Christ, a sign of our sanctification, a token of our allegiance and a foretaste of our eternal future in God's kingdom. The Sabbath is God's perpetual sign of His eternal covenant between Him and His people. Joyful observance of this holy time from evening to evening, sunset to sunset, is a celebration of God's creative and redemptive acts. (Gen. 2:1-3; Exo. 20:8-11; Luke 4:16) [182]

2.1.21   Stewardship:

We are God's stewards, entrusted by Him with time and opportunities, abilities and possessions and the blessings of the earth and resources. We are responsible to Him for their proper use. We acknowledge God's ownership by faithful service to Him and our fellow men, and by returning tithes and giving offerings for the proclamation of His gospel and the support and growth of His church. Stewardship is a privilege given to us by God for nurture in love and the victory over selfishness and covetousness. The steward rejoices in the blessings that come to others as a result of his faithfulness (Gen. 1:26-28; 1 Chronicles 29:14; Haggai 1:3-11).[183]

2.1.22   Christian Behaviour:

We are called to be a godly people who think, feel and act in harmony with the principles of heaven. For the spirit to recreate in us the character of the Lord we involve ourselves only in those things, which will produce Christlike purity, health and joy in our lives. This means that our amusement and entertainment should meet the highest

---

[182] Ibid.,Pp. 263-277
[183] Ibid. Pp. 281-297

standards of Christian taste and beauty. While recognizing cultural differences, our dress is to be simple, modest and neat befitting those whose true beauty does not consist of outward adornment but in the imperishable ornament of a gentle and quite spirit. It also means that because our bodies are the temples of the Holy Spirit, we are to care for them intelligently. Along with adequate exercise and rest, we are to adopt the most healthful diet possible and abstain from the unclean foods identified in the scriptures. Since alcoholic beverages, tobacco and the irresponsible use of drugs and narcotics are harmful to our bodies, we are to abstain from them as well. Instead, we are to engage in whatever brings our thoughts and bodies into the discipline of Christ, who desires our wholesome joy and goodness. (Romans 12:1; John 2:6; Ephesians 5:12-21).[184]

2.1.23   Marriage and The Family:

Marriage was divinely established in Eden and affirmed by Christ to be lifelong union between a man and woman in loving companionship. For the Christian, a marriage commitment is to God as well as to the spouse, and should be entered into only between partners who share a common faith. Mutual love, honour, respect and responsibility are the fabric of this relationship which is to reflect the love, sanctity, closeness and permanence of the relationship between Christ and His church. Regarding divorce, Jesus taught that the person who divorces a spouse, except for fornication and marries another, commits adultery. Although some family relationships may fall short of the ideal, marriage partners who fully commit themselves to each other in Christ may achieve

---

[184]   Ibid, Pp. 301- 322

loving unity through the guidance of the Spirit and the nurture of the church. God blesses the family and intends that its members shall assist each other toward complete maturity. Parents are to bring up their children to love and obey the Lord. By their example and their words they are to teach them that Christ is a loving disciplinarian, ever tender and caring, who wants them to become members of His holy body, the family of God. Increasing family closeness is one of the earmarks of the final gospel message. (Gen. 2:18-25; Matt. 19:3-9; 2 Cor. 6:14)[185]

2.1.24 Christ's Ministry in the Heavenly Sanctuary:

There is a sanctuary in heaven, the true tabernacle, which the Lord set up, and not man. In it Christ ministers on our behalf, making available to believers the benefits of His atoning sacrifice offered once for all on the cross. He was inaugurated as our great High Priest and began His intercessory ministry at the time of His ascension. In 1844, at the end of the prophetic period of 2300 days, He entered the second and last phase of His atoning ministry. It is a work of investigative judgment, which is part of the ultimate disposition of all sin, typified by the cleansing of the ancient Hebrew sanctuary on the Day of Atonement. In that typical service, the sanctuary was cleansed with the blood of animal sacrifices, but the heavenly things are purified with the perfect sacrifice of the blood of Jesus. The investigative judgment reveals to the heavenly intelligences, who among the dead are asleep in Christ and therefore, in Him, are deemed worthy to have part in the first resurrection. It also makes manifest who among the living are abiding in Christ, keeping the

---

[185] Ibid. Pp. 311-322

commandments of God and the faith of Jesus, and in Him therefore, are ready for translation into His everlasting kingdom. This judgment vindicates the justice of God in saving those who believe in Jesus. It declares that those who have remained loyal to God shall receive the kingdom. The completion of this ministry of Christ will mark the close of human probation before the Second Advent. (Heb. 8:1-5; Dan. 7:9-27; Num. 14:34)[186]

2.1.25   The Second Coming of Christ:

The second coming of Christ is the blessed hope of the church, the grand climax of the gospel. The Saviour's coming will be literal, personal, visible, and worldwide. When He returns, the righteous dead will be resurrected, together with the righteous living they will be glorified and taken to heaven, but the unrighteous will die. The almost complete fulfillment of most lines of prophecy indicates that Christ's coming is imminent. The time of that event has not been revealed, and we are exhorted to be ready at all times. (Titus 2:13; Heb. 9:28; Acts 1:9-11)

2.1.26   Death and Resurrection:

The wages of sin is death. But God, who alone is immortal, will grant eternal life to His redeemed. Until that day death is an unconscious state for all people. When Christ, who is our life, appears, the resurrected righteous and the living righteous will be glorified and caught up to meet their Lord. The second resurrection, the resurrection of the unrighteous, will take place a thousand

---

[186]   Ibid,Pp. 329- 3442 Ibid, pp. 347 - 363

years later. (Romans 6:15; 1 Tim. 6:15, 16; Eccl. 9:5, 6; Revelation 20:1-10; 1 Thessalonians 4:13-17) [187]

2.1.27 The Millennium and the End of Sin:

The millennium is the thousand-year reign of Christ with His saints in heaven between the first and the second resurrections. During this time the wicked dead will be judged; the earth will be utterly desolate, without living human inhabitants, but occupied by satan and his angels. At its close, Christ with the saints and the Holy City will descend from heaven to earth. The unrighteous dead will then be resurrected, and satan and his angels will surround the city; but fire from God will consume them and cleanse the earth. The universe will thus be freed of sin and sinners forever. (Rev. 20; 1 Corinthians 6:2, 3; Jeremiah 4:23-26; Revelation 21:1-5; Malachi 4:1) [188]

2.1.28 The New Earth:

On the new earth, in which righteousness dwells, God will provide an eternal home for the redeemed and a perfect environment for everlasting life, love, joy and learning in His presence. For here God Himself will dwell with His people, and suffering and death will have passed away. The great controversy will be ended, and sin will be no more. All things, animate and inanimate, will declare that

---

[187] Ibid. Pp. 371-388
[188] Ibid, Pp. 387-397

God is love; and He shall reign forever. Amen (2 Peter 3:13; Isa. 35; Revelation 21:1-7; Revelation 22:1-5; 11:15).[189]

2.2 Geographical Location Of Remoland

Remoland is an outstanding division of Ogun State of Nigeria. It is bounded on the East by Ijebu-Ode Local Government Area; on the West by Obafemi-Owode Local Government Area and some parts of Abeokuta territory; on the South by Lagos State and on the North by Ijebu North Local Government Area. The whole of Remoland is currently divided into three local government areas.[190] These are:

1. Shagamu Local Government Area
2. Ikenne Local Government Area
3. Remo Central Local Government Area

2.3 Population

According to the 1963 population census, Remoland had a population of 155,725 inhabitants. The population has been increasing as time goes on, and as at 1984, it stood at an estimated figure of 293,333 people.[191] Still on population, it was Malthus who said that human population is increasing at a geometric progression. Shagamu Local Government Area, which was carved out of the old

---

[189] Ibid. Pp. 403-413

[190] John O. Soriyan, A Comprehensive History of Saint Saviour's (Anglican) Church, Ikenne-Remo, Ogun State Nigeria (1898 - 1986) A Short History of Remoland-Earlier Times to Present Day. (Ibadan: African Press,1986), p.1.

[191] Ibid

Remo Local Council on the 23rd of September 1991, has a population of 203,350 as at 1997.[192] In the same way, Ikenne Local Government Area using the 1991 National Population Commission Census figure, which has been projected to 1998 based on 3% growth rate, has an estimated 72,980 inhabitants.[193] Remo Central Local Government Area, which came into existence on March 2, 2003, is still trying to settle down. There are thirty-eight different families founded under the group named REMO and they include:[194]

1. Offin
2. Ode-Ile (Now Ode-Remo)
3. Epe
4. Ilara
5. Iperu
6. Sonyinde
7. Ijagba
8. Ejokun
9. Ipara
10. Batoro
11. Isara
12. Oko
13. Emuren
14. Ikenne
15. Ilisan

---

[192] "Data on Sagamu Local Government" A Three paged Document on Sagamu Local Government Area received from the Information Officer of the LGA, May 16, 2003.

[193] Ikenne Local Government-Economic Blueprint. A Dawn of a New Era, (Abeokuta: OLAM-PRINTS, 2001), p. 1

[194] John O. Soriyan, p.2.

16. Akaka
17. Makun
18. Ikorodu
19. Ogunmogbo
20. Irolu
21. Eposo
22. Imota
23. Ogere
24. Agbowa
25. Idarike
26. Atakete
27. Are
28. Ideno
29. Latawa
30. Iresi
31. Ado
32. Igbogbo
33. Ode-Oko (now Ode-Lemo)
34. Ijesa
35. Isoso
36. Ipoji
37. Ibese
38. Ogija

2.4 Origin of Remoland

The people of Remoland who speak Yoruba language originally migrated from the Iremo Quarters of Ile-Ife many years ago. They settled in places which were quite conducive to their communal existence and development. Water and land for agricultural activities were the prerequisites for their existence and development.[195] According to late Rev. D. Onadele Epega of Ode-Remo, Olofin Odogbolu, the Ajalorun of Ife, led some families out of Ile-Ife in about 1450 A.D. to settle outside Ile-Ife in obedience to the Ifa oracle that was consulted that year. He went further to conclude that some thirty-eight families migrated from the Iremo Quarters of Ife to establish Remoland, which is now an important division of Ogun State of Nigeria.

The people of Remo derived their name from the territory of IREMO Quarters in Ile-Ife where they originally took off. As a matter of fact, they needed a name to give their new place of habitation a unique and distinct identity. They had also wanted to memorialize the name of their home of origin. It was therefore through the process of elimination without substitution that they adopted the name REMO from IREMO. Remo people are so fond and proud of their name. This has led them to append the word REMO to the name of their town or village as the last word. That is why today we have their names as Ilishan-Remo, Ikenne-Remo and Shagamu-Remo among others.[196]

2.5 Culture and Social Activities

The people of Remoland have a rich cultural heritage. There exist many cultural festivals such as Egungun, Oro, Agemo, Balufon and Eluku. These traditional activities are celebrated annually. These

---

[195] Ibid, p. 1
[196] Ibid. p.4

celebrations equally bring the people together and also give them a sense of belonging and direction. The Egungun festival for instance is celebrated annually to commemorate the high ideals which the ancestors had while they were living. This commemoration makes the Egungun festival one of the major events in the lives of people.[197]

2.6 Economic Activities and Revenues

Remoland as a whole is naturally endowed with good weather due to its excellent location within the rain forest region. This affords the people the favourable opportunity of engaging mainly in agricultural activities. The people of Remoland are involved in producing food crops like maize, cassava, rice, pineapples, cocoyam, cowpie, melon, etc. Some of their cash crops include kola nuts, oil palm, trees, rubber, timer, poultry, and fishery products among others. Remoland has the largest kolanut market in Nigeria.

Apart from the above-mentioned economic activities of the people, they are also occupied with blacksmithing, goldsmith work, block molding, mat making, traditional cloth weaving, (Aso Oke) Dyeing, soap making, pure water production and bread making. Tertiary economic work includes the activities of the West African Portland Cement PLC, Portland Electrical Repairs, Nucleic Industries Limited and CPI Moore Limited. Others include Pefac Associates Limited, Olusola Paper Industries Limited and the Balofun Animal

---

[197] Israel Lasisi. Oral Interview held on May 18, 2003 with Mr. Lasisi, a Mason from Ilisan who is working for Babcock University. He is 65 years old. The interview was held by 4.00PM after the Babcock University Alpha graduation exercise.

Feeds. All these contribute to the revenue base of the people. Other sources of revenue include the Statutory Allocation from the Federation Account, Internally Generated Revenue, loans and the Value Added Tax (VAT)

As a result of the existence of all the aforementioned natural endowments, agricultural parastatals like Agro-Services Cor-operation, Ogun State Agricultural Development Project, International Institute of Tropical Agriculture (IITA) and the Institute of Agricultural Research and Training (IART) are all based in Remoland. These organizations work with the indigenous farmers. They provide funds, agricultural equipment, improved seedlings, research and other extension services to the people.[198]

Other economic activities within Remoland apart from agricultural are industrial and commercial in nature. There are numerous commercial and community banks which are rendering banking services to the people. Even at Ogere, there is an International Market along the Lagos-Ibadan Express Way. Here economic activities are being carried out day and night. In addition to this, Artisans constitute another group of workers. These include Motor Mechanics, Radio/Television Technicians, Plumbers, Tailors, Masons and Photographers.[199]

It might be pertinent to mention here that the Nation's Express Ways transverse major sections of Remoland. Lucrative business

---

[198] Ikenne Local Government-Economic Blueprint. A Dawn of a New Era. p. 1

[199] Ibid. p. 3

activities take place at these road intersections. They all add to the revenue base of the people.²⁰⁰ Large deposits of lime stone at Sagamu has led to the establishment of the West African Portland Cement PLC, for the production of Portland Cement.²⁰¹ Apart from providing employment opportunities for the people of Remoland, it has also helped in developing this part of our nation.

2.7 Religions in Remoland

The people of Remoland are very religious. The people practice Islam, Christianity, and African Traditional Religion. It is interesting to note that all these co-exist in peace and harmony. It is equally pertinent to know that the International Headquarters of the Church of the Lord (Worldwide) is located within Remoland, and that is at Ogere.²⁰²

2.8 African Traditional Medicine and Remoland World View

It is relevant at this juncture to point out the importance of Remoland's worldview in the healing process. It is pertinent to point out here that the traditional worldview of the people is intrinsically connected to their healing process. With this understanding, E. Ikenga-Metuh opined that:

> African Traditional Religion is best understood against the background of traditional African worldviews. In

---

[200] Ibid. p. 2
[201] "Data on Sagamu Local Government" p.3
[202] Ikenne Local Government-Economic Blueprint. A Dawn of a New Era. p. 4

fact, religion consists of relationship between man and the spiritual beings in his worldview. Furthermore, a person lives his worldview because it is a means through which he makes sense of the universe. The assumptions of a people's worldview would therefore condition their notions of sickness and medicine and their healing practices[203]

As a result of the above assertion, the numerous belief systems of the people in Remoland coupled with their socio-religious festivals are rooted in their worldview. The belief systems of the people shall be briefly enumerated at this juncture and emphasis will be laid on their tutelary divinity of medicine. The people of Remonland as in all other parts of Yorubaland believe in the Supreme Deity or Supreme Being, called Olodumare, Olorun or Oluwa. Olodumare is Omnipotent, Omniscient and Omnipresent as well as immutable. He is pure, just and holy. He does not involve himself in any unethical behaviour. There are other divinities and spiritual beings who are closely associated with him in the discharge of his duties. These include Orisanla, Orunmila (Ifa), Esu, Sigidi, Cult of Egungun, and Osanyin.[204]

Among the people of Remoland, the tutelary divinity of medicine is called Osanyin-who has a very close relationship with Orunmila.

---

[203] E. Ikenga-Metuh. "The Healing Dimension of African Traditional Medicine and Healing." A Paper presented at the First Annual Conference of Religious studies, University of Ile-Ife, Ile-Ife, June 4-7, 1986, p. 1.

[204] Bolaji Idowu. Olodumare God in Youruba Belief (London: Longmans, 1966), Pp. 144-160

In Yoruba cosmology, some maintain that Osanyin is the younger brother of Orunmila while others hold that he is the servant, which Orunmila's wife bought for her husband. The important fact is that Osanyin is a very important figure with regard to the practice of medicine in Remoland.[205]

In the general Yoruba traditional belief, the Spirit of Osanyin can reside in a small calabash, which is covered with cowries, feathers, and blood. When someone comes for information, then Osanyin will speak in a ventriloquous manner which the servant of the deity and sometimes which the inquirer may understand. In as much as the traditional god of medicine throughout Yorubaland is Osanyin, the leader or head of the medicine men in each locality is known as the Egbeji Oloogun.

In the collection of ingredients as well as in the dispensing and application of medicine by the Egbeji Oloogun, the process is usually accompanied by some forms of rituals. These rituals are normally placed at cross roads, groves, or at specific sites, which have been prescribed by the divinity concerned.

Next to that is the practice of invoking God, the ancestors or the divinities in the process of medication. An example of invocation is cited below:

> God, here is my sacrifice may it be so you,
> the tutelary divinities of my father, I acknowledge
> you my father, may you accept my acknowledgement

---

[205] Ibid.

> I acknowlege you my father from whom I inherited the
> Medicine may you accept my acknowledgement
> I acknowledge Orunmila, the father of Ifa
> I acknowledge Osanyin the god of medicine,
> but, may it be sanctioned by Edumare.[206]

It must be pointed out however that the invocation of the ancestors with the practice of medicine is a common feature in the practice of medicine in many parts of Africa. It is an accepted practice that apart from God, the Creator, the divinity, the ancestors who were the first to practice the medicine and teachers are usually accorded honour.[207]

As mentioned earlier, there are basically two types of African traditional medicine. These are the explicable and the inexplicable forms of traditional medicine. Seventh-day Adventists in Remoland of Ogun State are aware of these two types of traditional medicine. As a result of their unique understanding of the word of God based on the Great Controversy themes, Seventh-day Adventist in Remoland of Ogun State practice, use and patronize traditional healers whose drugs are purely based on the explicable form of traditional medicine.

It is proper to point out here that herbalists and other traditional healers are quite knowledgeable and familiar with the medicinal value of various herbs. There are pure herbalists who are distinct from those who combine herbal remedies with divination, incantations,

---

[206] E. O. Babalola. "Abiku Concept Among the Owo (Yoruba) Community of Ondo State, Nigeria: A Socio-Religious Approach". PhD. Thesis Obafemi Awolowo University, Ile-Ife, 1987, p. 27.

[207] Ibid. p. 28

sacrifices and other mystical powers.²⁰⁸ According to Richard J. Gehman,

> Herbalists in traditional culture were familiar with the medicinal value of various herbs. To say that there were no pure herbalists is not true. Some herbal specialists freely give herbal medicine without any religious connotations.²⁰⁹

The use and practice of African traditional medicine among Seventh-day Adventist in Remoland is real. They apply the explicable form of traditional medicine based on their understanding of the Bible and the counsels of Ellen G. White.

---

²⁰⁸ Richard J. Gehman, <u>African Traditional Religion in Biblical Perspective</u>, (Kijabe: Kesho Publications, 1989), p 77.

²⁰⁹ <u>Ibid</u>, pp. 77, 78.

CHAPTER THREE

3.0 THE HISTORY OF THE PRACTICE OF TRADITIONAL MEDICINE FROM BIBLICAL TIMES TO CONTEMPORARY PERIOD AND ITS RELEVANCE TO SEVENTH-DAY ADVENTISTS

3.1 The Background To The Practice Of Traditional Medicine

Current medical literatures deal only perfunctorily with the health practices of the earliest man. This is partly due to the scarcity of medical and historical records. The Bible on the other hand gives a detailed account of some early activities of humanity that transpired for two millennia as recorded in the first eleven chapters of Genesis. Ancient Sumerian and Babylonian epics, which contain both legendary and fragmentary records, have not contributed so much into our understanding the health of the people at this time[210]

Numerous Creation theories and stories about the age of the earth abound. Some of them which hold the view that it took millions of years for our earth to be created include the Day-Age Theory, Theory of Evolution, Theistic Evolution, and Progressive Creationism.[211]

---

[210] Leo R. Van Dolson and J. Robert Spangler. Healthy, Happy, Holy. (Washington, DC: Review and Herald Publishing Association, 1975), p. 23

[211] Dayo Alao, ed. 90 Years of Adventism in Nigeria. 1914-2004-A Compendium. (Ikeja: The Adventist Publishing Ministry, 2004) p.

The Bible record, however informs us that man came from the hand of the Creator, about six thousand years ago[212] in a perfect condition. Man was mentally, physically and spiritually sound. Unfortunately, when Adam and Eve rebelled against God and chose to sin, a dramatic change which had adverse effects on their physical as well as other phases of their well being took place.[213]

The book of Genesis gives quite a definite account of social and individual life, and yet we have no record from that cosmogonic information of an infant being born blind, deaf, crippled, deformed or imbecile. There is not an instance upon record of a natural death in infancy, childhood or early manhood. There is no account of men and women dying of disease. Obituary notices in the book of Genesis run thus: "And all the days that Adam lived were nine hundred and thirty years; and he died; and all the days of Seth were nine hundred and twelve years: and he died; and all the days of Methuselah were nine hundred sixty and nine years: and he died" (Genesis 5:5, 8, 27). God endowed man with so great vital force that he has withstood the accumulation of disease brought upon the race in consequence of perverted habits, and has continued for six thousand years. This fact of itself is enough evidence to us the strength and electrical energy that God gave to man at his creation.

It took over than two thousand years of crime, abuse and various forms of indulgence to bring bodily disease upon the race to any great extent. If Adam, at his creation, had not been endowed with

---

143

[212] Ibid.

[213] Ibid.

twenty times as much vital force as men now have, the race, with their present habits of living in violation of natural law, would have become extinct. When Jesus Christ came, the human race had degenerated so rapidly that an accumulation of disease pressed upon that generation, bringing in a tide of woes and a weight of misery inexpressible. These adverse and unhealthy conditions of things in the world were not the work of a loving Father, but the work of sinful man. It has been brought about by wrong habits which include intemperance, and abuses, by violating the laws that God has made to govern man's existence.[214]

The violation of physical law, and the consequence, human suffering, have so long prevailed that men and women look upon the present state of sickness, suffering, debility and premature death as the appointed lot of humanity. Man came from the hand of his Creator, perfect and beautiful in form, and so filled with vital force that it was more than a thousand years before his corrupt appetites and passions, and general violations of physical law were sensibly felt upon the race. More recent generations have felt the pressure of infirmity and disease still more rapidly and heavily with every generation. The vital forces have been greatly weakened by the indulging the appetite and lustful passion.[215]

With the advent of sickness and diseases into the world, human beings sought for relief from their suffering. Our forebears were very curious about the environment they found themselves as exemplified

---

[214] Ellen G. White. <u>Fundamentals of Christian Education.</u> (Nashville, Tennessee: Southern Publishing Association, 1923), p.22

[215] Ellen G. White, <u>Fundamentals of Christian Education,</u> (Nashville, Tennessee: Southern Publishing Association, 1923), pp. 22-23

by the life of Adam and eve in the Garden of Eden. Our first parents therefore depended on plants and herbs as medicinal remedies in times of ill-health. The use of medicinal plants dates back to the Creation of man.[216] By experimenting with various plants, man was able to discover that God had made the plants and the herbs great chemists.[217] Closely connected to that is the fact that the magnificent diversity coupled with the vast varieties seen in nature attest to the numerous chemicals found in them. Man also found out that plants could be divided into four categories as either food plants, inedible plants due to their taste and colour, poisonous plants and medicinal plants.[218] It required great wisdom to distinguish between these plants and to utilize them appropriately. Some knowledge of the use of plants also came by observing animals that judiciously consumed them for food.[219]

God, the Creator also gave specific instruction on which plant should be used and how it should be applied as seen in some outstanding Bible passages.[220] As succeeding generations use these plants for either healing or preventive purposes, and as time passes,

---

[216] Anthony A. Elujoba. Pharmacognosy for Health and Culture: THE PHC JUNGLE CONNECTION. (Ile-Ife: Obafemi Awolowo University Press, 1999), pp 4-5

[217] Mervyn G. Hardinge. A Physician Explains Ellen White's counsels on DRUGS, HERBS AND NATURAL REMEDIES. (Hagerstown, MD: Review and Herald Publishing Association, 2001),p.123

[218] Ibid.

[219] Anthony A. Elujoba. Pharmacognosy for Health and Culture, p. 5

[220] 2 Kings 20:1-7

people began to write about them. The oldest herbal medicinal documents came from the ancient Near East, India and China.[221]

3.2 China:

China has one of the earliest records of the use of herbs for the treatment and cure of diseases. Chaulmoogra oil which is extracted from hydnocarpus Gaetn and used in the treatment of leprosy was recorded in the pharmacopoeia of Shen Nung, Emperor of China between 2730 and 3000 B. C.[222] Generally, all Chinese believed that two forces known as "*yin*" and "*yang*" which are two controverting factors contended that an imbalance in a person's *qi* (vital energy) will automatically upset that individual's "*yin*" or "*yang*" thereby causing illness. The function of the herbalist (physician) is to select medicinal plants to meet the patient's needs. Ginseng and Ephedra are two well-known plant materials from China.[223]

3.3 India:

In India, the "Ayurvedic" means knowledge of life. Medicine has its origin in the Vedas. This Vedas is the religious literature of the Indians and it is made up of four books. The Ayurvedic identifies three elements called "doshas" which pervade all nature. These doshas influence the body, mind, personality, the well-being and

---

[221] Mervyn G. Hardinge, A Physician Explains White's Counsels on DRUGS, HERBS AND NATURAL REMEDIES. p. 123

[222] Abayomi Sofowora. Medicinal Plants and Traditional Medicine in Africa. (Ibadan: Spectrum Books, 1993), p.9

[223] Norman Shealy. The Illustrated Encyclopedia of Healing Remedies, (Boston: Element Books Inc., 1998), pp. 18-21

health of individuals. It is significant to note that any imbalance in any of the doshas results in sickness and disease. Ayurvedic medicine on the other hand believes that the natural world is replete with plants, which have different properties. Therefore when someone is sick, a wise selection of these plants is made, and they will serve as medicines to cure the disease. The purpose of medication is to restore the balance of doshas. Once the doshas are balanced, it will in turn bring healing and health to the individual concerned.[224]

3.4   Egypt:

Egyptian herbal medicine was widely accepted and respected throughout the ancient Mediterranean world. Excavations from ancient Egyptian tombs indicated that as far back as 1500 B. C, Opium poppy (papaver somniferum L) and Castor oil seed (Ricinus Communis L) were used for medicinal purposes.[225] Indeed, archeological discoveries had shown that the ancient Egyptians had an impressive knowledge of medicinal plants. The Ebers papyrus, which was discovered by a German Egyptologist approximately one thousand years before the first advent of Jesus Christ, had records of medicinal plants and preparations. The seeds of Opium and Castor Oil were probably used for the same purposes both then and now.

According to Leo Van Dolson[226], the early Egyptians displayed a knowledge, which was both surprising and extensive in the fields

---

[224]   Mervyn G. Hardinge, p. 124

[225]   Abayomi Sofowora, Medicinal Plants and Traditional Medicine in Africa. P. 9

[226]   Leo R. Van Dolson and J. Robert Spangler, Healthy, Happy and Holy, (Washington DC: Review and Herald Publishing Association, 1975),

of pharmacology, anatomy and pathology. Many medical papyri dating from the first half of the second millennium B. C. have been discovered. The most outstanding were the Ebers and Smith papyri. The Ebers papyrus was 65feet long. It contained over 580 prescriptions and remedies for various diseases. This papyrus was written about 1570 B. C. from an older book.[227] Apart from this, the Smith papyrus contained detailed information on treating the wounds of the head, throat, clavicle, humerus, sternum, shoulders, spinal column and other parts of the human body. However, specific divisions of the Ebers papyrus included:[228]

(a) Invocation of the gods
(b) Recitals to be spoken while treating the patients
(c) Treatment for internal disease
(d) Prescriptions for disease of the eye
(e) Diseases of the skin and their various prescriptions
(f) Prescriptions for diseases of the extremities
(g) Treatment for women diseases.
(h) Prescriptions for keeping houses free of germs
(i) Prescriptions for heart diseases
(j) Blood Vessels and their treatment
(k) Surgical diseases and their treatment

This list demonstrates the extensive nature of Egyptian medical practice and knowledge. Describing the Egyptian physicians, Sten observed that the physician approached his patients as it is

---

p.29
[227] Leo R. Van Dolson and J. Robert Spangler, pp. 29-30
[228] Ibid, p. 30

currently being done today. A history was taken, and an examination performed. Such things as skin colour; sweating, shivering, odor, temperature, character of speech, character of quick and the rapidity of pulse were recorded. Palpitation of wounds and of the abdomen was widely described, and probing was done. He knew the pulse was found in many places in the body, the heart speaking through the vessels of the whole body. He was aware of the brain, heart, lungs, stomach, liver, gallbladder, intestines, urinary bladder, urethras, uterus, testicles and probably the spleen. His physiology recognized the heart as the blood's pump.[229]

Furthermore on the Egyptian herbal medication, Herodotus made some cryptic statements that the builders of the pyramids were made to consume large quantities of garlic and onions to enhance their endurance. Garlic was noted as an important healing agent to the ancient Egyptians just as they are to modern man. Some specific functions of garlic noted by the Egyptians include but not limited to the following:[230]

1. It aids endurance during hard labour.
2. It is used in treating asthmatics and bronchial-pulmonary cases.
3. It is used as gargle in rinsing the mouth
4. It is used internally to treat sore throats and toothaches.
5. It is used externally as a liniment to treat lung complaints.

---

[229] Sten. The Growth of Medicine, pp. 34-35, cited in Healthy Happy Holy, p. 30

[230] http://www.planetherbs.com/articles/HerbHist.html

6. It is used to protect the body against colds, flus, and other infectious diseases.
7. Garlic promotes healing and relieves pain.
8. It stimulates both digestive and sexual libido
9. It is used in treating insomnia and helps in preventing other parasites from entering the body.

The Egyptians were also known for other healing methods and techniques. They practiced various forms of spiritual healing, (chromotheraphy) or colour healing, massage, surgery as well as the extensive use of therapeutic herbs and foods. An interesting section of the Ebers Papyrus describes several charms and invocation, which were used to encourage healing by the Egyptians. One is used before taking any herbal remedy and it goes as follows: "Come Remedy! Come thou who expellest evil things in this my stomach and in this my limb!" [231] This was an example whereby the ancient Egyptian utilized the psychological aspects of healing to his best advantage.

The most renowned figure of Egyptian healing was named Imhotep. He was honoured as the first physician known by name. He was the physician and prime minister to King Zoser of the third Egyptian dynasty. His fame was so great that after his death he was elevated to the status of a god who was worshipped for his healing powers. As the first historically recorded physician, his statue is standing in the Hall of Immortals, and today it is also found in the International College of Surgeons in Chicago, United States of America.[232]

---

[231] http://www.planetherbs.com/articles/HerbHist.html p6
[232] Ibid.

Generally, the people of Egypt believed that disease and death were neither inevitable nor natural. Disease and death were caused by some influence, which might be natural, invisible but very often a part of the spirit world. A god, a spirit, or the soul of a dead person was believed to have been solely responsible for inflicting some irresistible misfortune of disease on human beings. With this development, it was left with the Egyptian Shaman-physician to discover what was responsible for that disease and to proffer the solution to that illness. This was normally done through the medium of some powerful magic through rituals, spells, incantations, talismans, amulets and divination. Physical healing with the use of herbs was only expected to assuage the disease or pain while magic in this situation was expected to provide the real cure.[233]

Along with other Mediterranean nations and India, Egypt was strongly involved with the magico-religious system of healing in addition to many practical cures which were achieved by the use of herbs, minerals and various animal parts. Historically, hygiene which was named after the ancient Greek goddess, Hygeia has been one of the most decisive aspects of health which Egypt has bequeathed to humanity.[234] Egyptian medicine went beyond the borders of the country to positively impact other nations around them. Amana tablets have the record of Egyptian physician being loaned to Assyria, Syria and to the Hittites. When the medical texts of the Greeks are compared with that of the Egyptians, scholars agree that the Greeks had learnt a lot from Egypt.[235]

---

[233] http://www.planetherbs.com/articles/HerbHist.html p. 7

[234] Ibid.

[235] Leo R. Van Dolson and J. Robert Spangler: Healthy, Happy Holy. P. 31

3.5 Middle East:

The code of Hammurabi was one of the earliest known written documents on the principle and practice of medicine from the Middle East. Thousands of years went before Avicenna, Ibn Sina (AD 980-1037) was able to codify the whole system of medicine known then in the Middle East. He was credited as being the first physician to distill essential oils from plants. As a prolific writer, his best-known medical book was the Cannon of Medicine which was in use in the medical field for many years. In the eastern part of Persia, Ibn Sina was popularly known as the "Prince of the Physicians." His medical influence was felt in Europe for many centuries.[236]

3.6 Greece:

Through the process of explorations, conquest and the desire to aid the sick, ancient civilizations borrowed and adopted the skills and knowledge of medicine and healing of many cultures to their own. The Greeks were experts in doing this especially in the area of amalgamating other people's ideas into their own. When Alexander the Great conquered and encompassed almost all of the then known world which included Persia, Egypt, India and others, he did so with the good intention of extolling the glory to Greece. All those nations, which Greece controlled, brought with them their own traditions and customs including their knowledge of healing.

History had it that a year before his death in 323 BC, Alexander the Great founded the city of Alexandria. It was there that exchange

---
[236] Mervyn G. Hardinge, p. 124

of knowledge between all the nations of the then ancient world took place. Alexandrian library contained up to seven hundred rolls of papyri. Greek legends further stated that any stranger who arrived Alexandria with any work not represented in their collection was detained until that work was copied and placed in the Alexandrian library.[237] Unfortunately, one of the greatest intellectual tragedies of the ancient world was the destruction of the Alexandrian library which once housed all the accumulated knowledge of the then known world.

Greece was indeed an important part of the world where medicine developed and flourished. The Greek religion in its earliest stages was a nature-culture religion. Asclepius, the Greek god of medicine was noted as a legendary physician who equally possessed miraculous healing powers. In ancient Greece, schools for the training of medical personnel were established.[238] Medical history had singled out Hippocrates (c. 460-370 B.C) as the first Greek to consider medicine as a science. He was the son of a physician, born on the Island of Kos off coast of Asia Minor, and he traveled to many countries researching and practicing medicine. His *materia medica* consisted of some 400 simple herbal recipes.[239] The emphasis of Hippocrates during his medical career was on the study of the patient rather than the disease. He initiated a new approach to the practice of medicine by pointing out that factors which cause disease include the environment, diet, climate and the individual's way of life. His

---

[237] http://www.plantherbs.com/articles/HerbHist.html

[238] Leo R. Van Dolson and J. Robert Spangler. Healthy, Happy, Holy. P. 40

[239] Abayomi Sofowora. Medicinal Plants and Traditional Medicine in Africa, p. 9

"oath" has been adopted by the medical professionals throughout the ages.[240]

The Oath of Hippocrates:

> I swear by Apollos, the physician, and Aesculepius and all the gods and goddesses that according to my ability and judgment, I will keep this oath and stipulation: To reckon him who taught me this art equally dear to me as my parents, to share my substance with him and relieve his necessities if required; to regard his offspring as on the same footing with my own brothers, and to teach them this art if they should wish to learn it, without fee or stipulation, and that by precept, lecture and every other mode of instruction, I will impact a knowledge of the art to my own sons and to those of my teachers, and to disciples bound by stipulation and oath, according to the law of medicine, but to none others.
>
> I will follow that method of treatment, which, according to my ability and judgment, I consider for the benefit of my patients, and abstain, from whatever is deleterious and mischievous. I will give no deadly medicine to anyone if asked, nor suggest any such counsel; I will not give to a woman an instrument to produce abortion. With purity and with holiness I will pass my life and practice my art. I will not cut a person who is suffering from a stone, but

---

[240] Leo R. Van Dolson and J. Robert Spangler. Healthy, Happy, Holy., p. 40

will leave this to be done by practitioners of this work. Into whatever houses I enter I will go into them for the benefit of the sick and will abstain from every voluntary act of mischief and corruption; and further from seduction of females or males, bond or free. Whatever, in connection with the professional practice, or not in connection with it, I may see or hear in the lives of men which ought not to be spoken abroad I will not divulge, as reckoning that all such should be kept secret. While I continue to keep this oath unviolated, may it be granted to me to enjoy life and the practice of the art, respected by all men at all times but should I trespass and violate this oath, may the reverse be my lot.[241]

Another famous doctor from Greece who made notable contribution in the field of medicine was Theophrastus of Athens. He was born in 370 A.D in the Island of Lesbos and he grew up and became very knowledgeable in the fields of Biology and Botany. He produced many manuscripts in these fields of learning but the most famous is the Historia Plantarium, which was later used as a standard textbook during his life time and for many years after his death. It is interesting to note that during this time various vegetables, myrrh, frankincense, aromatic roots and flowers were administered to combat diseases that plagued the people.[242]

---

[241] http://www.planetherbs.com/articles/HerbHist.html
[242] Abayomi Sofowora. Medicinal Plants and Traditional Medicine in Africa, p. 9

Galen, also a Greek physician of the second century A.D made a significant contribution in the area of traditional medicine. He was a prolific writer and his most outstanding publication was on herbal mixture and it was known as "De Simplicus." His most famous herbal mixture was called "theriac." This was made up of medicinal herbs, animal tissues, minerals and as the needs arose this preparation might also contain opium, wine and honey. As the years went by, other physicians have continued to add other ingredients to the original mixture of Galen and by the nineteenth century over 200 ingredients are contained in it.[243]

People who accepted his methods and also practiced such were known as "Eclectics." These people like Galen used herbal and mineral substances in combating diseases that plagued people during their time. Both allopathic as well as homeopathic systems of medicine are based on the principles and practices enunciated by Galen.[244] Generally the Greeks believed in the spontaneous healing properties of nature when applied rightly into human body. Contemporary health practices owe a lot to the Greek contributions in the areas of medicine. Specifically, the areas of humanitarian interest, professional code and ethical conduct present in today's medical work have come all the way from the Greeks.

The work of Alexander the Great in harnessing all the knowledge of the ancient world including their health and medical expertise led to similarities in herbal practices. Barbara Griggs had earlier noted that the drug inventions of these great Civilizations demonstrate

---

[243] Mervyn G. Hardinge, p. 123.

[244] Abayomi Sofowora, p. 10

remarkable similarities. A few representative examples of hundreds of herbs and their uses which are common to India, Mesopotamia, Egypt, Greece, Arabia and Rome are Castor oil plant, fennel plant, linseed or flax seed, asafetida, galangal, juniper and saffron. These have been briefly explained below:

Castor Oil Plant (Ricinus Communis), while the plant is poisonous, the expressed thick, viscid oil is used as a powerful laxative and purgative. Dose: one teaspoon to two tablespoons in the evening until condition improves for better.

Fennel Plant (Foeniculum vulgare), a member of the unbelliferae family, the stalks are eaten like celery while the seeds are used as a stomach carminative for the relief of intestinal colic and gas. It is also very beneficial for the liver, aiding regeneration of liver cells and therefore making it a pleasant flavouring in addition formulas with the many bitter herbs customarily used as cholagogues for the treatment of malfunctioning liver.

Linseed or Flax Seed (Linum usitatissimum) is used as a soothing demulcent, emollient, laxative, antitussive and pectoral. It is applied externally as a poultice for burns, scalds, boils and eczema rashes. It is also used as a cough medicine.

Asafoetida (Ferula assafoetide), which is the gum resin of the roots, has antispasmodic, expectorant and carminative properties, making it a good substitute for garlic and very useful to prevent and eliminate colic and gas and aiding digestion and assimilation. It is also a calm hysteria, nervousness, food, allergies and candidiasis.

Galangal (<u>Alpinia officinarum</u>) is used just like ginger as a carminative stimulant for dyspepsia. It is widely used as a condiment especially in cooking. A paste of the root mixed together with bloodroot has been used topically for periodontal disease such as gingivitis and cure skin rashes.

Juniper (<u>Juniperus communis</u>) The berries are used as a diuretic, antiseptic, carminative and anti-inflammatory. For chronic cystitis, backache and rheumatism, a teaspoon of the crushed berries are steeped in a covered cup of boiling water until it is cool enough to drink. Three cups are taken daily until the condition is restored to normal.

Saffron (<u>Crocus sativus</u>) This consists of the three fili from, deep orange-red stigmas attached to the upper part of the style. They give the appearance of loose threads. The flavour is aromatic and pleasantly bitter. A small pinch is typically added as a clouring and flavouring to food. It is also used for shock, depression and mental challenges.[245]

3.7 <u>The Romans:</u>

The Roman contribution to the development of medicine was in the areas of natural medication, administration and engineering. Pliny the elder who was born in Verona in A. D. 23 devoted two out of his 37 books to medical botany. He was among the first Romans who believed and also practiced natural healing. The establishment of hospitals was the other area in which the Roman Empire made

---

[245] http://www.planetherbs.com/articles/HerbHist.html

a significant contribution when it comes to medicine. Many of the hospitals and other allied medical institutions for the care of the sick and the outcast of the Middle Ages were initiated by the Roman people.[246] Concerning their administration and engineering contributions, Mustard surmises thus:

> Although the Greek code of personal hygiene served as a model for all times, it remained for the Romans to develop public health. With respect to the human body and personal hygiene, the Romans differed little from the Greeks, but in the fields of engineering and administration the Romans far surpassed the Greeks. A notable development was the Roman water supply, an excellent history of which was given by Sextus Julius Frontinus, the Roman water commissioner in the first century A.D. Frontinus relates in his classic treatise on the aqueducts of Rome that for over 400 years since the founding of the Empire, water was obtained in Rome from the Tiber or from private wells. In the fourth century B.C, however, the quantity and quality of the water increased markedly when the first large aqueduct, which transported water directly from the mountains to the city of Rome, was constructed. By Frontinus' time, aqueducts had been built which delivered many millions of gallons to the Empire[247]

Another important step, which the Romans took towards the progress of medicine, occurred in the year 466 B. C when Julius

---

[246] Ibid, p.41
[247] Ibid, pp. 40-44

Caesar granted citizenship to foreigners practicing doctors within the Romans Empire. Previous to this edict, Greek doctors were employed and maintained as skilled and knowledgeable slaves within the Roman Empire. As a result of their skill in healing the sick including emperors, in 23 B. C. Emperor Augustus, who was cured of liver inflammation, exempted the doctors from taxes.[248] Dioscorides, Born in Anazarbus, a town in present day Turkey was an outstanding medical personality of Rome. His <u>Materia Medica</u> consisted approximately of 80% plant medicines, 10% animal substances and 10% minerals. This is quite similar to a 1976 report which described the source of Western drugs as follows.[249]

A. Chemically synthesized 50%
B. Higher flowering plants 25%
C. Chemical substances 7%
D. Animal parts 6%

A close look at the work of Dioscorides shows a remarkable similarity to today's chemically synthesized drugs. The other significant aspect of his work was his arrangement of drugs according to their physiological effects on the human body. His classification includes the following:

1. Warming
2. Mollifying and softening
3. Astringent, bitter or binding
4. Diuretic

---

[248] http://www.planetherbs.com/articles/HerbHist.html.
[249] <u>Ibid</u>, p. 19

5. Drying
6. Cooling
7. Concocting
8. Sharpening
9. Making thin
10. Dilating
11. Gluing
12. Sleep inducing
13. Relaxing
14. Diaphoretic
15. Stopping of pores
16. Causing thirst
17. Checking
18. Cleaning
19. Decocting.
20. Hardening
21. Nourishing

By this type of classification, Dioscorides was able to raise herbal medicine to a new height.[250]

3.8 The Arabians:

Arabian physicians also researched into medicine, translated the original medical works of the Greeks into Arabic and also introduced new herbal drinks. These physicians traveled throughout Europe

---

[250] http://www.planetherbs.com/articles/HerbHist.html. pp. 20-21

preaching Christianity and practicing herbal medicine.[251] Finally, it must be noted that the work of Alexander the Great in harnessing all the knowledge of the ancient world including their health and medical expertise led to similarities in their herbal practices. This knowledge had been transported to our own time and people have built upon what had earlier been done in the field of medicine.

3.9 The Practice of Traditional Medicine in the Garden of Eden

Fundamental to the practice of traditional medicine in the Garden of Eden is the fact that herbs, which are important aspects of traditional medicine, were mentioned in the Bible right from the creation of our first parents, Adam and Eve. Herbs are nature's remedies which have been put in place by the Omniscient Creator for the benefit of man. There are herbs for every disease that a human body can be afflicted with.[252] Much has been written about herbs both in the sacred and the other literature down through human history to the present day. For instance, the Bible has this unique information:

> And God said, Behold I give you every herb bearing seed, which is upon the face of all the earth, and every tree in which is the fruit of a tree yielding seed; to you it shall be for meat.[253]

---

[251] Abayomi Sofowora. Medicinal Plant and Traditional Medicine in Africa, p. 11

[252] Jethro Kloss. Back to Eden. (California: Woodbridge Press Publishing Company, 1975), p. 168.

[253] Genesis 1:29

This provision of every herb was made for the sustenance of the newly created Adam and Eve and their descendants. We gathered from the inspired record that man was to eat the products of both fields and trees in the form of grains, nuts and fruits.[254] This original regulation concerning the diet of man revealed that it was not the will of God that man should slaughter animals for food. Even animals were not to prey on one another. The entrance of sin into the world, however, has led to the violent and painful destruction of life by both man and animals. The permission to eat the flesh of clean animals was not given to man till after the deluge. (Genesis 9:3). The clear and distinctive teaching of Scripture that death came into our world through sin shows clearly that God's original plan was that neither man nor beast should take the life of the other for food. [255]

Herbal medication was the first system of healing which mankind knew. During the creation of this world, God also made a beautiful garden, where He put the tree of life. The leaves of this tree were for the healing of all nations. The Creator told Adam and Eve to eat freely of that tree of life because it was designed to keep them well. That tree corresponds with the tree of life which the redeemed are going to eat in the paradise of God. When man was expelled from the Garden of Eden because of sin and he had no more access to the tree of life, God added herbs to man's diet when He said: "Thorns and thistles shall it bring forth to thee, and thou shall eat the herb of the field." (Genesis 3:18). God added herbs to the diet of man and He

---

[254] Francis D. Nichol. ed., The Seventh-day Adventist Bible Commentary, vol. 1, (Hagerstown: Review and Herald Publishing Association, 1977), p. 217

[255] Ibid.

expects man to eat these herbs to keep on being healthy.[256] Herbs are part of the remedial agencies which God has put in place for afflicted humanity. It is God's plan that man and woman everywhere should raise herbs in their gardens. People are also expected to gather herbs that grow wild everywhere and use them when the need arises.[257] Still on herbs which were added to man's diet after the entrance of sin, Francis D. Nichol says:

> The divine punishment provided also a partial change in diet. We evidently are to conclude that the quantity and quality of grains and nuts and fruits originally given to man were, as a result of the curse, reduced to such an extent that man would be required to look to the herbs for a portion of his daily food.[258]

3.10 The Practice of Traditional Medicine During The Old Testament

The Old Testament dates from the time of the creation of the world as recorded in Genesis, to God's dealing with Israel as a nation, including their captivity and return after exile. This period ended with Malachi, the last book of the Old Testament.

Apart from the use of herbs in the Garden of Eden, the other parts of the Old Testament are equally replete with incidents where

[256] Jethro Kloss. Back to Eden p. 169
[257] Ibid.
[258] Francis D. Nichol, ed. The Seventh-day Adventist Bible Commentary, vol. 1, p. 234.

various forms of natural and traditional medications were used for one purpose or the other. This was so because Moses, the greatest human leader that the Israelites ever had, taught them to clean their premises, wash their clothes, keep their bodies neat and abstain from lustful diet of flesh which they ate in Egypt. He went further and taught them to live on simple, nourishing food, and to use herbs for medication.[259] The Psalmist went further to educate the Israelites that the grass was caused to grow for the cattle, and the herbs for the service of man. (Psalms 104:14).

Specifically in the Old Testament, the Hebrew term "rapa" which means "to heal" or "to make healthy" appears 67 times. The cognates of this term are used in 19 different other ways such as repuah, 2 times; riput once; and marpe, 16 times.[260] When these words are considered holistically, we discover that the spiritual dimension of health is clearly manifested. The full meaning includes healing (Proverbs 12:18; Jeremiah 8:15); full restoration to spiritual soundness, Psalms 42:11; 43:55, and it also stands for the general well being of God's people.

However, shortly after the fall of man into sin, people have battled sickness, diseases, pain, suffering and oppression in their various forms which include physical, mental, emotional, psychological and spiritual. Indeed, sickness and oppression have constantly been a part of human experience since the entrance of sin. When man sinned by disobeying God, he came under the curse of sin and

---

[259] Jethro Kloss. Back to Eden. P. 168

[260] Lawrence O. Richards. Expository Dictionary of Bible Words. (Grand Rapids, Michigan: Regency Reference Library, 1989), p. 329

that curse included sickness, oppressions and sufferings humanity passes through today. It is in response to this suffering that man has understandably sought relief. Every human culture either ancient or modern has demonstrated evidence of man's pursuit of healing through variety of means, both natural and supernatural.[261] The quest for the wholesomeness of the human family has led to increasing demand in the call for a comprehensive approach in handling the spiritual, physical, social, and mental and even the psychological dimension of man.[262]

"The Hebrew term for being healthy or whole is *Shalom*."[263] This is also the word for peace which stands for soundness of the physical body as well as for the wholeness of the mind. In the Hebrew perspective of health, the body and the mind are closely related. These two aspects of health were accepted as gifts of God to His people. In view of this special gift from God, it was therefore considered a religious duty by the Israelite to remain healthy. Without good health, an Israelite could not participate fully in the activities of his immediate family and community. Due to ill health, an Israelite may also be ostracized.[264] This action is to prevent the spread of that disease. The isolation of the patient is also a measure in controlling air-borne and fly-borne diseases.[265]

---

[261] http://www.lff.net/about/issues/healingOT.htm

[262] Anthony O. Nkwoka. "Healing: The Biblical Perspective" <u>Africana Marburgensia</u>, XXVI, 1 & 2, 1993, p. 59

[263] Leo R. Van Dolson, <u>Healthy, Happy and Holy,</u> P. 32.

[264] <u>Ibid,</u> p.33

[265] <u>Ibid</u>, p. 35

Even though a very high estimate of health characterized the Hebrew thought, much emphasis was not placed on curative medicine. This lack of emphasis could be attributed to the fact that illness was seen as a divine judgment from God for the sin of the affected individual. The Old Testament further reveals God's willingness to use His supernatural power to heal the people of Israel from sickness and to deliver them from various oppressions. Yahweh reveals Himself as the "Healer" of His people when He emphatically declared:

> If you will give earnest heed to the voice of the LORD your God, and do what is right in His sight, and give ear to His commandments and keep all His statues; I will put none of the diseases on you which I have put on the Egyptians; for I, the LORD, am your Healer. (Exodus 15:26).

The Lord here sets forth an important declaration that He is the healer for His people. This was in contrast to the Egyptian physicians whose fame had spread all over the ancient Near East and who also claimed that their power to heal came from their gods. Their medical hand books, some which are over 4000 years old have divided diseases into three groups:

A. Those that can be treated medically
B. Those that can be arrested or controlled with known medical substances.
C. Those diseases that cannot be cured.

These grouping of diseases and their responses to the physicians have not changed. Modern medical science has made tremendous advancement since the days of Moses, and the surgeons today can incise, remove an organ, sow up the wound but healing will ultimately come from God. The same is applicable when the work of the physician is considered. The physician may administer certain medications which will eventually affect some ailments but the actual healing is controlled by a power under a process which no human doctor can control. God alone imparts healing as the greatest physician this world has ever known.[266]

3.11 The Practice of Traditional Medicine During the New Testament

The New Testament is the second part of the Bible which is made up of a collection of 27 different religious writings. The whole of the New Testament is less than one third of the Old Testament. The New Testament consists of the four Gospels, the Acts of the Apostles, fifteen epistles and letters from Paul, six general epistles from different individuals and the Apocalypse.[267]

The Gospels are books of faith written by several individuals on God's promises and provision for the salvation of man through Jesus Christ. The Gospels project the life, teachings and the ministry of Jesus Christ. The Acts of the Apostles presents the beginnings of the Christian churches. The letters and epistles of Paul were originally

[266] Francis D. Nichol, ed., The Seventh-day Adventist Bible Commentary, vol. 2, (Hagerstown: Review and Herald Publishing Association, 1978), pp. 574-575
[267] http://www.keymey.ca/htm20030221.htm

written to specific individuals and churches to meet specific needs, but through God's inspiration they are useful up to this day. The same is applicable to the general epistles of Peter, James, John and Jude. The book of Revelation, which is filled with symbols, portrays the final triumph of Jesus Christ and His Kingdom over the forces of evil.[268]

Throughout the New Testament, the use of medicine in general to cure the various diseases plaguing mankind was not given much attention. In the same way, the use of traditional medicine to achieve the same purpose of preventing disease or restoring man's health was not given the desired publicity. According to Sofowora:

> The Early Christians had little use for medicinal cures as they believed only in the power of the Holy Ghost. Furthermore, because they considered the majority of diseases to be heaven-sent punishments for the sin committed by man, they believed and propagated the idea that only repentance and prayer could alleviate the suffering of mankind. Thus, there was little progress in medicine at this time.[269]

This was also the concept held by the Hebrews during the Old Testament period. However, there seemed to have been some notable occurrences when the traditional and natural means of healing were used to cure people's disease. Specifically, from the New Testament,

---

[268] Don F. Neufield, ed., Seventh-day Adventist Bible Dictionary, (Hagerstown, MD: Review and Herald Publishing Association, 1979), p. 792

[269] Ibid.

traditional methods of healing were employed to cure maladies that plagued humanity. For instance, the same material that was used in creating man as recorded in the Old Testament became a substantial "material medica" used in healing in the New Testament by Jesus Christ. John 9:1-7 gives the full details of how Jesus used the clay, soil and water to restore a man born blind:

> And as Jesus passed by, he saw a man, which was blind from his birth. And his disciples asked him, Saying, Master, who did sin, this man, or' His parents, that he was born blind? Jesus answered, neither hath this man Sinned, nor his parents, but that the work of God should be made manifest in him, I must work the work of him that sent me, while it is day; the night Cometh, when no man can work. As long as I am in the world, I am the light of the world. When he had thus spoken, he spat on the ground, and made clay of the spittle, and he anointed the eye of the blind man with the clay. And said unto him, Go wash at the pool of Siloam (which is by interpretation sent). He went his way therefore and washed, and came seeing.

So the soil is not just a symbol of creation, it is also a symbol of healing, deliverance and restoration to life. Jesus Christ used it to restore the eyes of the blind. The use of soil for therapeutic purposes was another dimension of traditional medicine seen in the New Testament. On this issue, it should be emphasized that, it is also popular as an important agent of healing.

Oil is variously used in the Bible for healing, and for anointing both the living and the dead. The prophets, our Lord Jesus Christ, the disciples and all believers are enjoined to make use of the anointing oil for healing and deliverance. Specifically, let us consider what the Good Samaritan did to help the man who was wounded by robbers as recorded in Luke 10:33-34. The scripture says:

> But a Samaritan, as he traveled came where the man was, and when he saw him, he took pity on him,. He went to him and bandaged his wounds, pouring on oil and wine. Then he put the man on his own' donkey, brought him to an inn and took care of him.

The oil was a common household item of ancient Palestine. This oil was basically obtained from the trees (Leviticus 24:2); it was used for food preparation (1 Kings 17:12-13); and used equally for treating sores and wounds (Isaiah 1:6). This oil was a common material in every home and in the baggage of every traveler as seen in the case of the Good Samaritan. The cultivation of this important oil began in eastern Mediterranean about 6,000 years ago. Today, 99% of all olive oil in the world come from the Mediterranean area of Spain, Italy, Greece and from other nations. Spain is however, the world largest producer of olive oil.[270] In the region of Andalusia in Southern Spain, uniform rows of olive trees grow from old stocks, which were earlier imported to that country by the Phoenicians.

---

[270] Abayomi Sofowora, Medicinal Plants and Traditional Medicine in Africa, p. 9

It is noted that wherever the Phoenicians went, the olive trees followed.[271]

The best quality of olive oil is termed "extra virgin". It is one, which is obtained from mechanical extraction without being heated and has less than 1% acidity. Olive oils, which fall short of the above, are termed, "virgin olive oil", or first "olive oil". These are within the groups that have been refined by a chemical process with a little quality of extra virgin oil added to them to improve their flavour and colour.

Currently, science has discovered some of the essential properties of this oil. It contains a lot of vitamin E with no cholesterol. The oil is rich in mono-saturated "good" fat and antioxidants, which help in preventing the hardening of the arteries. It has also been noted that the Mediterranean people have the lowest rate of heart disease when compared with their fellow Western nations because of their liberal use of olive oil. The Vitamin E and polyphenols in the olive oil prevent oxidation of fatty acid, which in turn reduces the risk of arteriosclerosis and other forms of cancer. A recent study has demonstrated that foods fried in olive oil retain more nutritional value than those fried in other kinds of oil. Another study showed that women who consumed olive oil more than once in a day have a 45% reduced risk of developing breast cancer. In addition, the consumption of olive oil helps to prevent the formation of

---

[271] http:///www.giveshare.org/BibleSTudy/180.oliveoil.html

gallstones.[272] Olive oil is so versatile that its use includes but not limited to the following.[273]

A. Burned for lamplight (Matthew 25:1-9);
B. Babies are washed with it;
C. Squeaky hinges are lubricated with it;
D. Cosmetics are based on it;
E. Diamonds are polished with it;
F. Kings and Priests are anointed with it;
G. Fish, meat and wine are preserved in it;
H. Healing soap are made from it;
I. Hair tonic is made from it, (Luke 7:46)
J. It was an integral part of sacrifices;
K. Medical balm.

In our modern world, when the average person hears the word "oil" he thinks of petroleum oil. However, in Bible times the word "oil" means olive oil. It is considered the most versatile and useful fluid, which has been created by God. Writings in the *Signs of Times*, Chorles Mills the author of Vibrant Life Magazine gave an advertisement in the favour of longevity. This he did by sharing a recent study, which focused on the eating habits of 22,000 Greek people between the ages of 20 and 80 years. The study showed that these people used olive oil liberally and also consumed copious amounts of vegetables, fats, legumes and whole grains. All these contributed in lowering the possibility of suffering and dying from heart disease or cancer. Even though olive oil is rich in fat, the mixture

---

[272] Ibid
[273] Ibid

of the above mentioned food items contributed in making people on the Greek Island of Crete live longer and enjoy more vibrant health than their American and European neighbours.[274]

The Nigerian Tribune of Thursday, January 20, 2005 advertised this caption "OLIVE OIL PROTECTS AGAINST BREAST CANCER." The article corroborated our earlier information of recent scientific discovery that eating a Mediterranean diet made up of fruits, vegetables and olive oil can help prevent women from developing breast cancer. In a recent development, Dr. Javier Menendez of Northwestern University Feinberg School of Medicine in Chicago had confirmed that oleic acid found in olive oil blocks the action of a cancer-causing oncogene known as HER-2/neu. This oncogene is present in about 30 percent of breast cancer patients. Oleic acid, which has olive oil as its most important source plays two outstanding roles in the treatment of breast cancer. The first is that, it suppresses the action of the oncogene and secondly, it improves the effectiveness of the breast cancer drug, Herceptin, which works against HER-2/neu.[275]

An important product, which is made from the olive oil, is the "Pure Olive Oil Healing Soap". This hand milled olive oil soap is produced from the Holy Land olive oil and caustic soda. The formula for preparing this soap has been unchanged for two thousand years. This healing soap is hand-made with the same care, methods and ingredients which were used at the time of Jesus Christ

---

[274] http:///www.giveshare.org/BibleSTudy/180.oliveoil.html

[275] William G. Johnson, ed. Adventist Review of May 27, Your Big Fat Greek Diet by Charles Mills, (Hagerstown: Review and Herald Publishing Association, 2004), p. 21

and the prophets. The place of production is the town of Nablus in the Holy Land where soap factories dating back 250 years are still located. The person in charge of the soap production is an elderly woman who has been working through a process that has been handed from generation to generation. Indeed using soap made from olive oil makes you feel cleaner than chemically made soap. It is fragrance-free with 100% Pure Holy Land Olive Oil. This soap gently cleans, moisturizes and is ideal for extra-sensitive skin[276]

Still on the usefulness of olive oil, one perceptive writer urges its liberal use since it relieves constipation,[277] kidney disease,[278] and is beneficial for inflamed and irritated stomach.[279] Apart from being a laxative,[280] olive oil is better than animal oil or fat and it should be constantly used as a substitute for butter.[281]

3.12 The Practice Of Traditional Medicine In Contemporary Time

In our contemporary society, the use of traditional medicine to cure diseases is on the increase. An eminent medical personnel, Prof. Lateef A. Salako opines that:

---

[276] The Nigerian Tribune, Thursday, 20 January, 2005, p. 25
[277] http://www.bibleartistis.com/w-soap.htm
[278] Ellen G. White, Counsels on Diet and Food., (Washington, DC: Review and Herald Publishing Association, 1976), p. 360
[279] Ibid, pp. 360, 361
[280] Ibid, p. 350
[281] Ibid, p. 359

> In many parts of Africa, unofficial health care systems and operators exist side by side with the official system and include traditional herbal healers' medicine vendors and spiritual healers. These alternative systems are usually more readily accessible and cheaper than the formal system, and many patients seek treatment from these groups first, turning to the formal system only when they fail.[282]

Since the traditional healers are more readily available with their more acceptable and affordable products, they should be empowered through adequate training and orientation to handle the pandemic malaria. Malaria is a disease that affects over 300 million people around the world annually. Out of the above number, one to two million deaths occur every year. In Africa alone, Malaria is responsible for 9% of the total disease burden. On the other hand, severe and complicated cases of malaria are responsible for more than 85% of all in Africa. It is unfortunate that most of the death take place among children who are below five years old.[283] The solution for this problem can only come when the important role being played by the traditional healers are recognized by the government orientation and adequate training to diagnosis and treat the malaria disease with available medication.[284]

---

[282] Lateef A. Salako. World Health Organization - The Magazine of World Health Organization, 51st Year, No. 3, May-June, 1998, IX ISSN0043-8502, p, 24

[283] Lateef A. Salako. World Health Organization - The Magazine of World Health Organization, 51st Year, No. 3, May-June, 1998, IX ISSN0043-8502, p, 24

[284] Ibid

In view of the above, in 1977, the year in which WHO Traditional Medicine Programme was established the World Health Organization urged various National governments "to give adequate importance to the utilization of their traditional systems of medicine, with appropriate regulations, as suited to their national health system."[285] World Health Organization is aware that many aspects of traditional medicine are useful while others may not be so beneficial. This is why the organization is encouraging and supporting individual nations as they strive to discover safe and effective remedies and practices for use in health care delivery services. This does not mean approving the use of sub-standard products; neither will it amount to a blind endorsement of all activities called traditional medicine. It rather means that traditional medicine both in principle and practice will be objectively examined with an open mind to achieve the best result for the users. As a follow up on this, in 1991, a progress report on traditional medicine and modern health care was presented to the World Health Assembly for consideration. Five areas of concern which were emphasized in that report includes:

A. National programme development;
B. Health System and Operational Research;
C. Clinical and Scientific Investigation;
D. Education and training;
E. Exchange of information.[286]

---

[285] Ibid
[286] Xiaorui Zhang. Traditional Medicine and WHO as reported in World Health Organization- The Magazine of World Health Organization, 49th year, No. 2, March-April, 1996, IXISSN0043-8502.p. 4

Apart from this, the future programmes for traditional medicines were to focus on national policies to run this form of medicine, medicinal plants and acupuncture for the benefit of humanity.

3.12.1   National .Policy:

It is a known fact that there is an acute shortage of medical doctors and even pharmaceutical products. As a result of this, the teeming population in the developing nations of the world relies mainly on local medicinal products and the services of traditional practitioners to provide primary health care. Some of these practitioners include: traditional birth attendants, bone setters and herbalists. These traditional medicinal practitioners are not far fetched from the general populace. In the Federal Republic of Ghana, for example, the ratio of modern medical doctors to the general population is 1:20,000 while that of traditional practitioners is 1:200. In Swaziland, the figure stands at one modern medical doctor to ten thousand patients, whereas it is 1:100 for the traditional practitioners.[287]

Within the last few years, a growing interest in the use of traditional and alternative systems of medicine has been observed among the industrialized nations of the world. Some surveys carried out have the following revelations. In the United States of America, about one third of the general population uses alternative treatment in the form of herbal medicine.

In Belgium and Dutch, up to 60% of the people are willing to pay extra health insurance fees for alternative medicine which

---

[287]   Ibid.

would include herbal treatment, while 74% of the British people are in favour of complimentary medicine being made available at the national level. All these are indicators of the extent in which various countries have demonstrated their national interest in the alternative forms of treatment which include traditional medicine.[288]

---

[288] Ibid.

CHAPTER FOUR

4.0 THE PRACTICE OF TRADITIONAL MEDICINE AMONG SEVENTH-DAY ADVENTISTS

The practice of traditional medicine among Seventh-day Adventists in general and those in Remoland in particular is based on the growth and development of the SDA health message, experience gained from her health and medical institutions, and the general care delivery system of the Church based on divine revelations. At the Centre of all these is the inspiration and guidance which God had made available to the Seventh-day Adventist Church through the ministry of Ellen G. White. Her specific counsels on the health of the Seventh-day Adventist family and the validation of these counsels by recent scientific discoveries are available to confirm the above submission. Commenting on this, Stoy and Leilani Proctor surmised thus:

> The health and lifespan advantage of the Seventh-day Adventist Church have been traced to the way they live and eat. Since the 1800s, Seventh-day Adventists have practiced eight secrets of health that reduced their risk of heart disease and cancer, the two leading causes of premature death. By keeping these two killers at bay, Seventh-day Adventists enjoy greater health and

a longer life than the general population. The scientific confirmation has just been available in recent years, so how did they know before the scientist? From a woman named Ellen G. White. This visionary said God did not want people to suffer unnecessary illness and death and He inspired her to tell people how they could enjoy maximum wellness. Ellen G. White wrote with amazing simplicity and accuracy what has since been proved to be the best formula for health and longevity.[289]

4.1 Background of the Adventist Health Message:

The need for an improved health care delivery system was impressed on Ellen G. White after the death of her first son, Henry, in 1863. Henry died of pneumonia while he was just 16 years old. Another son of Ellen G. White died a few months after his birth. This fourth son called John died of erysipelas. As if that was not enough, in 1865, James White the husband of Ellen suffered a stroke which incapacitated him for three years. These are issues concerning disease and death, which took place within the White's family. At the same time, other families were equally experiencing one health problem or the other.

May 21, 1863 was a unique day in the medical history of the Seventh-day Adventists. It was on that day in the town of Otsego that God gave to the church through Ellen White a vision and instructions concerning health. This health message soon caught the

---

[289] http://www.nisbett.com/egw/mol/Chapter28.html

attention of many Seventh-day Adventist church members.[290] The health message was concerned with the physical wellbeing of the people, preventive medicine, causes of disease, care for the sick and the use of remedial agencies in taking care of the sick. The vision further stressed the duty of each person in making an intelligent decision concerning the health of the body and mind. In her own words, Ellen White described that first health vision at Otsego in the following words:

> I saw that it was duty for everyone to have a care for his health, but especially should we turn our attention to our health, and make time to devote to our health, that we may In a degree recover from the effects of overdoing and overtaxing of the mind. The work God requires of us will not shut us away from caring for our health. The more perfect our health; the more perfect will be our labor.[291]

4.2 Adventist Lifestyle Highlighted:

The message sent through Ellen White pointed out that caring for our health should be considered a special and sacred responsibility for all God's people. It is neither safe nor proper to request God to heal us while we continue violating the laws of health. Concerning the core principles of the comprehensive health message which God

---

[290] Dores E. Robinson, The Story of Our Health Message. (Nashville, Tennessee: Southern Publishing Association, 1965), p. 76

[291] Ibid.

sent to the SDA Church through Ellen White at Otsego, Douglas summarizes them as follows:[292]

1. Those who do not control their appetite in eating are guilty of intemperance.
2. The flesh of pig is not to be eaten in any circumstance.
3. Tobacco in any form is a slow poison.
4. Strict cleanliness of the body and home premises is important
5. Tea and coffee, similar to tobacco, are slow poisons
6. Rich cake, pies and puddings are injurious.
7. Eating between meals injures the stomach and digestive process.(This does not rule out the fact that anyone suffering any physical ailment such as stomach ulcer may not have the meal time table adjusted to meet such health needs.)
8. Adequate time must be allowed between meals, giving the stomach time to rest.
9. If a third meal is taken, it should be light and several hours before bedtime.
10. People used to meat, gravies and pastries do not immediately relish a plain, wholesome diet.
11. Gluttonous appetite contributes to indulgence of corrupt passions.
12. Turning to a plain, nutritious diet may overcome the physical damage caused by a wrong diet.
13. Reforms in eating will save expense and labor.

---

[292] Herbert E. Douglas. Messenger of the Lord-The Prophetic Ministry of Ellen G. White, (Mountain View, California: Pacific Press Publishing Association, 1998), pp.283-284

14. Children eating flesh meat and spicy foods have strong tendencies toward sexual indulgences.
15. Poisonous drugs used as medical prescriptions kill more people than all other causes of death combined.
16. Pure water should be used freely in maintaining health and curing illnesses.
17. Nature alone has curative powers. (This is where traditional medicine becomes very important to Seventh-day Adventists)
18. Common medicines, such as strychnine, opium, calomel, mercury and quinine, are poisons.
19. Parents transmit their weaknesses to their children, showing that prenatal influences are enormous.
20. Obeying the laws of health will prevent many illnesses.
21. God is too often blamed for deaths caused by violation of Nature's laws.
22. Light and pure air is required, especially in the sleeping quarters.
23. Bathing, even a sponge bath, will be beneficial on rising in the morning.
24. God will not work healing miracles for those who continually violate the laws of health.
25. Many invalids have no physical cause for their illness. They have a diseased imagination.
26. Cheerful, physical labor will help to create a healthy cheerful disposition.
27. Willpower has much to do with resisting disease and soothing nerves.

28. Outdoor exercise is very important to health of mind and body.
29. Overwork breaks down both mind and body, routine daily rest is necessary.
30. Many die of disease caused wholly by eating flesh food.
31. Caring for health is a spiritual matter reflecting a person's commitment to God.
32. A healthy mind and body directly affects one's morals and one's ability to discern truth.
33. All God's promises are given on condition of obedience to his revealed will.

These fundamental principles which have been enunciated above became the clear, sensible and pragmatic outline of what has become known throughout the world as the Seventh-day Adventist lifestyle. In the October 28, 1966 edition of the Time magazine, this astounding health and mortality between Seventh-day Adventists and the general public was referred to as "The Adventist Advantages"[293]

Writing earlier in 1905, Ellen White amplified these core principle in the book, The Ministry of Healing, where she made a classic statements which has galvanized millions of people around the world that "pure air, sunlight, abstemiousness, rest, exercise, proper diet, the use of water, and trust in divine power" are the true remedies.[294] Closely connected with these are positive attitudes toward life and living in hygienic environment.[295] For the Adventists

---

[293] Ibid.
[294] Ellen G. White. The Ministry of Healing. (Mountain View, California: Pacific Press Publishing Association, 1905), p. 127
[295] Ibid, p. 180

who were living at the time of these revelations, these principles were electrifying and it equally pointed out what was expected of them. Further, this philosophy of health has been simplified for application among all Seventh-day Adventist Church members and for all God's children through the acronym AH-NEWSTART. AH-NEWSTART means:

A	Attitudes
H	Hygiène
N	Nutrition
E	Exercise
W	Water
S	Sunlight
T	Temperance
A	Air
R	Rest
T	Trust in God

4.3 AH-NEWSTART

It is also known as the ten decisive factors or ten sure steps to health and happiness. The application of these ten factors to one's life is very simple. Apart from its simplicity in daily life application, making them the basis of one's life style will be a pleasant experience. The result would be vibrant health for all family members. These ten fundamental principles, if followed will lead to better, healthier and happier lives. They would be considered beginning with attitudes.

4.3.1 Attitudes:

In this respect, attitude stands for a manner of thought, feeling or behaviour. An attitude also has to do with positive disposition and positive thinking. All around us today are gloom, depression and negative thoughts. But one's attitudes towards problems could make a whole difference. Negative thinking spreads like wild fire to all facets of the society. It is not always easy to insulate oneself from the contamination of negative thinking which spreads through conversations, the print and electronic media.[296] In the midst of all negativity, we must maintain a positive attitude. Developing and adhering to positive thinking will ultimately lead into a higher attitude in life. Through inspiration, Solomon, the wise King of Israel said, "A merry heart doeth good like a medicine, but a broken spirit drieth the bones." (Proverbs 17:22). A happy, rejoicing heart even in the face of trouble or sickness, will release forces which would sooth and strengthen both body and mind. Solomon went further to instruct us that "A merry heart maketh a cheerful countenance; but by sorrow of the heart the spirit is broken. (Proverbs 15:13). Indeed, when the heart is merry, the face flows with joy and happiness while there is peace in the mind. On the other hand, when sorrow and anxiety are permitted to reign in the heart, resilience is weakened until finally the last resistance of the mind and body is broken.[297] It is therefore very important that we maintain positive attitudes in life for it will definitely affect how we think and what we say.

---

[296] Robert H. Schuler. Tough Times Never Last But Tough People Do, (Ibadan: Oluseyi Press, 1983), p. 14

[297] Francis D. Nichol. Seventh-day Adventist Bible Commentary, vol. 3, Hagerstown, MD: Review and Herald Publishing Association, 1977) p. 1004.

Pleasant words have been marked as one of the results of positive attitudes in life. Once more, the wise man opines that: "Pleasant words are sweet to the soul and health to the bones," (Proverbs 16:24). It is an established fact that pleasant words, arising from a positive disposition and attitudes in life are sweet but the precise relation between words, moods and health has remained a matter of scientific experimentation during our time. On the other hand, antagonistic, quarrelsome words bring ill-health both to the speaker and to the hearer.[298] Ellen White commenting on the influence of our words and actions said:

> There are few who realize how far-reaching the influence of their words and acts is. How often the errors of parents produce the most disastrous effects upon their children and children's children, long after the actors themselves have been laid in the grave. Everyone is exerting an influence upon others, and will be held accountable for the result of that influence. Words and actions have a telling power, and the long hereafter will show the effect of our life here. The impression made by our words and deeds will surely react upon ourselves in blessing or in cursing. This thought gives an awful solemnity to life, and should draw us to God in humble prayer that He will guide us by His wisdom. Those who stand in the highest positions may lead astray. The wisest err; the strongest may falter and stumble. There is need that light from above should be constantly shed upon our pathway. Our

---

[298] Ibid.

only safety lies in trusting our way implicitly to Him who has said, "Follow Me".[299]

Medical science also confirms that a positive attitude makes a wonderful difference in a person's physical condition.[300]

4.3.2 Hygiene:

This is the principle and practice of health with special emphasis on Cleanliness. To be clean in this respect is not limited to freedom from dirt and impurities in the environment but also includes Spiritual purities. Scrupulous cleanliness is needed for both our physical and mental health. Through the thousands of pores in our skin, impurities are constantly being thrown off from the body. The body should therefore be kept clean through regular bathing. The clothing should also be kept clean. It is the garments that we wear which absorb the waste materials from the body, and if these are not washed and changed regularly, these impurities will be reabsorbed into the body.[301]

Among the Hebrews, hygiene was an important health requirement. That was not just in their religious services but it was observed in all the affairs of their daily activities. There was always a distinction made between the clean and unclean among them. For

---

[299] Ellen G. White, Patriarchs and Prophets, (Mountain View, California: Pacific Press Publishing Association, 1958), p. 556

[300] Randell S. Skatu. "Health for Ministers and Their Wives" paper presented at the Ministerial Council of Seventh-day Adventist Church in Nigeria, Effurun, Warri Delta State, April 22, 1999, p. 4

[301] Ellen G. White. Ministry of Healing. P. 179.

someone who had a contaminating disease, the specific direction that was given by God through Moses stated as follows:

> Every bed whereon he lieth that hath the issue, is unclean; and every thing, whereon he sitteth shall be unclean. And whosoever toucheth his bed shall wash his clothes, and bathe (himself) in water, and be unclean until the even. And he that sitteth on (any) thing whereon he sat that hath the issue shall wash his clothes, and bathe (himself) in water, and be unclean until the even. And he that toucheth the flesh of him that hath the issue shall wash his clothes and bathe (himself) in water, and be unclean until the even. And whosoever toucheth any thing that was under him shall be unclean until the even; and he that beareth (any of) those things shall wash his clothes, and bathe (himself) in water and be unclean until the evening. And whomsoever he toucheth that hath the issue, and hath not rinsed his hands in water, he shall wash his clothes, and bathe (himself) in water, and be unclean until the evening. And the vessel of earth; that he toucheth which hath the issue, shall be broken and every vessel of wood shall be rinsed in water. (Leviticus 15:4-7, 10-12)

During the Exodus, the Israelites were almost continually in the open where impurities would have less effect on them than on people living in close houses. Even at that period, strict instructions regarding cleanliness were given concerning activities within and without their tents. For instance, no refuse was allowed to remain within the area of their encampment. The scriptures say:

> For the LORD thy God walketh in the midst of thy camp, to deliver thee, and to give up thine enemies before thee; therefore shall thy camp be holy, that he see no unclean thing in thee, and turn away from thee. (Deuteronomy 23:14).

Cleanliness is an integral part of our health responsibility. It was on February 5, 1854 that God gave Ellen White an important vision on the progressive step in the development of the health message with a special emphasis on hygiene. In a graphic description of that vision she wrote:

> I saw that God was purifying unto Himself a peculiar people. He will have a clean and a holy people in Whom He can delight. I saw that the camp must be cleansed, or God would pass by and see the uncleanliness of Israel and would not go forth with their armies to battle. He would turn from them in displeasure, and our enemies would triumph over us and we be left weak, in shame and disgrace. I saw that God would not acknowledge an untidy unclean person as a Christian. His frown was upon such. Our souls, bodies and spirits are to be presented blameless by Jesus to His Father, and unless we are clean in person, and pure we cannot be presented blameless to God. I saw that the houses of saints should be kept tidy and neat, free from dirt and filth and all uncleanliness.[302]

---

[302] Ellen G. White. <u>Patriarchs and Prophets</u>, p. 556

Still on personal hygiene, it is important that our bodies, teeth, hair and clothes be kept tidy at all times. Through inspiration, the apostle Paul said:

> I beseech you therefore brethren, by the mercies of God
> That ye present your bodies a living sacrifice, holy, acceptable Unto God which is your reasonable service. (Romans 12:1).

Apart from personal hygiene discussed above, keeping our environment clean is also important. Just after creation, the importance of environmental hygiene was put in its right perspective. The Bible made this very clear when it records: "And the Lord God took the man, and put him into the Garden of Eden to dress it and to keep it" (Genesis 2:15). This Garden of Eden was prepared as the dwelling place for man. The day to day care of that Garden was placed in the custody of Adam for him to 'dress and keep it." This instruction teaches us that right from creation, man had an important role to play in cultivating and keeping his environment neat and tidy. Man must use his physical and mental faculties to preserve his Eden-home environment up to the same perfect state in which he had received it from his Creator.

The Hebrew verb "to keep" is "shamar"[303] and it means "to guard", "to watch", "to preserve", "to observe", and "to hold fast." Since there was no record of sin as at that moment, every creature was in perfect harmony with one another, so the counsel to keep

---

[303] Francis D. Nichol. Seventh-day Adventist Bible Commentary, vol. 1, pp. 224

the garden was not against the attack of wild beasts. It was also not intended to be a warning against other human enemies who might plan to snatch the Garden of Eden out of Adam's hands. The assurance we have is that God does nothing affecting human beings without first informing man of his divine intentions (Amos 3:7). It is therefore certain that God must have kept Adam informed of his duty toward his immediate home environment and the dangers that might arise if he fails in keeping and dressing his environment as expected.[304]

In the light of these, our homes should not be dirty. This is because dirty environment invites rats, flies, cockroaches and other insects. At the community level, there should be properly prepared toilets for public usage. Lack of adequate public toilets breeds and leads to the spread of hookworm, typhoid, cholera, hepatitis, schistosomiasis and various other intestinal diseases. When community wastes are properly disposed, it will reduce the menace of rats, and roving dogs, which may carry rabies and other diseases.

Considering this environmental issue from another perspective, it is even discovered that poorly maintained vehicles pollute the air with exhaust fumes, which will ultimately end in causing breathing problems. Cutting of trees without replacing them is an effective way of reducing the production of oxygen and this could also lead to a reduction in rainfall.[305] Therefore, we must do our best to preserve our environment. Greater attention should be given in educating people on the sound principles of hygiene as it concerns diet,

---

[304] Ibid, pp. 224-225
[305] Randell S. Skau. "Health for Ministers and Their Wives" p. 4

exercise, treating the sick, and the home where we live and the place of work, than is currently being done. [306] Still on the importance of clean environment, Ellen White said:

> In the study of hygiene the earnest teacher will improve every opportunity to show the necessity of perfect cleanliness both in personal habits and in all one's surroundings. The value of the daily bath in promoting health and in stimulating mental actions should be emphasized. Attention should be given also to sunlight and ventilation, the hygiene of the sleeping room and the kitchen. Teach the pupils that a healthful sleeping room, a thoroughly clean kitchen, and a tastefully arranged, wholesomely supplied table, will go further toward securing the happiness of the family and the regard of every sensible visitor than any amount of expensive furnishing in the drawing room. That "the life is more than meat, and the body is more than raiment". (Luke 12:23), is a lesson no less needed now than when given by the divine Teacher eighteen hundred years ago.[307]

The end result of living in a clean and hygienic environment is good health while a dirty surrounding will leads to disease. So humanity has an important part to play to avoid disaster and disease.[308]

---

[306] Ellen G. White. <u>Education.</u> (Ontario: Pacific Press Publishing Association, 1952), p. 197.
[307] <u>Ibid</u>.
[308] P. Ade Dopamu, <u>Esu: The Invisible Foe of Man,</u> (Ijebu-Ode: Shebiotimo Publications, 2000), Pp. 213-214

4.3.3 Nutrition:

Nutrition is that branch of science that deals both with the amount of each nutrient necessary for the functioning of the body and also the amount contributed by different kinds of food. In simple terms, nutrition is the study of food and food items.[309] This study includes the right foods to be eaten, the quality and quantity of food, how healthy they are and where to get them. Nutrition, as a remedial factor of diseases, therefore, highlights on the kind of foods to be eaten in order to prevent and, if possible, cure the illnesses that man is facing today. But it is of great benefits to strive to choose a wide variety of whole food items nearest their natural state to readily supply the essential nutrients in promoting good health. In making such as choice, God's own designed food is the best in keeping one healthy.[310] Thus, Ellen G. White rightly states that grains, fruits, nuts and vegetables constitute the diet chosen for us by our Creator. These food items prepared in a simple and natural manner as possible are the most healthful and nourishing. They impact strength, a power of endurance, and vigor of intellect, that is not afforded by a more complex and stimulating diet. Seventh-day Adventist Church members started the Natural Health movement as a result of the divine revelation which God gave through Ellen G. White between 1863 and 1866.[311]

On September 1866, the Western Health Institute was opened. This medical institute also became an avenue for disseminating the

---

[309] Samuel Ebun Ayeni. You Can Be Healthier. (Somolu: Ayeni Nig. Ltd, 2001), p. 54

[310] Ibid.

[311] http://members.tripod.com/-csdachurch/egwmess.html

health principles espoused by the Church. Ellen G. White specifically taught that humanity should use natural means to achieve optimum health through the use of herbs, hydrotherapy, abstaining from animal fats, tobacco, alcohol, caffeine and many other harmful food items. She advocated the use of fruits, vegetables, nut and grains as being sufficient for man. In 1986, the US government through the National Health Federation named Ellen G. White for the President's Award posthumously. That was as a result of her pioneering work in Natural Health which the Natural Health Federation is valiantly preserving despite great opposition.[312] The use of tea, coffee and the sudden illness usually associated with it would now be considered.

4.3.3.1 Tea, Coffee and Sudden Illness:

The active ingredient in these universally cherished drinks is caffeine. This chemical is also found in cola nut. Caffeine produces nervous stimulation, which is closely followed by nervous depression. The habitual ingestion of these food drinks results in nervousness, tremors, sleeplessness and heart palpitation. In 1905, Ellen G. White said:

> Tea acts as a stimulant, and to a certain extent, produces intoxication. The actions of coffee and many other popular drinks are similar. The first effect is exhilarating the nerves of the stomach are excited; these convey irritation to the brain and this in turn is aroused to impart increased action to the hearts and short-lived energy to the entire system. Fatigue is forgotten; the strength seems to be increased.

---

[312] Ibid.

The intellect is aroused and the imagination becomes more vivid.[313]

In view of the above reaction, many people suppose that their tea or coffee is doing them a great good. On the contrary, this is a fatal mistake because tea and coffee do not nourish the body. Their effect is produced before there has been time for digestion and assimilation, and what seemed to be strength is only nervous stimulation. Finally, when the influence of that stimulant is gone, the unnatural forces abates, the system is left in a corresponding state of languor and debility. As the body becomes debilitated by their constant use, it gradually becomes more difficult to stimulate the energies to the desired point. Still on this thought provoking issue, Ellen G. White asserted that:

> Tea and coffee do not nourish the system. The relief obtained from them is sudden, before the stomach has time to digest them. This shows that what the users of these stimulants call strength, is only received by exciting the nerves of the stomach, which convey the irritation to the brain, and this in turn is aroused to impart increased action to the heart, and short-lived energy to the entire system. All this is false strength, that we are the worse for having. They do not give a particle of natural strength.[314]

---

[313] Ellen G. White, The Ministry of Healing, (Ontario: Pacific Press Publishing Association, 1942), pp. 326-327

[314] Ellen G. White, Testimony Studies on Diet and Foods, (Washington D.C: Review and Herald Publishing Association, 1971), p. 148

The second effect of tea-drinking is headache, wakefulness, palpitation of the heart, indigestion, trembling of the nerves, with many other evils. "I beseech you therefore, brethren, by the mercies of God, that ye present your bodies as a living sacrifice, holy, acceptable, unto God, which is your reasonable service." God calls for a living sacrifice, not a dead or dying one. When we realize the requirements of God, we shall see that He requires us to be temperate in all things. The end of our creation is to glorify God in our bodies and spirits, which are His. How can we do this when we indulge the appetite to the injury of the physical and moral powers? God requires that we present our bodies a living sacrifice. Then the duty is enjoined on us to preserve that body in the very best condition of health that we may comply with His requirements. "Whether, therefore, ye eat or drink, or whatsoever ye do, do all to the glory of God."[315]

She went further to warn that:

Tea and coffee is a sin, and injurious indulgence which, like other evils, injuries. These darling idols create an excitement, a morbid action of the nervous system; and the immediate influence of the stimulants is gone, it lets down below par just to that degree that its stimulating properties elevated above par.[316]

---

[315] Ibid.

[316] _____ Counsels on Diet and Foods. (Washington, DC: Review and Herald Publishing Association, 1976), p. 425

4.3.3.2   Validation of Medical Science:

The counsels of Ellen White concerning the dangers of using tea and coffee which was penned down in 1905 were validated through the writings of a medical doctor, H. A. Reimann in 1967. This medical expert stated that caffeine, xanthine alkaloid, mainly stimulate the cerebral cortex, the thalamus, the vasomotor and respiratory centers, and this evidently affects the thermal regulatory mechanism of the body. Furthermore, it reduces the cerebral blood flow. Some of the acute and chronic toxic effects on the human body are insomnia, irritability, cardiac palpitation, tremors, convulsion, flushing, anorexia, dehydration from diuresis, fever, albuminuria and epigastric discomfort. Still on the toxic effect of tea and coffee, Reimann declared:[317]

> Caffeinism is said to be current among intellectual workers, actresses, waitresses, nocturnal employees, and long-distance automobile drivers. Illness otherwise unexplained may be caused by excessive ingestion of xanthine alkaloids, including those in coffee, tea, cocoa and in some popular beverages.[318]

Again, the evil effects of these food drinks such as caffeine and tea, were clearly articulated by Samuel Vaisrub, M. D.; Senior Editor for the Journal of the American Medical Association. He noted in an editorial of that Journal that caffeine is a chemical known to

[317] The Ellen G. White Estate-General Conference of Seventh-day Adventists, Medical Science and the Spirit of Prophecy, (Washington DC: Review and Herald Publishing Association, 1971), p. 13
[318] Ibid.

precipitate some ectopic beats and also accelerate the heart rate. Caffeine raises the blood pressure, interferes with sleep, elevates the plasma levels of the fatty acids and causes a disproportionate rise in the blood glucose level in response to glucose loading especially in diabetes.[319]

4.3.3.3   Decaffeinated Coffee and Tea:

Some individuals prefer these decaffeinated food drinks as excellent beverages. It must, however, be pointed out that this group of coffee and tea are not one hundred percent free of caffeine. The irritating volatile oils, extractive matter, tannic acid and the vestiges of caffeine do cause abnormal stimulation of the nervous system, as well as lead to the inflammation in the gastrointestinal tracts. It is true that decaffeinated beverages must be considered the lesser of two evils; unfortunately, the decaffeination process used for many brands of decaffeinated beverages leaves behind traces of chemicals that might be more dangerous and harmful than caffeine.[320]

4.3.3.4   Alcohol, Brain Damage and Loss of Life:

Alcohol is another social drink, which is commonly used in most world societies. Its use has become customary at home, at work, organized parties and even during celebrations, alcoholic drinks are paradoxically used to "toast to your health and prosperity." Men and women of all social classes like alcohol in its various forms as

---

[319]   http://www.llu.edu/inf/legacy/LegacyBhtml.

[320]   Richard Hansen. <u>Get Well at Home—Complete Home Health Care for the Family</u>, (Maine: Shilo Medical Publications, 1995), pp. 268-269

wine, beer and other beverages because its intake makes them feel good. People depend on alcoholic drinks because that chemical is a psychotropic drug. This means that one of the major effects of alcohol in the body is its influence on the mind, usually by affecting the neurotransmitters. (Neurotransmitters are the chemicals, which control the liquid connection between the nerve endings.) [321]

Concerning alcohol, Ellen White stated in very strong words in 1885 that some people are "destroying reason and life by liquor drinking."[322] She further asserted that the use of liquor destroys the sensitive nerves of the brain and equally benumbs the sensibilities. Furthermore, on alcohol, she indignantly mentioned in 1891 that "moderate drinking is the school in which men are receiving an education for the drunkard's career."[323] She was distressed as she saw men and women committing slow suicide through the intake of the deadly poison known as alcohol. In 1905 through inspiration she wrote:

> Intoxication is just as really produced by wine, beer, and cider as by stronger drinks. The use of these drinks awakens the taste for those that are stronger, and thus the liquor habit is established. Moderate drinking is the school in which men are educated for the drunkard's career. Yet so insidious is the work of these milder stimulants that the high way to drunkenness is centered before the victim suspects his danger. Some who are never considered really

---

[321] William Dysinger. <u>Heaven's Lifestyle Today</u>. (Hagerstown, MD: Review and Herald Publishing Association, 1997), pp. 51-52

[322] Ellen G. White. <u>Testimonies for the Church</u>, vol. 5, p.44

[323] Ibid.

drunk are always under the influence of mild intoxicants. They are feverish, unstable in mind, unbalanced. Imagining themselves secure, they go on and on, until every barrier is broken down, every principle sacrificed. The strongest resolutions are undermined, the highest considerations are not sufficient to keep the debased appetite under the control of reason. The Bible nowhere sanctions the use of intoxicating wine. The wine that Christ made from water at the marriage feast of Cana was the pure juice of the grape. This is the "new wine . . . found in the cluster," of which the Scripture says, "Destroy it not; for a blessing is in it." Isaiah 65:8[324]

4.3.3.5 Confirmation by Medical Science:

The Spirit of Prophecy counsel on the dangers of alcohol has also been confirmed by medical science. Kurt Isselbacher, M. D., notes that alcohol is best known for its influence on the brain and it also affects almost all other organs of the body. Next, it has also been confirmed that prolonged high doses of alcohol could lead to pathological changes in peripheral nerves and other body tissues. It can lead to brain damage, loss of memory, judgment and learning. As drinking of alcohol continues, aggressions, antagonism, depression and psychosis may appear. Other consequences include gastritis, ulcers, pancreatitis and cardiac arrest.[325]

---

[324] _____ The Ministry of Healing. P. 331
[325] http://www.llu.edu/inf/legacy/LegacyBhtml

William Dysinger has clearly stated that alcohol as a drug is readily absorbed from the stomach into the blood and to all parts of the body. Its toxic effects are primarily noted in the brain and liver of every consumer. That is not all, according to him it works in the central nervous system as an anesthetic and kills some of the brain cells in the frontal lobe where judgment, self-control, psychological inhibitions and conscience are located. So alcohol is a depressant and causes poor reaction to time and loss of nervous reflexes and judgment. This has led to the loss of thousands of live around the world due to accidental deaths, suicides and other alcohol related murders. Drinking alcohol during pregnancy leads to stunted growth, mental retardation, malformed facial features and could also lead to lifelong heart problems.[326]

In his article on 'Health and Salvation" in the Journal of the Adventist Theological Society, Mervyn G. Hardinge maintained that electrophysiological studies indicate that alcohol, like all other anesthetics exert its first depressant action on the parts of the brain that are involved in discrimination, concentration, memory and sight as demonstrated below[327]:

---

[326] William Dysinger. Heaven's Lifestyle Today. (Hagerstown, MD: Review and Herald Graphics, 1997), p. 55.

[327] Mervyn G. Hardinge, "Health and Salvation" in The Journal of Adventist Theological Society, Vol. 3, No. 2, 1992, p. 104

FIG. I EFFECT OF ALCOHOL ON DIFFERENT PARTS OF THE HUMAN BODY

S/N	Special Senses	Actions
1	Sight	Blurred, deranged
2	Hearing	Dulled, out of tune
3	Taste	Dulled
4	Smell	Dulled
5	Touch	Dulled
6	Pain	Dulled, lost
7	Position	Deranged, imbalance
8	Direction	Distorted, confused

From the facts mentioned above in figure one above,[328] medical sciences have once again confirmed the health counsels of the Spirit of Prophecy and the evil consequences of this insidious poison.

4.3.3.6 <u>Fats Causing Heart and Blood-Vessels Diseases:</u>

Fats and carbohydrates supply the energy needed by the body to carry out its daily functions. Fats also function as protective pads especially for delicate organs in the human body. Fats could also cause problems when they are not used up because they can raise the cholesterol level and expose the individual to the danger of heart attack. The Levitical injunction is "eat no fat, of ox or sheep or goat."[329] Humanity would be better of and also enjoy better health

---

[328] <u>Ibid</u>.
[329] Leviticus 7:22-23.

if this injunction of the Omnipotent and Omniscient God through Moses is adhered to.

In 1868, Ellen White in the Testimonies to the Church warned overweight individuals of their being susceptible to acute attacks of disease, and even to sudden death if they continued consuming animal fats.[330]

Twenty-eight years later White wrote:

> Both the blood and the fat of animals are consumed as a luxury. But the Lord gave special directions that these should not be eaten. This is because their use would make a diseased current of blood in the human system. The disregard for the Lord's special directions has brought a variety of difficulties and diseases upon human beings. If they introduce into their systems that which cannot make good flesh and blood, they must endure the results of their disregard of God's word.[331]

All these demonstrate the adverse effect, which fats have on the blood vessels and heart. Let us now consider what modern medical science has discovered concerning the use of animal fats and the health of humanity.

---

[330] Ellen G. White. Testimonies for the Church, vol. 2, p. 61.
[331] _____ Counsels on Diet and Foods, p. 393.

4.3.3.7 The Witness of Medical Science:

Medical science has proved beyond reasonable doubt that coronary attacks and strokes are closely related to a type of fat almost exclusively found in flesh food. The American Heart Association in 1966 advices Americans and all who cherish vibrant health to control the amount of saturated fats they consumed because of its risk of causing heart attacks.[332]

Doyless, M. D. asserted that diet is one outstanding way to measure the prevalence and incidence of CHD (Coronary Heart Disease). And one effective method to be used in the control of cholesterol and enhance one's health is through vegetarians.[333] In order to achieve a balance vegetarian diet, nutritionists have recommended the following guide to good eating:[334]

A. Four servings of fruits and vegetables daily (Vitamins A and C should be included in high quantity).
B. Four servings of whole grain daily. (Wheat and cereal products
C. Two servings of Milk daily (preferably Soybeans milk)
D. Two servings of Protein-rich foods daily.

The food and Beverage Magazine has provided a comprehensive list of information why people in general and business executives in particular should be very careful when it comes to meat consumption.

---
[332] The Ellen White Estate, Medical Science and The Spirit of Prophecy, p. 15.
[333] http://www.llu.edu/info/legacy/LegacyB.html
[334] Ibid.

Fats from flesh food items harden the arterial walls and finally cause arteriosclerosis. This may eventually lead to myocardial attacks and cardiac thrombosis (stroke). It further contended that food items, which are rich in meat products such as meat pies, sausages, eggs, creams, and cheese, contribute significantly to fat-related heart diseases. Another danger, which may arise from consuming flesh products, is in the risk of getting certain kinds of cancer. It is a known fact that animals found in slaughter houses may contain benign or cancerous tumors.[335]

The other cause for alarm is the presence of methl lconlantrene, a substance formed when meat is heated to high temperatures, fried or grilled. This carcinogenic substance, even in small quantities develop malignant tumor. People who are in the habit of increasing their meat consumption are being advised to refrain from that harmful habit. On the other hand, they should eat more soybeans products, vegetables, nuts, and grains, as better alternatives. Commenting on soybeans, Sidi Osho emphatically opined that soybeans are a miracle crop, which is also the world's most valuable oil seed legume. It contains all the essential amino acids, linolenic acid and lecithin, which are phospholipids that contribute in lowering the blood cholesterol levels. In addition to the above, seven different food items are also derived from the soybeans as shown below:[336]

---

[335] Stephen Udeh, ed., "Why Business Executives Should Eat Less Meat" in Food and Beverage Magazine, Enhancing Life's Quality Through Informed Action, vol. 6 issue 67 (Lagos: Food and Beverage Centre, 2004), p. 15

[336] Sidi Osho, "Improving Human Nutrition Through Soybeans" in Food and Beverage Magazine, vol. 6, issue 66, p. 31.

FIG. II PRODUCTS DERIVED FROM SOYBEANS

PRODUCT	DESCRIPTION	USE
Sprouts	The tender sprouts of Soya beans. They are found in stores and can also be made at home	Can be used raw in salads and desserts. They are very rich in vitamins, enzymes, chlorophyll, as well as proteins with the advantages that when eaten raw, the maximum of all its nutritive properties are available.
Four	Composed of ground Soya beans. It can be found in stores, with or without the soybean fat.	In pastries, pasta and desserts. When added to wheat flour, it enhances its nutritional value. It allows one to replace eggs in pastries, with the advantage of not having cholesterol.
Milk	Is made of Soya beans which are grinded, cooked and filtered. In stores it is also known as soy drink.	Can replace cow milk with the advantage of containing animal fats or cholesterol. It is rich in essential fatty acids, especially linolenic. Its content of iron, vitamin B1 (thiamin) and Niacin is higher than that of cow milk. On the other hand, soymilk contains less calcium than cow milk. In the market there are some soymilk enriched with this mineral and vitamins A and D.

Milk	Is made of Soya beans which are grinded, cooked and filtered. In stores it is also known as soy drink.	Can replace cow milk with the advantage of containing animal fats or cholesterol. It is rich in essential fatty acids, especially linolenic. Its content of iron, vitamin B1 (thiamin) and Niacin is higher than that of cow milk. On the other hand, soyamilk contains less calcium than cow milk. In the market there are some soymilk enriched with this mineral and vitamins A and D.
Oil	High quality table oil with a neutral flavour. It has up to 6% polyunsaturated fatty acid.	Flavours salads, pastries and cooking in general.
Tofu	It is Soya cheese. It is prepared by adding a coagulant to Soya bean milk (for example: lemon) and applying pressure for several days until it acquires a semi-solid state.	It is used in the place of white cheese. It has neutral taste, which makes it very useful in many cooked foods. It must be seasoned with salt and consistency.
Meat substitute	It may contain Soya grains or may be combined with cereal flour or nuts. These are many kinds and taste: steaks, hamburgers, sausages, etc.	As a meat substitute, especially in transitional diets. It has all the advantages of meat in protein content, but without its inconveniences.

Sauce	Fermented Soya beans, water and marine salt. The fermentation process requires 6 to 12 months.	It is used moderately as a condiment.

Soya beans have a high protein and highly digestible oil contents of about 40% and 20% respectively. It is equally amazing that the protein content of soybeans is considerably higher than that of meat, diary products, fish or even eggs.[337] Although the protein content of Soya beans is slightly deficient in methionine and cystine, which are essential amino acids, these are easily rectified as nuts, legumes and cereals are combined with Soya beans food items.[338] As shown below, a comparative analysis of vegetable products based on Soya beans and those based on meat will shed further light on the importance of discarding meat food items with its saturated fats in favour of vegetable based ones.[339]

---

[337] Ibid.

[338] Ibid.

[339] George D. Pamplona-Roger, New Lifestyle-Enjoy It! Foods for Healing and Prevention, (Madrid: Editorial Safeliz, 1998), p. 115.

FIG. III COMPARISON OF SOYABEANS WITH MEAT PRODUCTS

S/N	TYPES OF FOOD	VEGETARIAN PRODUCTS BASED ON	MEAT AND ITS DERIVATIVES
1	Carbohydrates	Though they are fundamentally protein foods, they contain some Carbohydrates. This draws them nearer to the ideal proportion which should exist between the caloric nutrients (carbohydrates, fats, and proteins) Carbohydrates are necessary in all diets including weight loss diets. In their absence the body has to burn up fats and proteins, which results in ketonic bodies and other residual acids which alter the metabolism.	This food item do not contain carbohydrates, or only in a very small quantity (the viscera such as the liver). This makes a regimen based on meat unbalanced in the proportion of needed nutrients.
2	Fats	Contains much less fat than meat, and furthermore the fat is of higher nutritive quality, and fattens less.	Have a large amount of saturated fats, harmful to health and favour the increase of weight.

3	Proteins	The proportion of proteins is similar to or even superior to that of meat. Furthermore, the proteins in soybeans are complete.	Are good sources of complete proteins.
4	Cholesterol	No vegetable food contains cholesterol.	They are rich in cholesterol. It is recommended that no more than 300mg per day of cholesterol be ingested, a quantity that is easily reached and surpassed in meat foods.
5	Calories	As the same weight and quantity of proteins, vegetable foods provide fewer calories. This makes them especially suited to weight-loss diets.	The caloric content is high due to higher percentage of fat.

Finally, the scientific analysis of the physical endurance of pedaling a bicycle according to the diet one lives on has been shown below.[340]

---

[340] Ibid, p. 84.

FIG. IV DIFFERENT TYPES OF DIET COMPARED WITH ENDURANCE DURING PHYSICAL EXERCISE

S/N	TYPE OF DIET	NATURE OF ENDURANCE AT PHYSICAL ACTIVITY	RESULT
1.	A diet based on animal fats and proteins	Time of continued pedaling of a bicycle was 57 minutes	The results of the experiment executed in Sweden indicate that athletes who eat a meat diet rich in fats and proteins are the first to become tired when they carry on a sustained effort.
2	A mixed diet based on fruits, vegetables and animal products	Time of continued pedaling of a bicycle was 114 minutes	With a mixed diet including animal and plant foods, the resistance to fatigue as measured by a continuous pedaling of a bicycle, increased up to 114 minutes.
3	A diet based on vegetables, fruits and cereals which are rich in carbohydrates	Time of continued pedaling on a bicycle was 167 minutes	The best results for guaranteeing resistance are obtained by athletes whose diet is based on foods rich in carbohydrates, especially cereals (grains) and fruits.

From the facts so far showed above, it is evident that modern medical science not only validates Ellen White's counsels on the adverse effects of animal fats on the human body but also emphasizes the superiority of the vegetarian meal over the flesh based one. Finally, from the historical records of Genesis 5 and 11, the average age of the first ten Patriarchs from Adam to Noah was 912 years. After this period meat became a part of the diet of man. The next ten generations between Shem and Abraham lived an average of 317 years. A comparison of the two generations is shown below for emphasis.

FIG.V TEN GENERATIONS BEFORE THE FLOOD (ATE NON-FLESH FOOD)

S/N	Name	Age at Death in Years
1	Adam	930
2	Seth	912
3	Enosh	905
4	Cainan	910
5	Mahalalel	895
6	Jared	962
7	Enoch (before Translation)	365*
8	Methuselah	969
9	Lamech	777
10	Noah	950
	Average Life Span (Discounting Enoch)	912.2

*Enoch did not die, he was translated to heaven, the number of years he lived has not been added above.

FIG. VI TEN GENERATIONS AFTER THE FLOOD
(ATE FLESH DIET)

S/N	Name	Age at Death in Years
1	Shem	600
2	Arphaxad	438
3	Salah	433
4	Eber	464
5	Peleg	238
6	Rue	239
7	Serug	230
8	Nahor	148
9	Terah	205
10	Abraham	175
	Average Life Span	317

An objective analysis of these two generations reveals that following the flood, the life spans rapidly declined. The record of Genesis shows that the generation that consumed flesh diet lived shorter years.[341] The effect of excessive sugar on the human system and how it causes disease would be considered.

4.3.3.8 Sugar and Disease:

It was in 1890 that Ellen White specifically warned that the free use of sugar in any form tends to clog the human system and is also the cause of frequent illness.[342] Fifteen years after the above statement had been made, White also said:

---

[341] William Dysinger. Heaven's Lifestyle Today, p. 31.
[342] The Ellen White Estate, Medical Science and the Spirit of Prophecy, p. 16.

Far too much sugar is ordinarily used in food. cakes, sweet puddings, pastries, jellies, jams are active causes of indigestion. Especially harmful are the custards and puddings in which milk, eggs, and sugar are the chief ingredients. The free use of milk and sugar taken together should be avoided.[343]

4.3.3.9 Witness of Medical Science:

Sugar is a chemical substance which is derived from sugar-cane or beets. This substance is present in most refined food items as sweetening agents. During the processing of sugar-cane to sugar, minerals and vitamins are removed from it. The end product is the table sugar used all over the world. This sugar supplies only calories. Sugar could also lead to tooth decay. When deposits of food stick to the teeth after meal and germs act on them, plaque is formed. Excess sugar also decreases the protective strength of the white blood cells.[344]

Further witness on the adverse effect of sugar comes from John Yudkin who confirmed that sugar may be the etiological factor in arteriosclerosis or heart-vessel disease. Sugar raises the blood cholesterol level. Yudkin from his clinical investigations saw a higher association between sugar intake and sudden death from

---

[343] Ellen G. White, The Ministry of Healing, Pp. 302-303.
[344] Dave M. Nyekwere. End-Time Lectures. (Lagos: Update Communications, 1994), pp.154-155.

heart disease than fat intake and heart disease.[345] The incidence of diet-related diseases arising from high intake of sugar is on the increase worldwide. People are now more interested to consume "more quick to fix food and more food items away from home" as reported Rosemary Anyanwu. These food items have increased the consumption of energy dense nutrient but poor food items with high level of saturated fats and sugars.[346]

Numerous studies in recent times have confirmed that the shift in diet and life styles have led to a lot of chronic and debilitating health problems and life threatening conditions such as obesity. Other conditions that might follow obesity include:

A. Respiratory problems associated with chronic fatigue,
B. Arthritis aggravated by excess body weight might set in,
C. Diabetes will arise and lead to type 2 diabetes,
D. Cancer of the colorectal and prostrate will appear in males,
E. Cancer of the endometrial, cervical., ovarian and breast will appear in women,
F. Cardiovascular disorders such as hypertension, congestive heart failure, coronary artery disease, pulmonary thrombosis and stroke may occur.[347]

---

[345] The Ellen G. White Estate, Medical Science and the Spirit of Prophecy, p. 17.
[346] Rosemary Anyanwu, "Obesity, Health and Production: New Challenges for the Food and Beverage Industries", in Food and Beverage Magazine, vol. 6, issue 65, p. 26
[347] Ibid, pp. 26-27

As a result of the above health problems, accusing fingers are now being pointed at producers of soda and other sugar-filled drinks which make people fat and increase obesity. All these support the fact that the warnings of Ellen White over one hundred years ago are still relevant today. We must heed these counsels. Finally on nutrition, the food Guide Pyramid which is a demonstration of the major food groups should be taken into consideration to achieve a balanced diet.

FIG.VII THE VEGETARIAN FOOD PYRAMID[348]

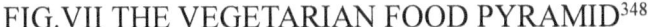

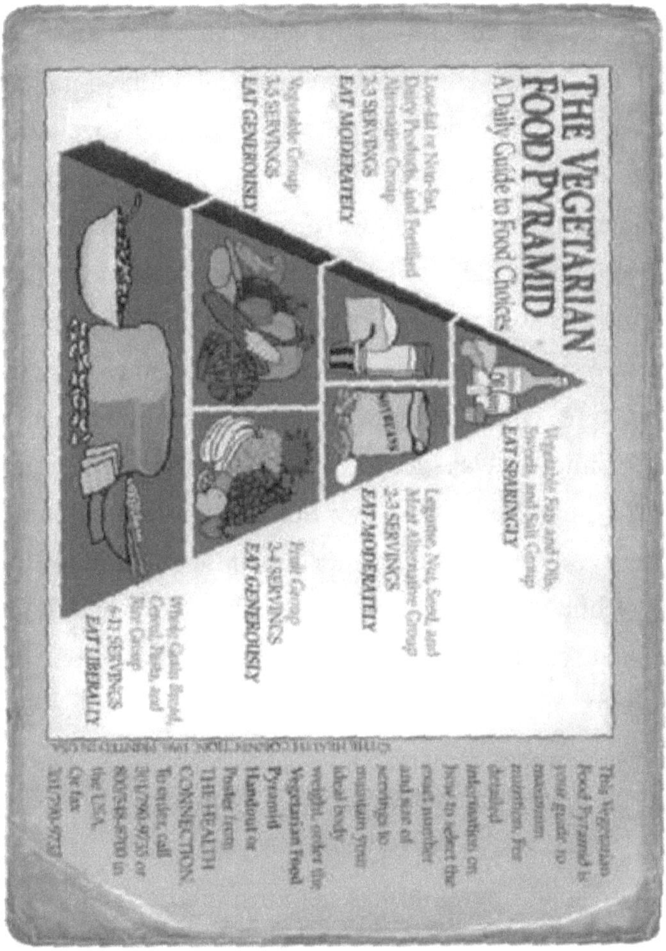

Every diet should include a variety of products as shown in the food pyramid

---

[348] The Vegetarian Food Pyramid Poster from THE HEALTH CONNECTION USA, 1999

Each of the above mentioned food groups provide certain nutrients, which the body needs on a daily basis. As a matter of fact, no single food group contains all the needed nutrients. In view of this, carbohydrates, which are the foundation, should be a major part of our diet; we must eat more of these. The fruits and vegetable groups should be consumed liberally. The protein groups should be eaten in very limited quantities. However, growing children should get adequate amount to help in their balanced development. Lastly, the fats and oils and sweets group must be consumed sparingly. This is because excessive consumption of these food items could contribute to high blood pressure, diabetes, strokes, cancers and other illnesses. One of the simplest ways to apply a sound principle in guiding us with the food pyramid is to center our diet on the food items at the base of the pyramid and to consume less of the foods at the top of the pyramid. While choosing food items within the group, one should endeavour to select from non fat and the lean food groups as often as possible for optimum health.[349]

4.3.3.10 Eating Right and Watching Calories:

The food guide pyramid has demonstrated a range of servings for each of the five major good groups we have. The number of servings needed in order to maintain a healthy body weight has also been indicated. The table below shows three different calorie levels (1,600, 2,200, and 2,800 calories), which are needed by three different groups of people.

---

[349] http://www.ring.com/health/food/FOOD.htm

FIG.VIII DAILY CALORIC NEEDS

	CHILDREN, WOMEN OLDER ADULTS	TEEN GIRLS, ACTIVE WOMEN, MOST MEN	TEEN BOYS, ACTIVE MEN
CALORIE LEVEL[1]	ABOUT 1,600	ABOUT 2,200	ABOUT 2,800
Milk & Milk products Group [2]	2 to 4	2 to 4	2 to 4
Meat & Meat Alternatives Group	2	2	3
Vegetable Group	3	4	5
Fruit Group	2	3	4
Bread & Cereal Group	6	9	11
Total Fat (grams)[3]	36 to 53 (grams)[3]	49 to 73 (grams)[3]	62 to 93 (grams)[3]

4.3.3.11 <u>Height and Weight Guidelines:</u>

It was Saint Francis of Sales (1567-1622) Bishop of Geneva who said: "In the control of appetite, we should think of the average. If the body is very fat, the weight is hard to carry, and it is too thing, it cannot carry us."[350] Since obesity is a current health problem around the world today, it is important that we watch our caloric intake. The

---

[350] George D. Pamplona-Roger, <u>New Lifestyle-Enjoy It! Foods for Healing and Prevention</u>, p. 111

guiding rules here is watch your weight, take in fewer calories and use more calories.[351] However, a height and weight guidelines chart has been provided below to aid us in controlling our weight through our daily caloric intake.[352]

---

[351] Ibid.

[352] http://www.ring.com/health/food/FOOD.htm

FIG.IX WEIGHT AND HEIGHT GUIDELINES FOR MEN AND WOMEN[353]

WEIGHT AND HEIGHT GUIDELINES

	WOMEN				MEN	
Height	Low	Midpoint	High	Height	Midpoint	High
4'10"	100	115	131	5'1"	123	145
4'11"	101	117	134	5'2"	125	148
5'0"	103	120	137	5'3"	127	151
5'1"	105	122	140	5'4"	129	155
5'2"	108	125	144	5'5"	131	159
5'3"	111	128	148	5'6"	133	163
5'4"	114	133	152	5'7"	135	167
5'5"	117	136	156	5'8"	137	171
5'6"	120	140	160	5'9"	139	175
5'7"	123	143	164	5'10"	141	179
5'8"	126	146	167	5'11"	144	183
5'9"	129	150	170	6'0"	147	187
5'10"	132	153	173	6'1"	150	192
5'11"	135	156	176	6'2"	153	197
6'0"	138	159	179	6'3"	157	202

The weight is measured in pounds

Apart from the height and weight, one's profession should equally have a contributing factor in determining the calories to be

---

[353] Ibid

consumed daily. Common sense and sanctified reasoning should guide us in making this important decision day by day.[354]

FIG. X DAILY NEED OF CALORIES ACCORDING TO PROFESSION

COMPARED WITH DAILY NEED OF CALORIES ACCORDING TO ACTIVITY[355]

Type of Activity	Professions	Calories Consumed Daily
Sedentary or Very Light	Office Workers, teachers	1,800
Light	Students, Salesmen, domestic labourers, (with electric appliance)	2,300
Moderate	Mechanics, carpenters, domestic labourers (without electric appliance)	2,800
Intense	Construction workers, farmers, miners, athletes	3,500+

---

[354] George D. Pamplona-Roger. <u>New Lifestyle-Enjoy It! Foods for Healing and Prevention</u>, p. 112.

[355] George D. Pamplona Roger, <u>New Lifestyle Enjoy It: Food for Healing and Prevention,</u> p.112

4.3.4 Exercise:

Exercise is the use of the muscles of the body for physical exertion for health improvement.[356] Exercise as a remedial factor is very important. But little interest is paid to it by so many people and so many have fallen sick from illnesses that would have been prevented. Our body is designed for movement. Contrary to what happens when man builds something, inactivity in the body leads to deterioration than does exercise. It has been demonstrated that persons who dedicate at least four periods of forty minutes each to physical exercise every week run a smaller risk of having a heart attack or circulatory diseases. Exercise combats arterial hypertension, prevents obesity and keeps the entire organism in good working condition. All members of the family should take part in this wholesome activity.

Recognizing still the importance of exercise to promote good health, Ellen G. White highlights that inactivity is a major cause of disease. Exercise quickens and equalizes the circulation of the blood, but in idleness the blood does not circulate freely, and the changes in it, so necessary to life and health, do not take place. The skin, too, becomes inactive. Impurities are not expelled as they would be if the circulation has been quickened by vigorous exercise, the skin is not kept in a healthful condition, and the lungs are not fed with plenty of pure, fresh air. This state of system throws a lot of burden on the excretory organs, and disease is the result.[357] Ministers, teachers, students and other brain workers often suffer from illness as a

---

[356] William Dysinger, Heaven's Lifestyle Today, p. 31
[357] Ellen G. White. The Ministry of Healing, p. 154

result of severe mental taxation, unrelieved by physical exercise. What these persons need is a more active life. Strictly temperate habits, combined with proper exercise, would ensure both mental and physical vigor, and would give power of endurance to all brain workers.[358]

Those who have overtaxed their physical powers should not be encouraged to forgo manual labour entirely. But labour, to be of the greatest advantage, should be systematic and agreeable. Outdoor exercise is the best, it should be so planned as to strengthen by use the organs that have become weakened; and the heart should be in it; the labour of the hands should never degenerate into mere drudgery.[359] Even those who have overtaxed their physical powers should not be encouraged to forgo exercise entirely. Invalids need exercise; inactivity has been noted as the greatest curse which could come upon invalids. Light employment and useful labour will strengthen their muscles and activate their minds to greater activities.

4.3.4.1   Why is Exercise so Important:

Being physically active offers many advantages. You can lose weight, become fitter, reduce stress levels, and improve sleep patterns, increase your life quality and expectancy, and reduces the rise of heart disease, diabetes and some forms of cancer. Overall, it makes you feel refreshed and happy! It is suggested that everyone should participate in some forms of exercise for 30 minutes 4 days a week, whether it be walking to the shops, running up and down the

---

[358] Ibid, p. 238
[359] Ibid.

stairs or going to a weekly aerobics class. Take the stairs, rather than lift, get off the bus one stop earlier and walk the rest of the way, park further away from the shops run up the stairs when you get to work. It can be difficult to fit exercise into your busy lifestyle, but every little bit helps. Therefore, go ahead and include exercise in your schedule since the advantages far out weight the disadvantages.[360]

4.3.4.2 How Exercise Affects Glucose:

Exercise consumes nutrients including glucose, and forces cells to draw on the glucose stored in muscles. Once this is depleted, the body turns it to sugar in the blood for energy. This would cause a drop in the blood glucose level where it is not for your liver, which under normal circumstances produces enough glucose to replenish the blood's supply. The demand for blood sugar can continue even when exercise has ended because muscles continue to remove glucose from the blood to restock their reserves. Diabetics should therefore, be extremely careful with vigorous exercise. Your doctor must be consulted before changing or starting fitness routine.[361]

Exercise doesn't have to be strenuous to be beneficial, but try to spend at least 30 minutes and engaged in some physical activity. While an individual may prefer walking, another may choose something more vigorous, such as biking, swimming, or even running, clearing the bush behind your apartment or even weeding your garden could serve the same purpose.

---

[360] http://www.hifit.co.uk/health-breaks/importance-exercise.htm
[361] http://www.ihj.com/ihj/story.jhtml:sessionid=XBDTB5F1C224DQFI BQNSCZQ?storyid=

The chart below shows the consumption of calories per hour for eight different physical activities.[362]

FIG.XI PHYSICAL ACTIVITIES AND CONSUMPTION OF CALORIES PER HOUR CHART

Physical Activity	Calories Consumed per Hour
Sleeping	65
Walking	250
Gymnastics	350
Tennis	450
Cycling	500
Swimming	650
Soccer	850
Racing	1,000

4.3.5   <u>Water:</u>

Water is generally known today as the universal solvent, and it is the creator's wish to provide it in abundance because of its healing power. It is observed that our bodies contain around 60% to 75% of water.[363] This proves the essence of water needed in the body. All parts of the body need water to have effective functions and to stay healthy. The kidney needs water to filter the blood and eliminate unneeded substances through the urine; the digestive system needs

---

[362] George D. Pamplona-Roger. <u>New Lifestyle Enjoy It! Food for Healing and Prevention</u>. P. 11.

[363] Ibid.

water so that the feaces are not too dry or hard, causing strain, the skin needs water to maintain itself firm and healthy elasticity; and even the bones should contain an adequate proportion of water to maintain their elasticity and hardness at different times. Water is needed for external as well as for internal uses. Water also promotes health and we are to drink it freely. About 8 to 10 glasses of water should be taken daily.[364] The chemical formula for this important liquid is H_2O. It is made up of two volumes of hydrogen and a volume of oxygen. Both of these gases are odourless. Inspite of the availability of many different kinds of liquids for drinking, water is still the only substance, which really quenches thirst.

4.3.5.1 Water is Essential to Life:

Water is as essential as well as a fundamental part of our lives. It had been ranked by experts as second only to oxygen as essential for life. The body of an average adult is 60% to 75% water. Water makes up 2/3 of our total body weight which is about 40 to 50 grams. A human embryo is more than 80% water. A new born baby is 74% water. On a daily basis our body replaces 3 quarts of water through its numerous functions. Every process in the body occurs in a water medium. The importance of water is seen in the fact that we can exist without food for 2 months or more, but we can only survive for a few days without water.[365]

---

[364] Ibid.

[365] http://www/information-entertainment.com/Fitness/fitwater.html

4.3.5.2 Water Aids Body Metabolism:

Water is the medium for various enzymatic and chemical reactions in the body. It moves nutrients, hormones, antibodies and oxygen through the blood stream and lymphatic system. The protein and enzymes of the body function more efficiently in solutions of lower viscosity. Water is the solvent of the body and it regulates all functions, including the activity of everything it dissolves and circulates.[366]

4.3.5.3 Water is necessary for Weight Loss:

Among its other benefits, water plays a major part in weight loss. Since water contains no calories, it can serve as an appetite suppressant, and helps the body metabolize stored fat; it may possibly be one of the most significant factors in losing weight. Water is the single most important nutrient one may consume every day. It is fat-free, cholesterol-free, low in sodium, and completely without calories. Also, drinking more water helps to reduce water retention by stimulating your kidneys. Studies have recommended that if you are overweight according to average height and weight comparison charts, you should add one glass of water to your daily requirement (of eight glasses) for every 25 pounds over your recommended weight. Dehydration leads to excess body fat, poor muscle tone, and size, decreased digestive efficiency and organ function, increased toxicity, joint and muscle soreness, and water retention. Water works to keep muscles and skin toned.[367]

---

[366] http://members.aol.com/SaveMoDoe2/importance.htm
[367] Ibid.

4.3.5.4 Water Helps the Digestive System Function Efficiently:

The digestion of solid food depends on the presence of copious amounts of water. Acids and appropriate enzymes both in the mouth and in the stomach break the food down into a homogenized fluid state which can pass into the intestine for the next phase of digestion. Constipation is a frequent symptom of dehydration. Increased water, along with increased fiber, will usually eliminate this problem. Gastritis, Duodenitis, pain from ulcers (as long as the ulcer is not perforated), and heartburn all decrease with increased water intake. Water eliminates toxins as well as other waste products from the body.[368]

4.3.5.5 Water Prevents Dehydration:

Dehydration is the loss of water from body tissues without replenishing it adequately. When the body is dehydrated, a type of rationing and distribution is activated to ration the available water in the body. Since the body has no reserve system, it operates a priority distribution system for the amount that has been made available. The body's signals of dehydration are frequently joint pains, stomach pains and cramps, back pain, low energy, mental confusion and disorientation. However, numerous disease symptoms respond to increased water intake.[369]

The "dry mouth" signal is the last outward sign of extreme dehydration. When the body tries to adjust to being deprived of

---

[368] http://members.aol.com/SaveMoDoe2/importance.htm
[369] Ibid.

water, our thirst mechanism is disabled. This dry mouth sign is actually the last outward sign of extreme decreases with age. The end result is increasing dehydration. Fortunately, when we begin to give the body more water, the thirst mechanism begins to work again, and this becomes more apparent when the bodies are fully hydrated. When we are getting sufficient water, we are often thirsty.[370] There is a need to daily replenish the water which the body looses in order to prevent dehydration. Indeed, an adult loses nearly 6 pints (12 cups) of water daily. Every adult loses ½ to 1 cup of water a day from the soles of the feet; another 2 to 4 cups are lost through breathing; perspiration accounts for the loss of another 2 cups; while 6 cups are lost in urine.[371]

4.3.5.6 Body Temperature:

Water helps to regulate our body temperature through perspiration. When we perspire, excess heat is dissipated and the body cools down.

4.3.5.7 Water is Needed for Breathing:

It is amazing that we need water in order to breath. As we take in oxygen and excrete CO^2 our lungs must be moistened by water. We lose about 1 to 2 pints of water each day just exhaling. Asthma is frequently relieved when water intake is increased. Histamine plays a key role in regulating the way the body uses and also distributes water and equally helps control the body's defense mechanisms. In

---

[370] http://www.laformechic.com/water.htm
[371] http://www.bottledwaterblues.com/Better Drinking Habits.cfm

asthmatics, histamine level increases with dehydration. Our best defense for the body is to close down the airways and the best way to do that is by drinking enough water.[372]

4.3.5.8 The brain needs water to function optimally:

Brain tissue is 75% water. Although the brain is only 1/50th of the body weight, it uses 1/20th of the blood supply. With dehydration, the level of energy generation in the brain is decreased. Depression and chronic fatigue syndrome are frequently results of dehydration. Migraine headaches may be an indicator of critical body temperature regulation at times of "heat stress."[373] Dehydration plays a major role in bringing on migraines. Dehydration causes stress and stress causes further dehydration.

4.3.5.9 Water is needed by the Kidneys:

The kidneys also need copious amounts of water to function properly in their work of filtration. The kidney removes wastes such as uric acid, urea, and lactic acid which must all be dissolved in water. When the body does not have sufficient water, these waste products are not effectively removed. Apart from causing pollution to the body, these wastes could damage the kidneys.[374]

---

[372] http://members.aol.com/SaveMoDoe2/importance.htm
[373] Ibid.
[374] http://members.aol.com/SaveMoDoe2/importance.htm

4.3.5.10 Body Joints Need Water to Work Well:

Water lubricates our joints. The cartilage tissues found at the ends of long bones and between the vertebrae of the spine hold a lot of water, which serves as a lubricant during the movement of the joint. When, the cartilage is hydrated, the two opposing surfaces glide freely, and friction damage is minimal. If the cartilage is dehydrated, the rate of "abrasive" damage is increased, resulting in joint deterioration and increased pain. The actively growing blood cells in the bone marrow take priority over the cartilage for the available water that goes through the bone structure. Rheumatoid joint pain frequently decreases with increased water intake and flexing exercises to bring more circulation to the joints.[375]

4.3.5.11 Adequate Water Intake is Needed During Pregnancy:

Adequate water intake is necessary by every pregnant woman. Morning sickness is a thirst signal for both the mother and the fetus. During the intrauterine stage of cell expansion, water needed for the growth of the fetus has to be provided by the mother. It has been observed that one of the first indicators for water needs for the fetus and mother is the morning sickness during the first trimester of pregnancy. The importance of water during pregnancy is further buttressed by the following:[376]

1. Water helps in carrying nutrients through the blood of the mother to the baby.

---

[375] Ibid.

[376] http://members.aol.com/SaveMoDoe2/importance.htm

2. Water helps in the prevention of bladder infections, constipation and bleeding, which are very common during pregnancy.
3. The more water one drinks the more water one retains.
4. Dehydration can trigger contraction and early labour. This should be prevented through adequate water intake.
5. Amniotic fluid which is mostly water is replaced continuously through out the day and night and as such more water is needed to keep the body healthy.
6. Hydration is so essential for the production of good breast milk.

4.3.5.12 Drinking Water and Other Beverages:

For the proper functioning of our body, there is the need to drink enough water and not just beverages that contain water. As a matter of fact, there is a difference between drinking pure water and taking beverages that contain water. Fruit juice, soft drinks, coffee and other drinks may contain substances that are not healthy. Some of the substances may even contradict some of the positive effects of the added water. For instance, caffeinated beverages stimulate the adrenal glands and end up robbing the body of necessary water. Soft drinks on the other hand contain phosphorus which can lead to depletion of bone calcium. Soda contains sodium. Fruit juices contain a lot of sugar which end up as a stimulant to the pancreas. Beer contains water but it also has alcohol in it which is both toxic and harmful to the body. These drinks which contain water will end up taxing the body instead of actually cleansing it.[377] A 12 ounce

---

[377] http://members.aol.com/SaveMoDoe2/importance.htm

of regular soda soft drink contains the equivalent of 9 teaspoons of sugar and plenty of calories. As one takes beverages the water reserve in the body is reduced. The habit of taking beverages may also lead one to lose his taste for water.[378]

4.3.5.13 How Much Water Should We Drink?

The quantity of water we may take will depend of the activities we are engaged in on a daily basis. An individual who is not active will need a half ounce of water per pound of body weight per day. This will amount to some 8 ounce glasses of water in a day if your weight is 160 pounds. For every other 25 pounds of excess ideal body weight, one 8 ounce glass of water will be added. However, an active athletic individual needs 13-14 8 ounce glasses of water daily if the weight is 160 pounds. As a rule, the more physical activity one engages in, the more water one needs. The water intake, however, should be spread throughout the day. One should not plan to drink more than 4 glasses of water within any given hour. When properly followed, after a few weeks the bladder will calm down while the urination will be less frequent but in larger amounts.[379]

4.3.5.14 Water is Needed both Internally and Externally:

Even our earth seems to be unique among all known celestial bodies. For instance, it has water, which covers three-fourths of its surface and constitutes 60-70% of the living world. Water regenerates and redistributed through evaporation, making it seem endlessly

---

[378] Ibid.

[379] http://www.cpft.edu/ete/modules/waterq/wqwaterimport.html

renewable. So water will always be with us. Actually, only 1% of the world's water is usable to us. About 97% is salty sea water, and 2% is frozen in glaciers and polar ice caps. Thus, that 1% of the world's water supply is a precious commodity necessary for our survival. Dehydration (lack of water) will kill us faster than starvation (lack of food).[380]

Since the plants and animals we eat also depend on water, lack of it causes both dehydration and starvation. The scenario gets worse because water that looks drinkable can contain harmful elements, which could cause illness and death if ingested.

To be in optimum health, we must, therefore, drink pure and clean water and also use the same for external purposes. It is therefore not surprising that in 1905 Ellen White said:

> In health and in sickness, pure water is one of heaven's choicest blessings. Its proper use promotes health. It is the beverage which God provided to quench the thirst of animals and man. Drunk freely, it helps to supply the necessities of the system and assists nature to resist disease. The external application of water is one of the easiest and most satisfactory ways of regulating the circulation of the blood. A cold or cool bath is an excellent tonic. Warm baths open the pores and thus aid in the elimination of impurities. Both warm and neutral baths soothe the nerves and equalize the circulation.[381]

---

[380] Ibid.
[381] Ellen G. White, The Ministry of Healing, p. 11

But many have never learned by experience the beneficial effects of the proper use of water, and they are afraid of it. Water treatments are not appreciated as they should be, and to apply them skillfully requires work that many are unwilling to perform. But none should feel excused for ignorance or indifference on this subject. There are many ways in which water can be applied to relieve pain and check disease. All should become intelligent in its use in simple home treatments. Mothers, especially should know how to care for their families in both health and sickness.[382]

Another important property of water is its powerful cleansing effect. Water works wonders both in the body and out of the body to keep it clean. Dr. Kloss still went further to discuss some basic rules, which should be applied when using water for bathing.[383] Some basic rules for bathing have been shared below:

1. Always use the thermometer when possible in preparing bathing water for the sick. Test the water by placing the elbow on it when thermometer is not available.
2. Room temperature where bath is taken should be between 70 and 85°F. Patients and invalids require warmer temperature.
3. Extremely hot or cold baths should not be used for old or nervous patients.

---

[382] Ibid

[383] Jethro, Kloss. Back to Eden, (California: Woodbridge Press Publishing Company, 1997), pp. 108-124.

African Traditional Medicine

4. Never take a cold bath when you are extremely fatigued. It is always better to begin with tepid water and later increase to the cold water.
5. Cold bath should not be taken during menstruations.
6. Pure and soft water should be used for baths.
7. Patients should exercise before and after bathing.
8. Hydrotherapic treatments are best given to patients about three hours after their breakfast.
9. Cleansing baths should be taken once every three or four days.

All the above-mentioned rules for bathing should be applied appropriately for optimum well-being. Appropriate care and measures should equally be taken for foot bath, leg bath, eye bath, ear bath and nose bath. Finally, Kloss divided baths into seven different classes depending on the temperature of the water.

1. Very cold bath — 32-$55°F$
2. Cold bath — 55-$65°F$
3. Cool bath — 65-$80°F$
4. Tepid bath — 80-$92°F$
5. Warm bath — 92-$98°F$
6. Hot bath — 98-$104°F$
7. Very hot bath — $104°F$ and above

The condition of the patient will ultimately influence the temperature of the bath.[384]

---

[384] Ibid, p. 124

4.3.6   Sunlight:

What a dull place this earth would be if there was no sunlight. Therefore, God made sunlight to bring a wealth of beauty into our lives. Not only does sunshine make our flowers grow, but it adds green chlorophyll to the leaves and colours to the gardens. Energy from the rays of the sun also acts on certain substances in the skin, changing them to vitamin D, one of the vitamins required by the body. The sun is full of health-giving energy to keep our bodies alive and healthy. The precious sunlight not only warms us, and the world all around us, but it is necessary in making us grow strong and healthy. It produces food for us and for all the living things God has created.[385]

Concerning sunlight, Ellen G. White states that for us to make our home the abiding place of health and happiness we must place them above the miasma and fog of the lowlands, and give free entrance to heaven's life-giving agencies. Dispense with heavy curtains, open the windows and blinds and allow no vines, however, beautiful, to shade the windows and permit no tree to stand so near the house as to shut out the sunshine. The sunlight may fade the drapery and the carpets, and tarnish the picture frames; but it will bring healthy glows to the cheeks of both the old and young in every home.[386]

The sun, created by God is to provide light and energy for planet earth. The energy from the sun is what sustains all forms of life in our planet. Life cannot exist here without sunlight. For instance,

---

[385] Ellen White. The Ministry of Healing, p. 11
[386] Ibid, p. 275

solar energy (electromagnetic energy from the sun) shines down on earth, where light is produced. On the other hand, it also produces heat which is used by plants in photosynthesizing chemical energy whose end products are food and oxygen and other living creatures which do not go through the photosynthetic process, get their food from plant and metabolism, food is transferred into energy.[387] This energy is demonstrated in many outstanding ways such as work energy which enables us to move our muscles in accomplishing our daily activities. It is also seen in the production of energy which enables living organisms to make enzymes and hormones.

Finally, this energy is demonstrated in the production in electric currents for nerve cells and all other body activities.[388] The importance of light could be seen in the fact that it was the first thing God made during creation week. The power we derive from the sun and its general benefits to mankind has led many throughout history to worship it. Many ancients nations and civilization worshipped the sun personified as one or more of the gods of their land. God on the other hand has warned his people against sun worship. Despite the divine warning, Israel still followed the nations around them to worship the sun god as recorded in several passages in the scripture (2 kings 21:5; 23:5, 11).

4.3.6.1 Types of Light:

There are three types of light: Ultraviolet (UV)—short waves which constitutes 5 per cent of light; visible light (54 percent). The

---

[387] William Dysinger. Heaven's Lifestyle Today, P. 68.
[388] Ibid.

other one percent is a combination of cosmic rays, gamma rays, x-rays, radio rays, and electric waves. Ultraviolet rays of the sun are responsible for the production of vitamin D in the skin. This vitamin D is needed so much in calcium metabolism and bone production.[389]

4.3.6.2 Benefits of Sunlight:

Sunlight is a disinfectant. The ultraviolet radiation present in sunlight serves as a disinfectant which is capable of destroying numerous pathogenic organisms. Two hours of exposure to the sun's UV rays will kill most bacteria even through most glass windows.[390] Sunlight assists the body which has been wounded or injured to get quicker healing. It is also essential in healing different diseases. During the WORLD WAR II, wounded soldiers were healed while many others survived much better when their wounds including broken bones were exposed to the healing properties of sunlight. Even ancient Egypt used light for healing various diseases which modern scientists recognized just towards the end of 1700's.

4.3.6.3 Sunshine Boosts Immune System:

Apart from disinfecting our environment by killing germs and harmful organisms, the light from the sun also makes the neutrophils more efficient in destroying germs inside our bodies. The availability of sunshine also aids in increasing the number of lymphocytes

---

[389] Ibid, p. 68

[390] George D. Pamplona-Roger. New Lifestyle Enjoy It! Food for Healing and Prevention. P.11

circulating in our bodies and through this process the human immune systems is strengthened. It normalizes blood pressure and decreases blood cholesterol.

Sunlight is equally beneficial to diabetics. Sunlight lowers blood sugar, by stimulating the beta cells of the pancreatic organ system to be more efficient in the production of insulin. The second positive effect which sunlight has for the diabetic patient is through the stimulation and production of glycogen synthesize, which helps the liver remove glucose from the blood and stores it as glycogen.[391]

4.3.6.4 Sunlight Aids Body Metabolism:

This is achieved through the action of sunshine in acting as a stimulus of the thyroid gland which in turn increases thyroxin's production. When thyroxin is produced in large quantities, there would be a corresponding increase in body metabolism, more calories are burnt up which invariably is a distinct advantages in weight reduction.[392] Premature infants usually suffer jaundice. Exposing such infants to the healing sunlight will aid in altering the bilirubin in the blood of the infant who is infected with jaundice. This action will enable the jaundice to be excreted through the kidney and also prevent brain damage of the new born baby. The aged also need the healing powers of the sun on their body for optimum health and longevity.[393]

---

[391] William Dysinger. Heaven's Lifestyle Today, p. 68
[392] Ibid.
[393] Ibid.

4.3.6.5 Sunlight, Body and Cancer:

The use of the sun for all age groups must be controlled. According to Dysinger sunlight is an excellent example of the natural law which says that "many things are good on small amount, but more is not always better." Moderation is an important law of health. Sun provides wonderful benefits but its favourable effect on health does not require long exposure.[394] Exposure of the body to sunlight must be carefully done because, first the ozone layer that covers our planet and filters the ultraviolet rays is decreasing. This decrease has led to more intense solar radiation, which is adversely affecting the inhabitants of earth. In Nigeria and many other African countries, exposing the body to sunlight from sunrise up to 10:00 a.m could be very beneficial to the health of the individual. After this period, exposing the body to the hot sun could be very harmful.[395]

A lot of discussions by photo-biologists (scientists who research into the effect of light on living organisms) have been going on for a long time on the health hazard and benefits of sunlight. In Atlanta U. S. A., the importance of sunlight for the health of various people has been the focus of intensive research in a wide variety of scientific fields for many decades. The purpose of the International Light Symposium in Atlanta was to assess in detail the broad range of bio-positive effects-especially those of ultra-violet radiation (UVS)-and the risks related to sunburn[396] It is, however, important to

---

[394] Ibid, p. 69

[395] Samuel Ebun Ayen, You Can Be Healthier. (Somolu: Ayeni Nig. Ltd., 2001), p. 54

[396] http://66.218.71.225/search/cache?p=import6ance+of+sunlight&ei= UTF-8&b-11&u=tanni

note that the risk of skin cancer from sun exposure is much smaller than the public has been led to believe while the risks of vitamin D deficiency or insufficiency, which are seldom mentioned, are now known to be very substantial. Insufficient vitamin D at crucial times of life or for prolonged period appears to increase the risk of several cancers, including breast and bowel cancer, diabetes, high blood pressure, schizophrenia, multiple sclerosis and many other chronic diseases including tooth decay.[397]

Why are people not dissuaded from enjoying the sun for optimal health. It has been frequently reported that those who are regularly exposed to ultraviolet radiation (UVR) due to their occupation have a reduced risk of developing melanoma or any skin cancer. The reasons appear to be two fold: first-they develop a tan that blocks the penetration of UVR so it cannot lead to melanoma: and secondly—they produce lots of vitamin D. Both links have been demonstrated to keep the body fit and well protected against the attack of this dreaded skin disease.[398] It is true many people believe that ultraviolet light is harmful. It must be pointed out however, that our bodies need at least a small amount of UV light in order to function properly on a daily bases. Therefore, the moderate exposure to sunlight in the course of everybody activity is beneficial to mankind while the excessive exposure to UV should be avoided.[399]

---

[397] http://www.healthresearchforum.org.uk/sunlight.html
[398] http://www.shirleys-wellness-café.com/sunabth.htm
[399] http://www.gcrio.org/ozone/ozoneFAQs.html

4.3.7 Temperance:

Temperance in a simple term is defined as the proper or moderate use of those things that are good to the body and abstinence from those which are harmful to the body. It is observed that the human being is the only being which voluntarily destroys its health with toxic substances.[400] Ellen G. White cautions and draws the attention of all in relation to the importance of temperance by stating that thousands of people in positions of trust and honour are indulging in habits that mean ruin to their soul and body.

Ministers of the gospel, statesmen, authors, men of wealth and talent, educators, men of vast business capacity and power for usefulness are in deadly peril because they do not see the necessity of self-control in all things. They need to have their attention called to the principles of temperance, not in a narrow or arbitrary way, but in the light of God's great purpose for humanity. Could the principles of true temperance thus be brought before them, there are very many of the higher classes who would recognize their value and give them a hearty acceptance. All are therefore called upon to embrace the health and temperance reform.[401]

Temperance has also been called the third law of health and well being. Closely connected to temperance is abstemiousness. To be abstemious "is to be moderate or sparing on the use if certain

---

[400] Ellen G. White, The Ministry of Healing, P. 275

[401] _____ Counsels on Health and Instructions to Medical Missionary Workers. (Ontario: Pacific Press Publishing Association, 1951), pp. 517-518

things, including an excess use of even good foods."[402] That which is harmful should be avoided, and many of those things which are good should be used in moderation. Maintain a balance of rest and exercise, not too much or too little. Regularity in scheduling and the daily routines of life will greatly aid in keeping you in the best health. Try to have a set time for rising, morning worship, prayer, drinking your water, mealtime, quitting time in the afternoon, family worship, evening walk time, bedtime etc. Maintaining simple routines simplifies life, relaxes the mind and helps us work more efficiently. This involves abstaining from eating or drinking what is too hot or too cold, because both upset the stomach and weaken the digestive organs.[403]

4.3.7.1 Conditions for Temperance:

There are two important conditions, which should encourage every child of God to embrace the Christian virtue of temperance; these include the sense of shame and the sense of honour.

4.3.7.2 The sense of Shame:

This is praiseworthy emotion that causes one to fear the disgrace or embarrassment connected with something degrading and base, and since grave sins of intemperance are degrading and base—for when they occur the animal in us is master and not human reason—the sense of shame in a special way pertains to the virtue of temperance. We are not speaking of the shame of embarrassment

---

[402] http://www.pathlights.com/nr-encyclopedia/00print4c.htm
[403] Ibid.

that follows a base action when detected by others (this could be caused by pride), but the fear of any action that helps one to avoid that debasement.[404]

This sense of shame one must note is not a virtue but a passing protective emotion, and a God-given inclination placed in the human mind to deter one from the excesses of life. The presence of this sense of shame should be cultivated in the lives of the children and will most likely impact them throughout their lives.[405]

4.3.7.3 The Sense of Honour:

Unlike the sense of shame, the sense of honour is an appreciation and reverence for the spiritual beauty connected with the practice of the virtue of temperance. While the sense of shame is based on fear, the sense of honour is a love for the beauty of temperance. One is a fear of the disgraceful; the other is a reverence for the sacred and beautiful. The spiritual beauty of temperance consists in a man's conduct being well proportioned to right reason. It is poles apart from the base and ugly actions that temperance repels. Here, too, training must start early. For the wise man through inspiration had said: "Train up a child in the way he should go, and when he is old, he will not depart from it." (Proverbs 22:6)

In his discourse on Christian Temperance, Paul A. Duffner maintained that there are different species of temperance. These include temperance which concerns the sense of taste on one hand

---

[404] http://www.rosary-center.org/1151n5.htm
[405] Ibid.

and the sense of touch on the other. The sense of taste is closely connected with abstinence. Abstinence on its own is a special virtue under temperance which moderates the appetite for food and drink according to the dictates of reason which is enlightened by the Holy Spirit.

The sense of touch has been closely associated with chastity. Chastity is that moral virtue that controls the desire for pleasure connected with the sexual powers according to the guidance of reason as led by the Holy Spirit.[406] The second purpose of this virtue in using it within God's plan of marriage is both lawful and virtuous. Duffner concludes that we need the gift of the Holy Spirit to control all our faculties and to apply the sound principles of abstemiousness in restraining our passions.[407] It is essential to note that intemperance of any form is a violation of the laws of our being. Through the indulgence of appetite, people violate the sound principles of life and health. God's command for self-control is clear and must be adhered to for optimum health and well being. The scriptures inform us that:

> For the grace of God that brings salvation has appeared to all men, teaching us that, denying ungodliness and worldly lusts, we should live soberly, righteously, and godly in the present age, looking for the blessed hope and glorious appearing of our great God and Saviour, Jesus Christ, who gave Himself for us, that He might redeem us

---

[406] http://www.rosary-center.org/1151n5.htm
[407] Ibid.

> from every lawless deed and purify for Himself Himself His own people, zealous for good works. (Titus 2:11-14)

It is God's desire that we enjoy abundant life. Self-control and moderation are therefore very important to achieving and sustaining a healthy body.

4.3.8 Air:

Air is a free blessing from God to all creatures. It is constantly available to us without money and without price. So many today have not taken advantage of its abundance on the surface of the earth. We need a constant supply of pure air into our bodies to keep healthy our lungs and keep our voices speaking clearly. Pure, fresh air promotes the appetite, improves the circulation, purifies the blood, refreshes the body, aids in the digestion of food, helps us sleep soundly, and helps sick people to get well. Its influence upon the mind impacts a degree of composure and serenity. The lungs throwing off impurities need constant supply of fresh air. Sleeping rooms should equally have free circulation of air day and night for optimum well-being of the occupants.[408] Fresh air as the breath of life is a special blessing from God to all creatures. The Genesis account for the creation of man says: "And the Lord God formed a man of the dust of the ground and breathed into his nostrils the breath of life, and man became living being" (Genesis 2:7)

It has been noted that from the eagerly awaited first cry of a new born baby child to the last gasp of the dying, life is completely

---

[408] http://www.rosary-center.org/1151n5.htm

dependent on breathing in adequate oxygen and exhaling carbon dioxide. Air is a mixture of gasses that surround the earth which also make up our atmosphere. Pure, fresh air consists of 21% oxygen and 78% nitrogen by volume. Other gases such as argon, carbon dioxide and water vapour are also present in air [409]

4.3.8.1   Air Pollution and Health:

Sometimes, the air we breathe is not pure. It may be polluted with so many particles; some are visible while some are microscopic. It may contain thousands of chemical and biological substances emitted into the atmosphere by natural sources or human activities. In addition, these chemicals may react in the atmosphere to produce other pollutants.

Substances that foul the air are called pollutants which include ground-level ozone (O_3), particular matter (PM) sulphur dioxide (SO_2), carbon monoxide (CO), nitrogen oxide (N), volatile organic compound (VOCs), hydrogen sulphide (H_2S), Sulphates and nitrates. Additional air pollutants of concern include toxic metals (lead, mercury, manganese, arsenic and nickel), benzene, formaldehyde, polychlorinated biphenyl's (PCB), dioxins and other persistent organic compound. Still on this group are dust from construction sites, individual wastes, and toxic fumes from vehicles and smoke from various other sources.[410]

---

[409]   http://www.hc-sc.gc.ca/hecs-sesc/air-quality/faq.htm
[410]   http://www.bcas.net/Env.Features/HumanHealth-december2002/15%20to%2030.htm

4.3.8.2 Air Pollution Adversely Affects Our Health:

These pollutants cause cough, nausea, fatigue, headache, sneezing, skin rashes and it is the most outstanding enemy of the asthmatic patient. Furthermore, particles and gasses in the air can be a source of lung irritation. Chronic exposure to pollutants in the air we breathe can damage deep portions of the lung even after symptoms such as coughing or a sore throat disappear. Ozone damages the alveoli (individual air sacs in the lung where oxygen and carbon dioxide are exchanged). The health effect of pollution can trigger off any other ailment in the human system.[411]

4.3.8.3 Relationship between Indoor and Outdoor Air:

As intelligent being we must endeavour to minimize our exposure to air pollution. This could be achieved by limiting our outdoor activities when it is obvious that pollution levels are high. Indoor air quality is important to human health because most of us spend over 80% of our time indoors. Occupants of indoor environments may be exposed to a variety of pollutants originating from human activities such as, combustion from heating and cooking, consumer products, furnishing, building materials and outdoor air. The quality of indoor air depends both on the quality of outdoor air and on the strength of emissions of indoor sources. In most inhabited spaces there is a continuous exchange of air with the outside. Therefore, all contaminants of the outdoor air are likely to be present indoors

---

[411] Ibid.

except ones which reacts with the surfaces of objects within a house and is thus greatly reduced in concentration.[412]

4.3.8.4 How to Improve Indoor Quality Air:

Since we spent most of our time indoors, either at home or in the place of work, it is pertinent that we become knowledgeable on how to improve the quality of the air where we stay. This could be accomplished by doing the following: [413]

1. Maintaining our heating, cooling and air conditioning systems.
2. Keeping our carpets and flooring dust free.
3. Maintaining a relative humidity below 50% to prevent the growth of mold.
4. Avoiding the use of chemical as cleansing agents when natural cones are available.
5. Making sure that there is a steady supply of fresh air. This is because the more the air can circulate the better.
6. Avoid smoking indoors. (Smoking outside is however not being advocated nor encouraged by this work.)
7. Using home appliances, which emit heat and smoke less often.

In the same manner we can improve the quantity of the outdoor air by retracing from indiscriminate burning. Since the car is a principal source of air pollution; we can walk, cycle or even join the public means of transportation while going to places. Even if we

---

[412] http://www.hc-sc.gc.ca/hecs-sesc/air-quality/faq.htm
[413] Ibid

must drive, we can greatly contribute to the quality of the outdoor air by reducing the speed of the vehicle, turning off the vehicle's air conditioning unit and by driving fuel-efficient vehicles.[414] Spending a day in a big city can make someone to inhale up to 17,000 pints of air containing some 20 billions of particles made up of dirt, dust and chemicals. Every city air is polluted by carbon monoxide and hydrocarbons (mostly from vehicles Sulphur oxides (burning coal and fuel oil) nitrogen oxides from stream power plants and automobiles, and photochemical oxidants. All of these are harmful to the health of humanity.

4.3.8.5 Adverse Effects of Smoking:

Apart from dirt and dust, the most outstanding air hazard to health is tobacco smoking. The smokes directly damage the lungs of smoker as well as constitute health hazards to others who come in contact with the smoke that goes into the atmosphere. Smoking causes not just chronic bronchitis, emphysema, lung cancer, and respiratory infections but also about 30% of all heart diseases.[415]

Actually, smoking destroys the defense mechanism, which the creator has put in man. Air is important to life that's the human body, for instance, less numerous defense mechanisms for protecting the lungs, to start. In the first place, the hairs in nose, serve the purpose of trapping the largest particles that pass through nostrils. Following that, the air is brought in contact with the nose lining, which warm

---

[414] http://www.bcas.net/Env.Features/HumanHealth-december2002/15%20to%2030.htm
[415] Ibid.

as well as muster it. In the back of the nose and throat the air comes in contact with other organs such as the adenoids and tonsil, which are special immune system organs that commence the work of destroying germ and virus that might be contained in the air. There is an also mucus-producing cell whose function is to provide mucus to trap foreign object. The bigger tubes of the respiratory tract are lined with ciliated cells which move dust and other unwanted particles out of the lung. (AIR-7). Smoking is so dangerous and harmful that it will paralyze and cause the death of those essential cilia cells. With this development, the best option is coughing or sneezing. Coughing in this situation produces a rush gear, which is up to the speed of 600 miles per hour. And this is a common occurrence to clear the respiratory tract of foreign bodies.[416]

4.3.9   Rest:

Rest means a period of inactivity to enable someone relax, sleep, to be still or refrain from one's routine duty. This period of cessation from our daily work should be cultivated and cherished for the reward of all aspects of our health. According to Ellen G. White, some people who make themselves sick by overwork need rest and freedom from the cares of this world.[417]

Fatigue from mental or physical exertion is a normal biological reaction. Its manifestation is observed in decreased ability to perform assigned responsibilities. Prolonged muscular activity leads to a point where the muscles are unable to contract. In this situation, a

---

[416] Ibid
[417] Ellen G. White, The Ministry of Healing, p. 236

thoroughly physically fatigued person will have limp and relaxed muscles and this is known as hypotonic fatigue. On the other hand, a mentally or emotionally tired person will experience muscle tenseness, which is known as hypertonic fatigue. The common factor, which affects them, is that both sets of people feel "tired" at the end of day.[418]

Problems arise when people do not differentiate between hypotonic and hypertonic fatigue. The individual who has been engaged in a hard work during the day will easily fall asleep when it is night. The wise man says, "The sleep of a laboring man is sweet' (Ecclesiastes 5:22). On the other side is the educated person whose duty involves decision making, attending committees and board meeting. The person in this second group feel tired too at the end of the day but her muscles are tense and sleep does not come so easily like the one who spent his time in physical exertion. What the second group needs is not primarily sleep but some physical exertion to work off the nervous tension.

Chronic hypertonic condition can lead to irritability, poor judgment and less efficiency. When individuals in this category cannot perform up to expectation, they resort to spending longer hours at the place of work and post of duty yet the work is not done satisfactorily. What such individuals need is rest, which will come after physical exertion had taken place. Those activities, which cause the muscles to relax act like tranquilizers that lead to sound sleep, rest and recuperation. When people get enough rest, they think more clearly and complete their work more efficiently within a record

---

[418] Dysinger, p. 69

time.[419] Our rest should be both restorative and recuperative. When we sleep, the neurons cleanse themselves of accumulated metabolic wastes while vital organs in our body rest. The heart rests between each beat, the lungs relax between each breath while the stomach rests between each meal. The central nervous system is equally recharged during sleep.[420]

4.3.10 Trust in God:

When we trust someone, we have perfect confidence that the person we trust will be our friend at all times and in all situations. If we can trust a person that much, how very much more we can trust our Saviour for He alone, is worthy of complete trust. God does not want us to be sick. But since sin has entered the world due to the disobedience of our first parents, and has distorted the perfect health bestowed upon them by God, He desires to renew a healthful state in us. Thus, He requires our confidence and faith in Him, which will benefit both mental and physical health. Many people seek this faith in God by finding time to read the Bible.[421]

Others develop complete confidence in God by including in their daily busy schedule a time to pray to the Creator. Indeed, medical research has confirmed that religion has a positive influence in a person's health. For example, the Israeli Ischemic Heart Disease Project has revealed that Orthodox Jews who prayed

---

[419] Ibid, pp. 69-70

[420] http://www.projectrestore.com/library/health/rest.htm

[421] George D. Pamplona-Roger. Enjoy It, p. 13

daily experience fewer heart attacks than people who rarely attend the synagogue.[422] Numerous others get connected to the Divine healer through daily private periods of meditation.[423] All these have been found to contribute to the over all wellbeing of man.

---

[422] Leo Van Dolson & Robert Spangler. Healthy, Happy, Holy, p. 17

[423] George D. Pamplona-Roger, Enjoy It, p. 13

CHAPTER FIVE

5.0 THE IMPACT OF THE PRACTICE AND USE OF AFRICAN TRADITIONAL MEDICINE AMONG SEVENTH-DAY ADVENTISTS

5.1 <u>Herbal Medicine</u>

The use of medicinal plants and herbs, which is of great importance to the health of individuals and communities, is on the increase. Up to 70,000 different species of medicinal plants and herbs have at one time or the other been identified for medicinal purposes.[424] According to the World Health Organization, (WHO) traditional medication involves the use of herbal medicines, animal parts and minerals. However, herbal medicines are the most widely used of the three mentioned above due to such factors as their availability, accessibility, functionality, and cost effectiveness.[425] Herbs, herbal materials and herbal preparations are all used in handling the menace of diseases ravaging humanity.

Finished herbal products are made up of one or more herbs. Sometimes the term mixture herbal product could be applied when

---

[424] Xiaorui Zhang. Traditional Medicine and WHO as reported in World Health Organization- <u>The Magazine of World Health Organization</u>, 49th year, No. 2, March-April, 1996, IXISSN0043-8502.p. 4

[425] Ibid

the finished product contains more than one herb. Herbal medicines therefore are:

> Finished, labeled medicinal products that contain as active ingredients aerial or underground parts of plants, or other plant materials, or combinations therefore, whether in the crude state or as plant preparations. Plant materials include juices, gums, fatty oils, essential oils, and any other substances of this nature. Herbal medicines may contain excipients in addition to the active ingredients.[426]

It is equally important to add that in some countries, herbal medicines may include by their tradition, natural organic or inorganic active ingredients which might not necessarily be of plant origin.[427]

The use of traditional medicine in contemporary time cannot be over-emphasized. Right from childhood, many people use medicinal plants to treat all manner of ill health and diseases with much effectiveness. In Nigeria, mothers from the Yorubaland and Igboland respectively, for example, give two or three drops of squeezed leaves of "effirin" for their children to drink in the case of abdominal cramps. To treat fever, people commonly search for the leaves of the tree, vernonia amygdalina (bitter leaf).[428] Traditional Medicine is the most popular way of treating ailments in our contemporary time. This is due to its availability, efficaciousness and in most cases they are free of charge. According to Ebenezer O. Olapade:

---

[426] General Guidelines for Methodologies on Research and Evaluation of the Traditional Medicine World Health Organization, 2000, p. 3

[427] Ibid, p.21

[428] Ibid.

Traditional medicine is practiced all over the world and the WHO has estimated that about 80% of the rural population depends on this method for their health care delivery system.[429]

Some medicinal plants are used both as food and medicine. A few of these healing gifts from nature which include bitter leaf, pawpaw, coconut, aloe Vera, lemon, garlic, ginger, guava, neem, passion fruit and sweet Annie would be considered here. As a result of divine counsels members of the Seventh-day Adventist Church eat these natural food items for good health and longevity. A liberal use of these natural fruits, legumes and green leafy vegetables are being used by the Adventists as recommended by White in her writings.

Bitter Leaf:

This is an evergreen tree known as *vernonia amydalina*. People from the eastern part of Nigeria call it "Olugbu" while it is called "Ewuro" in Yoruba and "Shiwaka" in Hausa lands respectively.[430] The most distinctive feature of bitter leaf plant is its bitterness. Every part of this plant is bitter. The leaves, the stems, root and bark. In the Eastern part of Nigeria, the Igbo people use it mostly as vegetable while in Yorubaland it is usually applied as a medicine. Bitter leaf is useful in toning the vital organs of the body such as the liver and kidney. The liver is involved in the excretion of bile and in the formation of glycogen in the human body. It is also essential

---

[429] Isabel Carter, ed, Footsteps, No. 48 September, 2001, p. 2
[430] Ebenezer O. Olapade, ed., Traditional Medicine in Nigeria. (Ibadan: Toyin Okebunmi Printers, 1998), p. 1.

in the metabolism of fats and proteins. Refined food items, sugar and alcohol may all contribute in weakening this important organ and also make it susceptible to infection.[431] The kidneys on the other hand aid the system in eliminating waste products. It secrets urine which flows into the urethras. So a dysfunctional kidney causes a general disorganization in the normal functions of the body. Bitter leaf is essential in the care of these two important organs of the body.

This leaf contains yernodalin, venomygdin and saponin.[432] To get the maximum medicinal benefits from bitter leaf, it should be consumed fresh. Cooking reduces the potency of the most plants including bitter leaf. The Igbo people eat a lot of bitter leaf after squeezing and throwing away the bitter chemicals of the vegetables and this is complete with thorough cooking. At the end of the exercise what the people consume seems to be mere chaff with little or no medicinal value. It must be noted that vegetables generally are better consumed in their raw or fresh state while half cooked vegetables are better than over cooked ones. Fresh vegetables contain fiber, simple and complex carbohydrates, vitamins and minerals which are of great biological value to the human body though eaten in small quantities.[433] In view of this, vegetables and especially bitter leaf should be consumed liberally for maximum health. Some of the many uses of bitter leaf are highlighted below:

---

[431] Anselm Adodo, <u>Nature Power</u>. (Akure: Don Bosco Traininig Centre, 2000), p. 33

[432] Ibid, p. 34

[433] Anselm Adodo, <u>Nature Power</u>, p. 34

A. Treating boils: Boils are brought to a ripe state quickly with the use of a poultice of bitter leaf. This poultice made up of ground bitter leaf and a few drop of red palm oil. When applied, it helps painful hard boils and abscesses to form pus. With the use of a plaster or bandage this bitter leaf poultice could be left on the boil over night to relieve the pain, soften the hardness and also helps the puss to gather quickly for emission. This type of poultice is efficient not only as a pain reliever but also act as a protector against infection.[434]

B. Stomach-Ache: Bitter leaf is also beneficial in handling the problem of stomach-ache. The tender stem of bitter leaf is chewed like a chewing stick and the bitter water is swallowed. An alternative is to grind a handful of the leaves in a mortar and the juice is pressed and a pinch of salt is added to this juice before it is sipped by the individual with the stomach ache. This treatment always brings immediate relief.

C. Diabetes: Diabetes is a medical disorder, which results in the body's inability to absorb carbohydrates, which is caused by a deficiency of insulin, and this leads to high level of sugar in the blood and urine.[435] Herbalists have been treating diabetics for a very long time with bitter leaf. This leaf in addition to reducing the sugar level in the system

---

[434] George D. Pamplona. Enjoy It-Foods for Healing and Prevention. (Madrid: Editorial Safeliz, 1998), p. 97

[435] Elizabeth Kafaru. "The Use of Bitter Leaf" The Guardian, February 6, 1997, p. 29

also helps in restoring the pancreas to an effective state. Some ten handful of bitter leaf are squeezed and mixed with ten liters of water. A glass of this juice is taken three times daily for a month for a wonderful relief of the above health problem.

D. Prostate Cancer: This is a health problem experienced by some men who are over forty years. Difficult and painful urination are among its commonest symptoms. Drinking the juice of bitter leaf as mentioned above will increase the flow of urine and at the same time reduces the pain. The same treatment could be applicable to alleviate general weakness of the body, stroke, pneumonia, insomnia and even arthritis.[436]

5.3 Pawpaw:

This is another important plant whose leaves, fruits and roots are useful to man. There are 22 different types of trees that make up the pawpaw genus but the most famous is known as *Carica papaya*. These fresh leaves are used as soap, the fruits are eaten as food while the dried leaves seed and roots are items for curing various diseases. Every part of the tree seems to be very important to man. The pawpaw when eaten fresh improves digestion and expels the worms in the human body. The ripe fruits are rich in vitamin A, B, and C. [437] Vitamin C which is also known as ascorbic acid is water soluble. It is easily eliminated from the body and this makes its constant supply

---

[436] Longman Dictionary of Contemporary English
[437] Anselm Adodo, Nature Power, pp. 36-37

in our daily food very essential to health. This vitamin is reasonably present in a limited range of food item mostly in their fresh forms. Prolonged storage and heat can destroy this vitamin and its absence in our diet could lead to scurvy, which manifests itself in swollen and bleeding gums.[438]

The vitamin B complex is also a water-soluble substance present in pawpaw. First among this complex chemical is vitamin B_1, which is also known as thiamin. It is present in the green pops of the pawpaw, green leafy vegetables and cereals. A deficiency of this substance in the body causes *beriberi*. This is a disease, which is prevalent in any population that feeds predominating on polished rice and white bread. The next member of the B complex family is Riboflavin, which is more popularly known as Vitamin B_{12} Its deficiency in the body causes a skin disease known as Pellagra. This is a skin disease which makes the skin becomes rough.

Vitamin A on the other hand is a yellow, pale, fat-soluble substance, which is equally soluble in water. Its plant and animal sources include pawpaw, carrots, garden eggs, tomatoes on one hand and eggs, animal liver, and fish liver oil on the other hand. People who are deficient of Vitamin A suffer from a disease called night blindness whereby such people cannot effectively adjust to darkness when light is suddenly switched off.[439]

Externally, the fresh leaves of pawpaw could be used as soap for bathing the body. In this process the fresh leaves are squeezed

---

[438] Ibid., pp. 38-39
[439] Samuel E. Ayeni. <u>You Can Be Healthier</u>, p. 21

together and used to scrub the body as it foams like any other soap. It could also be used in healing wounds. The white milky sap of the unripe pawpaw contains papain which is a chemical substance used in healing and treating chronic wounds and ulcers. This chemical is obtained by making a slight cut on the unripe pawpaw fruit and allowing the white juice to drop.[112] For the treatment of malaria fever and jaundice, yellow pawpaw leaves are squeezed out and a glassful is taken three times a day for a week. The same dosage of the fresh green leaves of pawpaw is good for the treatment of diabetes and diabetes induced hypertension. Inhaling the smoke of the dried and burnt leaves of pawpaw also brings instant relief during an attack of asthma. On the other hand, the dried and ground brown pawpaw leaves mixed with palm kernel is an excellent remedy to combat convulsion in children. This preparation is rubbed on all parts of the child's body to arrest this abnormal situation and to reduce high body temperature as a result of fever.[440]

Still on the benefit of pawpaw, the roots are useful in treating bronchitis and piles. The treatments involve boiling the roots of pawpaw and drinking half a glass for three and two times in cases of bronchitis and piles respectively.[441]

Pawpaw is a wonderful natural remedy for the treatment of intestinal worms, dirty wounds, indigestion, boil, infected wounds, and burns. To treat intestinal worms, the latex of the unripe pawpaw is collected while the fruit is still attached to the tree. The fluid is

---

[440] Samuel E. Ayeni. You Can Be Healthier, pp. 20-21

[441] Isabel Carter, ed, Footsteps, No. 48 (MiddleSex: Tear Fund, September, 2001,) p. 8

collected in a stainless clean cup after several vertical incisions have been made on the fruit with a stainless knife. These materials must be free from rust so the papaine in the chemical being collected will not be contaminated. Care must be taken to prevent the chemical from touching the eyes as this is very painful when it comes in contact with the eye. The dosage for adults is four teaspoons of fresh latex before break fast each day for a week. For babies between 6 months and 1 year, they should be given half a spoon of the latex. For the treatment of mild amoebic dysentery, a teaspoon of fresh pawpaw seeds should be chewed three times daily for a week. In serious cases such as dysentery, one tablespoon of grinded pawpaw seeds is taken three times daily for seven days. Open boil, infected wounds, and burns also have a solution from pawpaw. A stainless steel knife is used to cut an unripe pawpaw. Then a slice of the unripe pawpaw is further cut out and placed on the wound. This could be held in place with a clean bandage and allowed to stay on the wound for three to four hours. This is repeated four times a day until all the infected pus had disappeared.[442]

Apart from being a wonderful source of medicine for the well being of a man, ice cream, cake muffins, pies and wine could equally be produced from this wonder fruit. Pawpaw ice cream could be made with the following ingredients.

    A. Two cups of pawpaw puree
    B. Two cups of leafy cream
    C. Half a cup of milk
    D. One cup of sugar

---

[442] Anselm Adodo: <u>Nature Power</u>, pp. 40-41

All these are mixed and refrigerated for human consumption.[443]

Pawpaw cream cake production

A. 1 two-layer white cake mix
B. 2-3-ounce softened package cream cheese
C. 1 cup flavored butter
D. 2 teaspoon of vanilla
E. ¼ to ½ cup pawpaw pulp
F. 2 cups of confectioner's sugar
G. 5 egg whites
H. 2 leaping tablespoon corn starch
I. ¼ cup granulated sugar

All these are mixed appropriately and baked in a 350-degree oven for 5 minutes.[444]

Pawpaw also makes an excellent dry or white wine. In order to get pawpaw wine the following ingredients would be needed:

A. 2-3 pounds of ripe pawpaw
B. 2 ibs. Q granulated sugar
C. 7 ptq of water
D. 1-1/2 tablespoons of citric acid
E. ½ teaspoon of peptic enzyme
F. 1 teaspoon of grape tannin

---

[443] Ibid.
[444] Isabel Carter, ed, "Natural Remedies" Published in Footsteps, No. 48, September, 2001,) p. 8

All these are mixed as specified in the wine production procedures, they are boiled, chilled and finally the extraction of the wine takes place for human consumption.[445] It is always a common occurrence to be served with these kinds of fruit drinks in the homes of Seventh-day Adventists. Instead of running to the nearby liquor seller for alcoholic beverages. This is an advantage which Seventh-day Adventists have as a result of obeying the counsels of Ellen G. White. The next medicinal plant to be considered is coconut.

5.4   Coconut:

The Scientific name for common coconut is <u>cocos nucifera</u> and it belongs to the palm family known as <u>Arecaceae</u>. Coconut is one of the most valuable plants to man since it is a major source of food, drink, shelter and medicine.

5.4.1   History and Origin:

This tree was first mentioned in 545 AD by an Egyptian monk called Cosmos Indicopleustes who visited western India and Ceylon. In his book, <u>Topographia Christiana</u> he described coconut as the great nut of India. In the same manner, the mahavasma, an ancient chronological history of Ceylon described the coconut planting activities in that land which took place as far back as 589 AD. It was Marco Polo who described the coconut which he saw in Sumatra, Madras and Makabar in India as "<u>nux indica</u>", which

---

[445]   http://www.post-gazette.com/food/20030918pawpaw0918fnp2.asp

means the Indian nut as far back as 1280 AD. [446] In view of the above, the coconut tree seems to have originated from the Southern Asian Peninsular. And it is cultivated on all tropical regions around the world today. In all probability, the peoples of India and Southern Asia were the first to cultivate coconut trees and emigrants from these countries introduced this plant to other tropical lands.[447] Today, members of the Seventh-day Adventist Church plant this important tree around their homes for its many benefits.

5.4.2   Coconut oil:

The oil of coconut has been used for centuries as a source of food for health and general well being in many traditional communities around the world. Virgin coconut oil has an important role to play in maintaining a well balance, nutritious diet. Recent medical research has shown that our daily nutritional intake should include at least 30% fats or oil.[448]

Further findings in human nutrition have shown that replacing other cooking oils with virgin coconut oil is more beneficial to man. This is because coconut oil has antiviral, antibacterial, antimicrobial and anti-protozoal properties which are needed for a healthy body.[449] In addition to containing saturated fats (92%), triglycerides (62%), it also has lactic acid (50%) which is essential in maintaining the body's immune system. The other source or lactic acid is a mother's milk. So tropical coconut oils and mother's milk are the richest food

---

[446]   http://www.post-gazette.com/food/20030918pawpaw0918fnp2.asp
[447]   http://www.winemaking.jackkeller.net/pawpaw.asp
[448]   http://www.siu.edu/-ebl/leaflets/coconut.htm
[449]   http://www-ang.kfunigraz.ac.at/-katzer/engl/Coco nuc.html

source of medium chain fatty acids which are available for man. The medium chain fatty Acids (MCFA) help to increase metabolism, they are more easily digested; they are processed directly in the liver and from there they are converted into energy. There is therefore less stress and strain on the liver, pancreas, digestive organs and more important the MCFA provides the body with a quick source of energy that it needs.[450] More incredible health benefits of coconut oil include:

A. Helps you lose weight, lowers cholesterol
B. Reduces your risk of heart disease and other diseases.
C. Helps those with diabetes, thyroid, chronic fatigue
D. Improves digestive disorders
E. Boost your daily energy
F. Rejuvenates your skin, prevents wrinkles.[451]

Other areas in which the other parts of the coconut are used include treating fibroid, bronchitis, hepatitis and skin diseases. The bark of the plant is dried, burnt into ashes and mixed with an appropriate quality of palm kernel oil. This preparation could then be used for the treatment of black spots, rashes, scabies and measles. Half a glass of palm kernel oil is mixed with two-desert spoons of the burnt power or ashes. The ashes mixed with water could also be used as mouth wash and goggle in case of toothaches.[452] The water in the coconut is an excellent agent. It is one of the best natural antibiotics available to humanity. This water strengthens the

---

[450] http://www.coconut-connections.com/
[451] Ibid,
[452] http://www.coconut-connections.com/, p.2

immune system and assists the body in resisting diseases. To prove the effectiveness of coconut water, whenever anyone takes an over dose of any drug coconut water is usually administered to neutralize the adverse effect of such drugs on the body of the individual.[453]

Another important part of the coconut which is equally beneficial to man is the white pulp of the immature coconut. This part of the coconut is very useful for the memory. Individuals suffering from loss of memory, forgetfulness and other forms of memory defect should mix the pulp inside the immature coconut with a little honey. This preparation should be taken liberally to effect a positive change in these memory defects.[454]

5.5   Aloe Vera:

Aloe is the general name given to a variety of plants from *the Liliaceae* and *Aloeaceae* family. There are over 325 species in this genus. Some better known species include Aloe Ferox, Aloe Rerryi, Aloe barteri, also called Aloe Vera. This Aloe Vera is the most common of the Aloes found in Nigeria and some neighbouring countries around our nation. It grows well in flowerpots and other containers around the home. A balanced measure of sunshine and water is needed for it to survive. In any conducive setting Aloe Vera may grow up to seven feet.[455] Seventh-day Adventists have flower pots and gardens where Aloe Vera and other medicinal plants are grown for medicinal and other purposes.

---

[453]   http://www.mercola.com/2001/mar/24/coconut-oil.htm
[454]   Anselm Adodo. Nature Power, pp. 42-45.
[455]   Ibid, pp. 43-45.

5.5.1 History of Aloe Vera:

The history of Aloe Vera is a very old one since it had been in use from time immemorial. Wall paintings of ancient Egypt showed that it was used by the Egyptians to treat catarrh. As a native of Southern and Northern Africa, Aloe Vera came to Greece in the 4th Century B. C. and to China in the 11th Century A.D.[456] Among the Hebrews, Aloe Vera was used as an ingredient for preparing various chemicals. The substances could be used for embalmment or for other preservatory activities.

Further historical documents from the Egyptians, Romans, Greeks, Algerians, Moroccans, Athenians, Indians and Chinese report of the numerous uses of Aloe Vera both as medicine and cosmetic. Cleopatra, tradition holds attributed for irresistible charm and beauty to the judicious use of Aloe gel. History also had it that Aristotle persuaded Alexander the Great to conquer Socroto, a land off the East coast of Africa for the singular purpose of obtaining Aloe Vera which was a wound healing medicine for his soldiers. Other ancient records described the application of this miracle plant to include skin care, protection against fire scald, sun, the healing of wounds, relieving of insect stings and bites bruises, scratches, acne allergic conditions, eczema and other damaged skin.

However, Aloe Vera was almost abandoned as the seat of civilization moved to the temperate regions of the world where the freezing winter periods could not allow the plant to survive. Initially only the powdered sap was used in these regions. The situation

---
[456] Ibid, p. 44

however, took a dramatic turn in 1942, when Rodney M. Stockton, a chemical engineer, suffered severe sunburn during a holiday in Florida. The sunburn was healed miraculously with aloe Vera. Five years later, he successfully commenced a project to commercially produce Aloe Vera ointment. Since then, research activities on this healing plant have been undertaken in the former Soviet Union, Europe, Africa and America.

Among the Jews, Aloe Vera was used as an ingredient for embalming the Dead. The body of Jesus Christ was wrapped with linen soaked in Myrrh and Aloes. The Holy Bible says:

> Nicodemus brought a mixture of Myrrh and Aloes about seventy-five pounds. Taking Jesus' body, the two of them wrapped it, with spices in stripes of linen. This was in accordance with Jewish burial.
> (John 19:39-44)

Aloe Vera has been recognized for millennia for its healing properties, and a great amount of research is currently going on in many parts of the world on this miracle plant. This amazing plant has been used by many indigenous cultures of various civilizations because of its healing and medicinal properties. Some of these have been briefly outlined in this section.

5.5.2   Maintenance of Skin Elasticity:

Researchers have observed that when an extract of Aloe Vera gel is applied on the skin, it stimulates growth of fibroblasts. Fibroblasts are key cells that help in the manufacture of collagen, a protein that has been recognized to be responsible for maintaining skin elasticity.[457]

5.5.3 Anti-Viral Activity:

It has been observed that Aloe Vera has very high anti-viral properties. A compound known as acemannon has been extracted from aloe. This action of this acemannon is such that it envelops various viruses and germs thereby preventing them from attaching to other cells in the human body. [458]

5.5.4 Accelerated action of healing

It accelerates healing in the digestive system. This is another benefit derived from using Aloe Vera. Regular internal consumption of Aloe Vera has contributed positively to the healing of several disorders to the gastro-intestinal tract such as ulcerative colitis, esophagitis, peptic ulcer, rheumatoid arthritis, osteoarthritis, mouth lesions and even sore throat.[459]

5.5.5 Strong antioxidant and immuno-stimulant:

Aloe Vera is so versatile that among its many properties is the production of anti-oxidative compound. This was isolated from a methanolic extract of Aloe Barbadensis. Closely connected to this is

---

[457] Anselm Adodo, Nature Power, p. 46
[458] Ibid.
[459] Ibid.

the production of immuno-stimulatory poly saccharides from Aloe Vera. These actions of activation may seem to be the single most important component from the juice of Aloe Vera.[460]

5.5.6 Aloe Vera is also used for the treatment of burns.

This is normally achieved by harvesting, washing and skinning through the leaf to enable you have access to the juice that flows from the leaf. The treatment involves rubbing the juicy side of the Aloe Vera leaf all over the site of the burn. This should be repeated four times daily to effect the desired healing. The method described above could also be used in treating other wounds and ulcers.[134] Still on the external use of aloe Vera, Winston J. Craig posited that: "To date, there are no known adverse reactions or side effects with the tropical use of aloe gel.[461]

5.5.7 Raw or Processed Aloe Vera Gel:

Recent studies have demonstrated that aloe Vera gel facilitates the healing of wounds, damaged skin tissue and also reduces redness and swelling associated with a burn. However, the best way to use aloe Vera is to apply it fresh without any dilution. Fresh aloe gel is known to be effective for the treatment of many skin ailments and care should be exercised in using some aloe Vera creams and ointments. This is because there is doubt regarding some of these preparations, while some products that claim they contain

---

[460] http://www.petspourri.com/herbs01.htm

[461] http://www.petspourri.com/herbs01.htm

aloe actually have so little of the aloe Vera gel that they have no therapeutic value at all.[462]

5.6 Early Health and Medical Publications:

As a result of the importance of the health message, which God had given to the Church, the need arose to have same disseminated to the people in printed forms. This led to Mrs. White's first health publication titled, "An Appeal to Mothers".[463] This was a booklet on the subject of health and it was addressed to mothers as the managers of homes. The mothers are the ones who are always in constant touch with the children and youth since the fathers are most of the time outside in search of daily bread for the family. In her publication, Ellen White gave reasons for the imbeciles, dwarfed forms, crippled limbs and deformities of every description. She maintained that they were the results of crimes and sins and the violation or nature's laws by man.

In that little pamphlet, Mrs. White showed the relationship of diet to the spiritual and physical life of the people. She finally appealed to mothers to return to the edenic diet. In order to strengthen the moral perceptions of children and youth the use of animal food items must be dispensed with while the use of grains, vegetables and fruits as articles of food should be encouraged.[464] Up to the present moment, many Seventh-day Adventists around the world, including those at

---

[462] Ibid

[463] Dores E. Robinson. The Story of Our Health Message. (Nashville, Tennessee: Southern Publishing Association, 1965), p. 76

[464] Ibid., Pp. 89-91

Remoland, are vegetarians as a result of the counsels of Ellen G. White.

Another book that was prepared and published during the later part of 1863 and early part of 1864 respectively was the forth volume of Spiritual Gifts. This book traced the history of man from creation. It pointed out that the violation of health principles had led to disease and deformity. Further violation of the laws of health by the human family led to the perversion of appetite as seen in the antediluvians, the people of Sodom and Gomorrah, and even among the children of Israel during the Exodus. The story of Nadab and Abihu were other illustrations of the evil effects of intemperate living.[465]

The next health publication was titled "Health or How to Live". There were actually six pamphlets designed to handle the issues of diseases and their causes. Each pamphlet was devoted to the several questions and issues of food, baths, drugs, air clothing and proper exercise respectively.[466] Over the years, articles on health have been written and published in the "Signs of the Times" as well as "The Review and Herald magazines". The Testimonies for the Church often contained balanced advice on healthful living. Subsequent health publications included:[467]

The Health Reformer (1866)
The Pacific Health Journal (1904)
Health (1932)

---

[465] Ibid, p. 91
[466] Dores E. Robinson. The Story of Our Health Message, pp. 106-107
[467] Ibid, pp. 430- 437

Christian Temperance and Bible Hygiene (1890)
Healthful Living (1896)
The Ministry of Healing (1905)
Counsels on Health (1923)
Medical Missionary (1932)
Counsels on Diet and Food (1938)
Temperance (1949)
The Story of our Health Message (1943)

5.7 Endorsement of Adventist Lifestyle:

Among the many individuals who spoke out in support of the health principles enunciated by Ellen White was a famous physician, John H. Kellogg. He was amazed that what Ellen White wrote and said was almost wholly ignored by medical personnel and the world at large at that time. He specifically supported and endorsed what Mrs. White had written with the following under listed points:[468]

- In 1863 health reform was almost totally ignored by Adventists and the world at large.
- The few people who were advocating reform included with their insights the most disgusting errors.
- No one before Ellen White's message had presented a systematic and harmonious body of hygienic truths, free from patent errors, and consistency with the Bible and the principles of the Christian religion.

---

[468] Herbert E. Douglass, Messenger of the Lord-The Prophetic Ministry of Ellen G. White, (Mountain View, California: Pacific Press Publishing Association, 1998). Pp. 283-284.

- Thousands changed lifelong habits after reading these messages because they recognized not only the inherent harmony of these truths, but also their divine endorsement.
- Ellen White's principles have stood the test of time and experience.
- Many of the principles ridiculed or ignored in 1863, had become accepted in 1890 and beyond.
- Remarkable scientific discoveries since 1863 had only fortified these principles, without "the overthrow of a single principle."
- Divine guidance is "as much needed" in distinguishing truth from error as "in the evolution of new truths."

Years of reflection have given unmistakable evidence of the divine insight and direction given through a person who has no claim to scientific knowledge. The organization of hygienic principle so harmonious, so consistent, and so genuine which arose from the confused and error tainted mass of ideas is an indication that God is in total control of the health message which was presented by Ellen White.

5.8 Relationships between Health and Gospel Messages:

Ellen White linked the health principles and practices which God had revealed through her with other Bible based truths. This was a demonstration that the health message was an integral part of the "everlasting gospel" recorded in Revelation 14:6. Three outstanding ways by which these linkages or relationships have been discernable are on the humanitarian, evangelical and stereological principles.[469]

5.8.1   The Humanitarian Principles:

In so many ways, by precept and example, Ellen White emphasized that the goal of the health reform messages which God had sent through her to the church was a means for lessening the miseries and sufferings of humanity. All who would accept it wholly will enjoy sound and vibrant health.[470] In her book, A Call to Medical Evangelism and Health Education, Ellen White said:

> Medical missionary work brings to humanity the gospel of release from suffering. It is the pioneer work of the gospel. It is the gospel practiced, the compassion of Christ revealed. Of this work, there is great need, and the world is open for it. God grant that the importance of the medical missionary work shall Be understood, and that new fields may be immediately entered.[471]

Still on the principle of teaching health reforms, the servant of God had instructed that health education should be an integral part of preaching the gospel in towns and cities. Cooking schools should be held where those who are interested are further taught how to prepare wholesome food. Since people are being advised to drop

---

[469] Herbert E. Douglass. Messenger of the Lord-The Prophetic Ministry of Ellen G. White, P. 292

[470] Ibid.

[471] Ellen G. White. A Call to Medical Evangelism and Health Education, pp. 46-48

their old ways of eating and drinking, special care must be taken in teaching them how to prepare appetizing and balanced food. This is a humanitarian work of the highest order.[472]

5.8.2 The Evangelical Principle:

Ellen White was instructed that the health reform which had been communicated through her was to be a bridge through which the gospel will be taken to all other people no matter their status, gender or location in the world. This health message had been variously called "door opener"[473] "great entering wedge"[474] "prejudice remover against evangelical work",[475] and the "right hand of the gospel"[476] among other names. Concerning Seventh-day Adventist health-care institutions, Ellen White wrote "The great object of receiving unbelievers into the medical institutions or sanitarium is to lead them to embrace the truth".[145] In order to achieve this, members who are leading the medical missionary work should not lower the standard of the medical work. If it is lowered, those who come to hear other Bible messages may conclude that these messages are of little importance. This will discourage them and they would be placed in a position which is harder to win for the Lord Jesus Christ.[477] In view of this, one of the objectives of our medical centers is not just

---

[472] _____ Testimonies for the Church, vol. 9 (Oklahoma: Academy Press, Inc. 1947). P. 112

[473] _____ Evangelism. (Oklahoma: Academy Press Inc. 1947), p. 513

[474] _____ Testimonies for the Church, vol. 9 P. 112

[475] Ibid, Vol. 7, p. 56

[476] Ibid, Vol. 1, p. 560

[477] _____ Testimonies for the Church, vol. 1

to handle the physical maladies but also to care for the spiritual life of the patients.

5.8.3 The Soteriological Principle:

Theologically, soteriology has to do with the doctrine of salvation as espoused through Jesus Christ. Through the vision revealed to her, Ellen White also made it clear that the health message was given to prepare a people for the coming of the Lord. When men and women have formed characters which God can endorse by accepting in principle and practice the revealed health messages, then they are ready to be included into God's family. The balanced health message is a work that will bring great satisfaction and joy to the Father and Son because it is a work of saving perishing souls.[478]

Even though the medical institution should not be established with the intent of not making gains, it should be so well organized that those who visit there will appreciate eternal things and also correctly value the redemption which had been purchased by Jesus Christ. These three fold principle has been guiding the Seventh-day Adventist Church in her welfare and humanitarian services, in imparting health principle through her educational and medical institutions, and in the great task of preaching the everlasting gospel of Jesus Christ to a perishing world.

---

[478] _____ A Call to Medical Evangelism and Health Education, p. 47

5.8.4 Health Care Institutions:

Sequel to the plethora of publications on sound medical principles and practices is the call to establish health care institutions. Ellen White was the advocator who was making this clarion call for the church to own medical institutions. With her encouragement and support, the General Conference Session of 1866 voted to build a sanitarium. This became a reality with the establishment of the Western Health Reform Institute located at Battle Creek, Michigan was built. It was opened in September 5, 1866 to the public. This institution afforded Seventh-day Adventists in general the opportunities of learning in the shortest possible time the health principles which will afford them the privilege of standing without any feebleness among all other people the effectiveness of this institution which became a channel for preaching the gospel encouraged the Seventh-day Adventist to establish more in other parts of USA and beyond.[479]

Other medical and health care institutions were later established such as the great Battle Creek Sanitarium, Glendale Sanitarium, Paradise Valley Sanitarium, Loma Linda Medical Centre and others. And as the church expanded her activities to other parts of the world, the health and medical work also followed. It is therefore not amazing that the early Adventist Missionaries to Nigeria, who realized the positive effect of the medical ministry in their home churches, incorporated same in their missionary and evangelistic activities. Therefore, similar health institutions were established in different parts of Nigeria with the coming of the Seventh-day

---

[479] _____ A Call to Medical Evangelism and Health Education, p. 47

Adventist in 1914. As a rule, these health care institutions were to offer both medical and surgical services. However, there was to be included in their program an emphasis on temperance, diet, exercise, and all other aspects of healthful living. The Spiritual dimension of the patients was also of paramount importance in the health philosophy of the church. It was part of the objectives set for these health care institutions to develop adequate plans to train doctors, nurses and other health professionals to serve in the denomination's medical institutions.

On the issue of training workers, Seventh-day Adventist health professionals are to be well trained and fully qualified in their various disciplines. These professionals are to be so prepared that they can pass their qualifying examinations with superior grades. They are also to be evangelists and experts in communicating the love of Christ to their patients. This led to the establishment of schools of nursing in most hospitals. A school of medicine was also opened in Battle Creek, Michigan, but in 1906 it was moved to Loma Linda in California, USA.[480]

5.9   Churches and Health Relationships:

Sound health education is not only the duty of health professionals centered in hospitals, clinics and outpost health centers, but it is also an integral part of the activities in each local church. All churches are to be agents of health information, education and healing for the community in which it was located. Every local church is meant

---

[480]   http://www.aims-ministry.org/sge5.html

to be a "solid base" for wholistic health evangelism. In fact, White correctly notes that:

> The medical missionary work should be a part of the work of every church in our land. Disconnected from the church it would soon become a strange medley of disorganized atoms. The minds of men must be called to the scriptures as the most effective agency in the salvation of souls, and the ministry of the word is the great educational force to produce this result. Those who disparage the ministry and try to conduct the medical missionary work independently are trying to separate the arm from the body.[481]

The other point is to note the close relationships between the church in her effort to preach the gospel as well as in promoting health education. The Seventh-day Adventist Church believes on the wholistic nature of man. Man, created in the image of God, has multiple dimensions of mental, physical, social and spiritual aspects which are all united as a whole. These different phases of man are not distinct and independent parts on their own, but they are interconnected, and dependent on one another for balance and the optimum health of man. This concept was evident in the balance ministry of Jesus Christ as well as in the prayer of the Apostle Paul for all God's people (Matthew 4:23; 1 Thessalonians 5:23). As a result of this, spiritual realities can only be partially understood as long as sickness exists in the body. On the other hand, depression and mental sorrow can result in symptoms and actual disease. In the same way, the gospel team and the health professionals are to be

---

[481] _____ Testimonies for the Church, vol. 6, pp. 288-289

united and interconnected in the discharge of their duties.⁴⁸² On this issue Ellen White writes:

> The gospel ministry is needed to give permanence and stability to the medical missionary work; and the ministry needs the medical missionary work to demonstrate the practical working of the gospel. Neither part of the work is complete without the other.⁴⁸³

---

[482] http://www.aims-ministry.org/sge5.html
[483] _____ Testimonies for the Church, vol. 6, P. 112

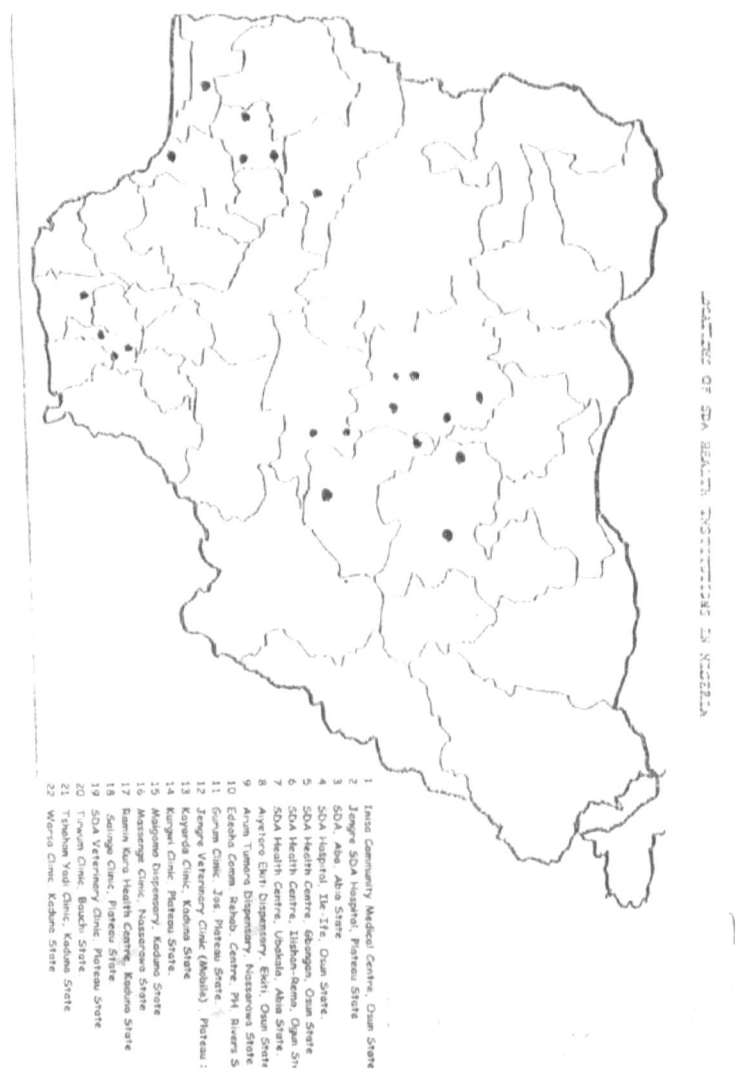

FIG. XII LOCATION OF SDA HEALTH INSTITUTIONS IN NIGERIA

Specifically, there are 22 medical institutions being operated by the Seventh-day Adventist Church in Nigeria. The hospitals, clinics, dispensaries and health centers operated by the Seventh-day Adventist Church in Nigeria as at 2004 are as follows:[484]

1. Inisa Community Medical Centre, Osun State.
2. Jengre Seventh-day Adventist Hospital, Plateau State.
3. Seventh-day Adventist Hospital and motherless Babies Home, Aba, Abia State.
4. Seventh-day Adventist Hospital, Ile-Ife, Osun State.
5. Adventist Health Centre, Gbongan, Osun State.
6. Babcock University Medical Centre, Ilishan-Remo, Ogun State
7. Adventist Health Centre, Ubakala, Abia State.
8. Aiyetoro Ekiti Dispensary, Ekiti, Osun State.
9. Arum Tumara Dispensary, Nassarawa State.
10. Edeoha Community Rehabilitation Centre, Port Harcourt, Rivers State.
11. Gurum Clinic, Jos, Plateau State.
12. Jengre Veterinary Clinic (Mobile) (Jengre Hospital), Plateau State.
13. Kayarda Clinic, Kaduna State.
14. Kurgwi Clinic, Plateau State.
15. Maigamo Dispensary, Kaduna State.
16. Massenge Clinic, Nassarawa State.
17. Ramin Kura Health Centre, Kaduna State.

---

[484] The General Conference Corporation of the Seventh-day Adventists. Seventh-day Adventist Yearbook 2004, (Washington DC: Review and Herald Publishing Association, 2004), p. 399

18. Salingo Clinic, Plateau State.
19. Seventh-day Adventist Veterinary Clinic, Plateau State.
20. Tirwum Clinic, Bauchi State.
21. Tshohon Yadi Clinic, Kaduna State.
22. Warsa Clinic, Kaduna State.

Among all the earlier listed medical institutions, expatiation would be made on the ones at Ile-Ife, Osun State; Jengre, Plateau State; and the one located at Aba in Abia State.

5.10   Seventh-day Adventist Hospital, Ile-Ife:

This is the oldest and the largest health institution being operated by the church in Nigeria. When the call was made to establish a medical institution in Nigeria, it received both a positive and inspiring response. It was Dr. G. A. Madgwick that was charged with the responsibility of locating a favourable site for this project. Madgwick arrived Nigeria in 1939 and without delay he visited Lagos, Ibadan and Ile-Ife in search of a spot to establish the institution. It was at Ile-Ife that the Oni, Sir Adesoji Aderemi gave 45 acres of land, $1,000 for the project and promised to give more land if the need arises.[485]

With that generous donation and support from the king, the project commenced in 1940. In 1941, when it was almost completed, the British soldiers took it over and converted it into a military hospital

---

[485] Don. F. Neufield, ed. Seventh-day Adventist Encyclopedia, (Washington DC.: Review and Herald Publishing Association, 1976), pp. 617-618

to care for the casualties from the Second World War. In 1944 it was handed over to the church. It is currently a 130-bed hospital. The positive influence of this hospital was felt not only at Ife but within the whole Western Region of Nigeria. In 1949, for instance, this hospital performed 850 operations, and rendered services to 33,886 out patients. The institution's positive influence was felt at such places as Ondo, Omuo, Arandun, Ayetoro, Ugbo, Inisa, Erumu, Ilishan-Remo, which was later blessed with the establishment of smaller medical center.[486] Still on the unique services being rendered by the hospital, it even served the needs of a University teaching hospital. According to Babalola:

> Because of the high reputation of this hospital, Ile-Ife University Teaching Hospital used the hospital as the basic training school for its medical students until 1975 when the Western State of Nigeria Government took over operation of all private hospitals in the State, including the Seventh-day Adventist Hospital, Ile-Ife.[487]

---

[486] Abraham A. Kuranga, "Seventh-day Adventism in Nigeria, 1914-1981: A Study in the Relationship Between Christianity and African Culture from the Missionary era to the Introduction of African Leadership", PhD.Dissertation, Miami University, 1991, p.65

[487] David O. Babalola, On Becoming a Conference: The Story of the Seventh-day Adventist Church in Yorubaland 1914-2002. (Ibadan: OSB Design Limited, 2002) p. 165

FIG. XIII MEDICAL DIRECTORS OF SDA HOSPITAL, ILE-IFE (1940-2002)

George Madgwick	1940-1942 (Pioneer Medical Director who assisted in laying the foundation of the building)
G. W. Allen	1944-1947
Sherman Nagel (Jr.)	1947-1963
Arthur Zeismer	1963-1968
A. M. Owens	1968-1970
M. T. Oliverio	1970
L. Marter	1970-1972
J. C. Jay	1972-1974
Kenneth L. Kelly	1975

Nigerian Government Take Over—1975-1987[488]

S. A. Daniyan	1987-1990
Greg Saunders	1990-2002
H. N. Gible	2002-present[489]

---

[488] Dave M. Nyekwere, "A Study of Medical Institutions of the Seventh-day Adventist Church in Southern Nigeria as an Instrument of Evangelization 1940-2000." (PhD Dissertation, University of Port Harcourt). 2003

[489] David O. Babalola, On Becoming a Conference: The Story of the Seventh-day Adventist Church in Yorubaland 1914-2002. p.170

FIG. XIV SEVENTH-DAY ADVENTIST HOSPITAL, LE-IFE STATISTICS[490]

Items/Date	2000	2001	2002	2003	October 2004
Total Admission	1,454	2,903	2,665	2,012	1,560
Total Out Patients	8,793	15,945	16,148	16,099	13,617
Total Surgeries	647	1,238	1,174	955	559
Laboratory Investigation	4,738	10,802	11,749	10,861	11,031
Ultra Sound Examination	286	2,000	2,182	3,412	1,920
X-Ray Examination	2,814	1,971	5,057	5,725	5,057
Live Birth	149	191	209	153	135
C/Sections	42	85	80	62	63
Bed Occupation	24%	58%	44.4%	35%	22%

5.11 Seventh-day Adventist School of Nursing, Ile-Ife:

This school was established in 1944 to train Nurses who will enhance optimum development of the spiritual, mental, emotional growth and physical well-being among the general populace. Other objectives of establishing the school included developing in students' competence in both theoretical and practical aspects of nursing, providing a balanced education to meet community health needs; and inculcating the love of God in students to enable them demonstrate compassion as they alleviate suffering among the

---

[490] H. N. Gible. Quinquennum Report for Seventh-day Adventist Hospital, Ile-Ife, 2001-October 2004" presented at the Seventh Reorganization Session of the Seventh-day Adventist Church in Nigeria, Owerrinta, December 1-4, 2004, p. 103

people.[491] On May 1, 1950 another great achievement was recorded and that was the addition of the school of midwifery to the existing nursing school. The dental unit was added to the existing facility in 1973.[492] The greatest achievement of this school of nursing in recent time has been her affiliation with Babcock University of which the Nursing and Midwifery Council is in full support.

FIG. XV STATISTICS OF STUDENTS WHO GRADUATED 1994-2004[493]

S/N	SET YEAR OF ADMISSION/ GRADUATION	NO. OF CANDIDATES	NO. OF CREDITS	PERCENTAGE	NO ENTERED
1	Oct. 1994-Nov. 1997	16	5	100	
2	Oct. 1995-Nov. 1998	12	1	92	13
3	Oct. 1996-May, 1999	3	3	100	
4	Oct. 1996-Nov, 1999	20	2	100	
5	Oct. 1996-May, 2000	4	Nil	100	
6	Oct, 1997-Nov, 2000	18	1	100	
7	Oct, 1997-May, 2001	7	1	100	
8	Oct, 1998-Nov, 2001	19	1	95	20
9	Oct, 1998-May, 2002	8	1	100	
10	Oct, 1999-Nov, 2004	20	-	67	30

[491] Ibid.² Abraham A. Kuranga, "Seventh-day Adventism in Nigeria, 1914-1981: A Study in the Relationship Between Christianity and African Culture from the Missionary ear to the Introduction of African Leadership, PhD. Dissertation, Miami University, 1991, p.65

[492] ³ R. A. Ajaiyeoba. "Principal-Seventh-day Adventist School of Nursing, Ile-Ife, Osun State. Report presented at Owerrinta during 7th Reorganization Session of the Seventh-day Adventist Church in Nigeria, 2004

[493] Ibid

11	Oct, 1999-May, 2003	17	-	89	19
12	Oct, 2000-May, 2004	40	4	87	46
13	Oct, 2000-may, 2004	15	1	88	17
14	Oct, 2001-Nov, 2004	56	Awaiting	Awaiting	

5.12 Seventh-day Adventist Postgraduate Medical Education:

Apart from providing a wholistic system of medical care, producing highly trained and functional nurses, the Seventh-day Adventist Hospital, Ile-Ife, which is an affiliate of Adventist Health International (AHI) has also established a Postgraduate Medical Education programme to prepare young people in Africa to serve primarily their fellow Africans and people from other parts of the world.

FIG. XVI SOME POSTGRADUATE MEDICAL EDUCATION STUDENTS AT SDA HOSPITAL ILE-IFE, OSUN STATE, NIGERIA.[494]

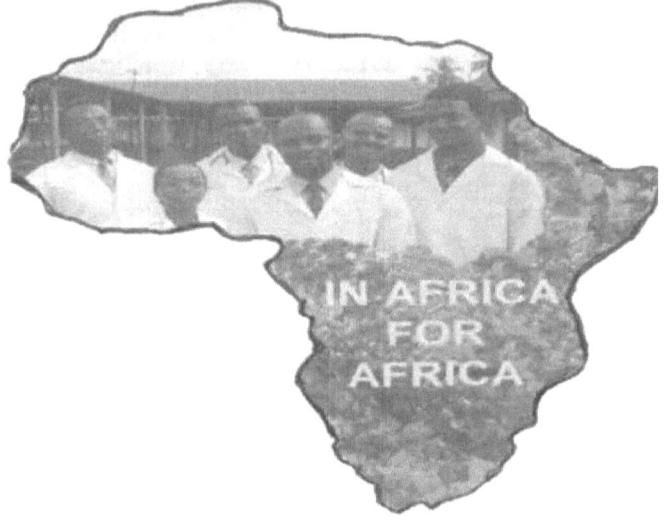

The Postgraduate Medical education involves training in the following areas:

A. Short term clinical rotations for medical and allied health students and residents.
B. Housemanship programme.
C. Four-year family medicine residency programme.

---

[494] Dave M. Nyekwere, p. 161

The short-term clinical provides opportunities for nationals and international students to be exposed adequately to the study and practice of medicine in a typical tropical African setting. The housemanship programme lays emphasis on providing qualitative health care delivery system in the whole of Africa; encouraging community health education through personal responsibility, and providing both compassionate and competent medical services with limited resources. The residency programme on the other hand prepares medical personnel with broad based knowledge on medical, surgical, and community skills to work in either the rural or urban communities in Africa. In all these training at Seventh-day Adventist Hospital, Ile-Ife, and emphasis is always made on following Christ's method of healing the sick.[495]

5.13 Adventist Hospital, Aba:

This medical institution was established in 1984 as an Adventist Health Centre with funds from the Adventist Development and Relief Agency (ADRA) in Sweden. This institution did so well that in 1989, it was pronounced a full fledged hospital. It is also a medical institution that had enlisted the services of more indigenous medical doctors than others.[496] The chart below explains it better:

---

[495] E. E. Enyinna. Medical Director Seventh-day Adventist Hospital, Aba, 2005.

[496] Dave M. Nyekwere, p. 66

FIG. XVII MEDICAL DIRECTORS OF THE SEVENTH-DAY ADVENTIST HOSPITAL AND MOTHERLESS BABIES' HOME, ABA[497]

S/N	NAME	POST HELD	PERIOD OF ENGAGEMENT AS EMPLOYEE
1	DR. E. E. ENYINNA	MEDICAL OFFICER	1984-1990
2	DR E. N NZOTTA	AG. MEDICAL DIRECTOR	1984 (APRIL-DECEMBER)
3	DR. N.P. MOSQUEDA	MEDICAL DIRECTOR	1985-1990
4	DR. E. E. ENYINNA	MEDICAL DIRECTOR	1991-1999
5	DR. G.C. NWANKWO	AG. MEDICAL DIRECTOR	1999-2000
6	DR. PETER OPREH	AG. MEDICAL DIRECTOR	1999-2000
7	DR. E. E. ENYINNA	MEDICAL DIRECTOR	2005-PRESENT
8	DR. IFEYICHUKWU OMORDIA	MEDICAL OFFICER	1992
9	DR. OLGA BOYCAN	MEDICAL OFFICER	1988-1989
10	DR. K. O. KALU	MEDICAL OFFICER	1992-1997
11	DR. O ISIGUZO	MEDICAL OFFICER	1998-2000
12	DR. A. C. NJOKU	MEDICAL OFFICER	1997-1999
13	DR. A OLAJIDE	MEDICAL OFFICER	1999-2000
14	DR. BOB OGU	MEDICAL OFFICER	

---

[497] E. E. Enyinna, Medical Director, SDA Hospital and Motherless Babies' Home, Aba 2005 Yearend House Committee Report

15	DR. BOB DURU KINGSLEY	MEDICAL OFFICER	2000-2001
16	DR. EMELE NWAUBANI	MEDICAL OFFICER	6 MONTHS
17	DR. DOUGLAS	MEDICAL OFFICER	2000-200
18	DR. LARRY	MEDICAL OFFICER	2002-
19	DR. OSASA, M.	MEDICAL OFFICER	2001-2002
20	DR. UDENSI	MEDICAL OFFICER	2002-2003
21	DR. OBINNA WADIBIA	MEDICAL OFFICER	2003
22	DR. OGUGUO	MEDICAL OFFICER	2003-
23	DR. VINCENT GINIKANWA	MEDICAL OFFICER	2001-2004
24	DR. HART	MEDICAL OFFICER	
25	DR. OGU	MEDICAL OFFICER	2003-2004
26	DR. ONYEWUCHI	MEDICAL OFFICER	2002-2004
27	DR. ONYEMACHI	MEDICAL OFFICER	2002-2003
28	DR. CHIOMA OJIABO	MEDICAL OFFICER	2003
29	DR. ENWEREJI	MEDICAL OFFICER	2005 (7 MONTHS)
30	DR. B. C. AJUNWA	MEDICAL OFFICER	2004-PRESENT
31	DR. EUNICE KALU	MEDICAL OFFICER	2005-PRSENT

FIG. XIX SEVENTH-DAY ADVENTIST HOSPITAL AND MOTHERLESS BABIES' HOME, ABA-IMMUNIZATION DEPARTMENT—JANUARY-DECEMBER, 2005[498]

MONTH	T.T	BCG	OPV	DPT	MEASLES	YELLOW FEVER	VIT A	ORAL POLIO	HBV	MONTH TOTAL
JAN.	37	26	74	48	10	-	-	-	-	195
FEB.	30	23	64	41	7	-	-	-	-	165
MARCH	38	39	100	61	20	-	-	-	-	258
APR.	34	34	94	64	26	18	22	-	45	337
MAY	49	51	126	87	17	17	16	-	39	402
JUNE	44	21	72	71	18	-	-	-	23	249
JULY	36	19	61	63	10	-	-	-	32	221
AUG.	49	40	28	81	14	8	-	81	74	375
SEPT.	34	13	-	69	17	-	-	45	62	240
OCT.	29	28	26	66	6	6	-	66	43	270
NOV.	52	64	-	96	5	22	-	157	47	443
DEC.	33	26	-	73	11	12	-	50	45	250
TOTAL	465	384	645	820	161	83	38	399	410	3405

---

[498] E. E. Enyinna, Medical Director, SDA Hospital and Motherless Babies' Home Aba, Report Presented at the 2005 Year end House Committee Report

FIG. XX SEVENTH-DAY ADVENTIST HOSPITAL AND MOTHERLESS BABIES' HOME, ABA-FAMILY PLANNING DEPARTMENT JANUARY-DECEMBER, 2005[499]

INJECTABLES

MONTH	ORAL	IUCD INSERTION	DEPO. P	NONS	CHECK-UPS	REMOVAL	MONTHLY TOTAL
JAN.	-	1	5	1	2	-	9
FEB.	1	-	2	-	3	1	7
MARCH	-	4	1	1	3	1	10
APR.	-	1	6	-	2	2	11
MAY	-	2	1	-	2	1	6
JUNE	-	2	2	-	3	-	7
JULY	-	-	6	1	-	1	8
AUG.	-	1	-	-	1	1	3
SEPT.	1	-	2	-	1	-	5
OCT.	-	2	1	1	2	-	6
NOV.	-	1	1	-	1	-	3
DEC.	-	-	2	-	4	-	6
TOTAL	2	14	29	4	24	8	81

5.14 Seventh-day Adventist Hospital Jengre, Plateau State:

The medical work of the Seventh-day Adventist Church in northern Nigeria started with the arrival of J. J. Hyde and his family in 1932. Mrs. Hyde who accompanied the husband on his missionary journey to Nigeria was already a trained nurse who had earlier worked at Stanborough Hydro in Watford, England. With this experience she commenced medical missionary work on arrival to Jengre. Within

---

[499] Ibid

two years of their coming. Pastor Hyde reported that their house was turned into a medical center. Their store was made the waiting room and a general place of worship; their dinning room was turned into the treatment room; while their bedroom metamorphosed into the examination room.[500] Their medical work was helping greatly in the establishment of the gospel propagation. It was a successful but taxing assignment and in 1934 Hyde observed the following:

> We are very thankful that we are permitted to open our work here in Nigeria on a strong medical foundation. not many stations have been more generously treated in this respect than has our station, and Mrs. Hyde finds her nursing skill taxed in handling the many cases that come to her. Our people are primitive pagans, Mohammedans,

Hausas, or Fulanis. They are all very shy people on the one hand because of their dislike for Christianity. Under such circumstances the medical side of our work proves to be invaluable.[501]

It was in 1947 that the leaders of the Seventh-day Adventist work in West Africa appointed J. Ashford Hyde, a medical doctor and son to the Hydes, to enlarge the health services of the church in Northern Nigeria. He swung into action and in the following year, a ward was established with a special grant of $2, 500.00. A new ward with threatre and maternity section was equally put in place in 1971.[502] In 1952, the medical institution was granted the certificate to operate

---

[500] Ibid.

[501] Dave M. Nyekwere, p. 97

[502] Ibid, p. 66

as a full fledged hospital. Apart from the fact that the hospital is located in Jengre, a Muslim community, religion was not a barrier in getting the medical services being rendered by the hospital. As many as 275 people visited the hospital daily. In 1965 alone, the outpatient department recorded that 35,000 people had received medical treatment at one time or the other within that year.

FIG. XXI JENGRE SEVENTH-DAY ADVENTIST HOSPITAL, STATISTICS 2001-OCTOBER, 2004[503]

Items/Date	2001	2002	2003	October 2004
Out Patients/Attendance	11,309	10,180	6,510	4,884
Admission	3,033	2,757	1,714	1,004
Delivery	274	248	130	114
X-Ray Examination		15	88	199
Ultra Sound Examination		450	427	409
Spiritual Contacts and Health Education			4,205	15,063
Laboratory Investigation	31,116	28,948	15,.351	10,693
Major Operations	254	187	108	82
Minor Operations	376	292	178	110
Immunization Service	38,247		5,384	19,869
Ante-natal Care	1,470	1,464	1,090	698
Death	173	194	119	56
Veterinary Services	17,079	9,815	14,324	8,152

---

[503] Ibid, p. 103

All these hospitals provide a time every morning for devotionals. This time is normally set aside for both the staff, students (where they are available), and patients to share the word of God and to pray together. It is interesting to note that both indigenes and missionaries accept the fact that wisdom to excel in the medical institutions, as well as healing and relief from distress come from God, the great healer.

CHAPTER SIX

6.0 DATA ANALYSIS AND PRESENTATION OF FINDINGS ON THE PRACTICE AND USE OF AFRICAN TRADITIONAL MEDICINE AMONG SEVENTH-DAY ADVENTISTS IN REMOLAND OGUN STATE

6.1 Introduction

This study undertook the examination of the practice and use of African traditional medicine among Seventh-day Adventists in Remoland of Ogun State. The instrumentation, validity of instruments, questionnaires, interviews and data collection had been treated under methodology and instrumentation earlier on this work, attention will now be focused on the population, sampling procedures and analysis of the responses from the questionnaire. The researcher visited all the designated churches in Remoland for the purpose of distributing the questionnaires and conducting the interviews. This was done between May and August 2004, May to July 2005 and finally in December, 2005. The data collected with the questionnaires were analyzed using simple frequency table, electronically processed on the statistical package for social sciences (SPSS Inc., USA).

6.2 Population

The population of the research was representative of all the Seventh-day Adventists in Remoland of Ogun state. This represents an approximate group of 7,000 members in 27 different congregations, which are located in different parts of Remoland plus the MA Pastoral students of Babcock University which was considered as a separate congregation for the purpose of this work. About 80% of this population is literate, with divergent conceptions on the subject under discussion. Below is the data of the Seventh-day Adventist churches in Remoland with their current memberships.

FIG. XXII THE MEMBERSHIP OF THE 28 DIFFERENT SEVENTH-DAY ADVENTIST CONGREGATIONS IN REMOLAND OF OGUN STATE

S/N	CONGRGATIONS	MEMBERSHIP
1	Church 1, Ilishan	298
2	Church 2, Ilishan	692
3	Beautiful Gate	197
4	Town Planning	143
5	Ikenne Church 1	85
6	Ikenne Church 2	55
7	Aiyegbami, Shagamu	195
8	Sabo, Shagamu	120
9	Makun, Shagamu	290
10	Iperu branch	81
11	Irolu	152

12	Pioneer Church, Babcock University	1,404
13	Heirs of the Kingdom Chapel	320
14	Prince Emmanuel Chapel	240
15	Feeders Chapel	145
16	Living Spring chapel	222
17	New creation chapel	198
18	Ogden Hall Worship Center	190
19	White hall Worship Center	150
20	Siloam Valley Chapel	140
21	Nyberg Hall Worship Center	230
22	Pre-degree Worship Center	382
23	Grace Chapel	598
24	Ilara Branch	143
25	Ijesha Branch	50
26	Odogbolu Branch	70
27	Esperon Worship Center	150
28	MA Students (Pastors)	60
	TOTAL	7,000

*The membership is made up of the baptized and Sabbath school members.

6.3 Sampling Procedures

The sample is the portion of the population being surveyed or interviewed. The sample for this study is made up of 9 different congregations with a membership of 3,702.

FIG. XXIII SUMMARY OF POPULATIONS, SAMPLES AND RETURNS

S/N	CONGREGATIONS	POPULATION NUMBER	NO OF RETURNED QUESTIONAIRES	% OF RETURNS
1	Aiyegbami, Shagamu	195	27	13.84
2	Beautiful Gate, Ilishan	200	39	19.50
3	Grace Chapel, BU	548	67	12.26
4	Ikenne (I&II)	140	16	11.42
5	Makun. Shagamu	290	21	7.24
6	PG Students (Pastors)	60	42	70.00
7	Pioneer Church, BU	1,459	35	2.39
8	Sabo Church, Shagamu	120	18	15.00
9	Township II	690	37	5.36
	TOTAL	3,702	302	8.16

6.4 Questionnaire Analysis

The Oxford Advanced Learners' Dictionary (6TH Edition) has defined questionnaires as a written list of questions that are answered by a number of people so that information can be collected from the answers. Indicated below is the analysis of the responses from 302 respondents on the 41 questions contained in the questionnaire. Each response has been objectively presented using the frequency tables.

Bar charts, pie charts and histograms with their various percentages have been selectively used to report these responses.

6.5 Frequency Tables on the Practice and Use of African Traditional Medicine Among Seventh-day Adventists in Remoland of Ogun State

FIG. XXIV FREQUENCY TABLE ON THE GENDER OF RESPONDENTS

Gender?

		Frequency	Percent	Valid Percent	Cumulative Percent
Valid	Missing Variable	6	2.0	2.0	2.0
	Male	192	63.6	63.6	65.6
	Female	104	34.4	34.4	100.0
	Total	302	100.0	100.0	

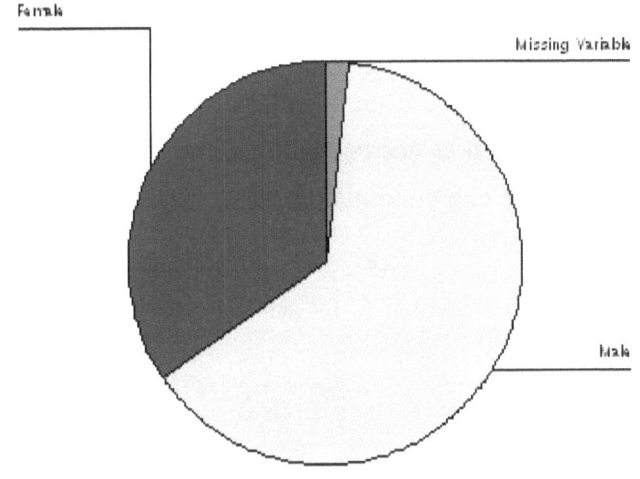

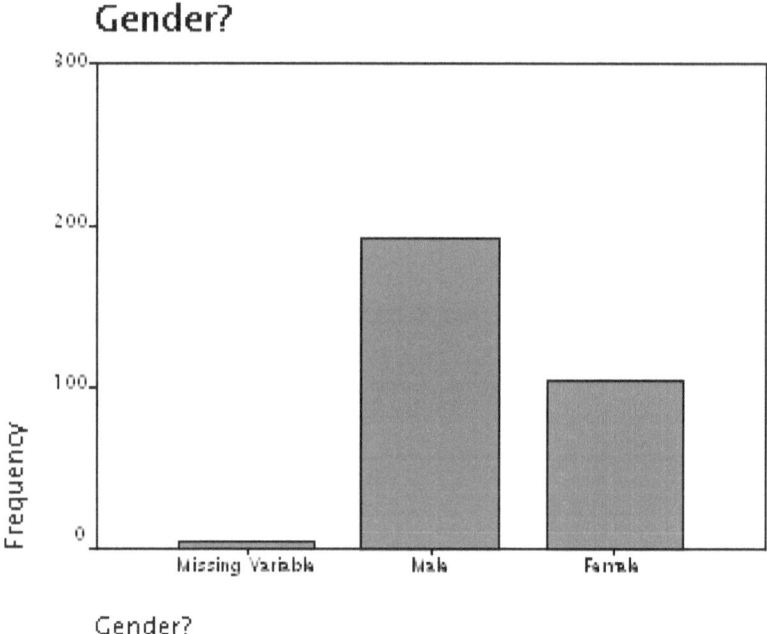

According to the responses, out of the total 302 people who responded, 192 were Males, 104 were Females while 6 individuals gender were not indicated. These represent 63.6%, 34.4% and 2.0% for men, women and missing variable, respectively. These statistics also demonstrate that more men took part in responding to these questions than women as has been ably demonstrated on the above frequency table, pie chart and histogram.

African Traditional Medicine

FIG. XXV FREQUENCY TABLE ON THE AGES OF RESPONDENTS

Age?

		Frequency	Percent	Valid Percent	Cumulative Percent
Valid	Missing Variable	6	2.0	2.0	2.0
	13-19 years	71	23.5	23.5	25.5
	20-29 years	93	30.8	30.8	56.3
	30-39 years	58	19.2	19.2	75.5
	Above 40	73	24.2	24.2	99.7
	Do not know	1	.3	.3	100.0
	Total	302	100.0	100.0	

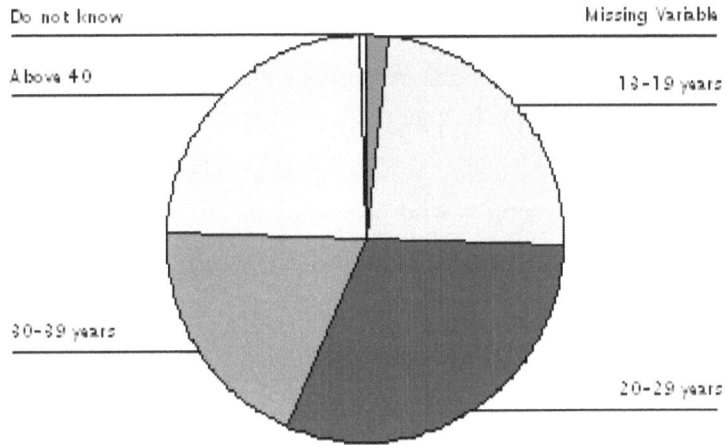

Age?

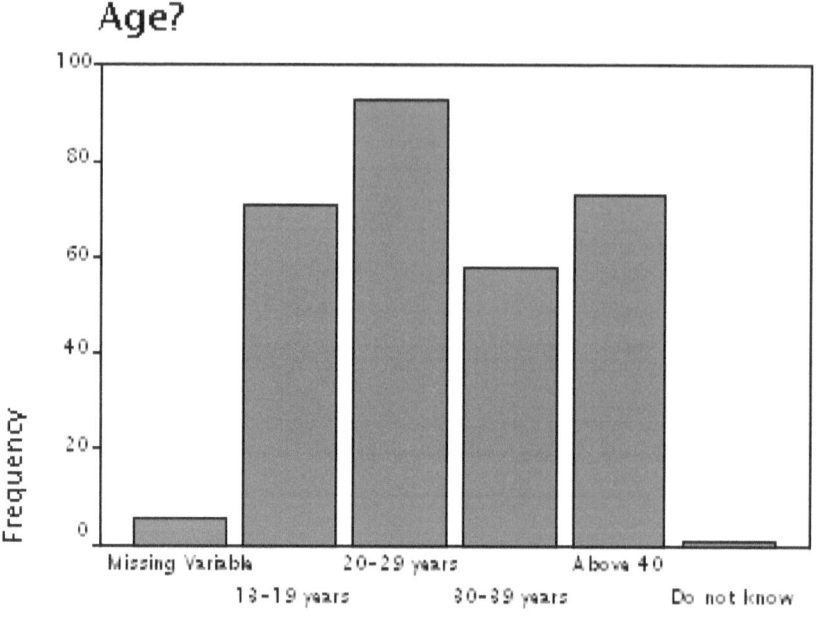

Age?

From the above frequency table and charts those who are between 20 and 29 years old participated more than others in responding to the questionnaire. This is a direct result of the numerous students from Babcock University who took part in this exercise. 73 adults who are 40 years and above equally took part in responding to the questionnaire.

FIG. XXVI FREQUENCY TABLE OF TRIBES/ETHNIC GROUPS OF RESPONDENTS

Tribe/Ethnic Group?

		Frequency	Percent	Valid Percent	Cumulative Percent
Valid	Missing Variable	21	7.0	7.0	7.0
	Igbo	106	35.1	35.1	42.1
	Yoruba	139	46.0	46.0	88.1
	Hausa	7	2.3	2.3	90.4
	Edo/Delta	5	1.7	1.7	92.1
	Middle Belt	1	.3	.3	92.4
	Others	23	7.6	7.6	100.0
	Total	302	100.0	100.0	

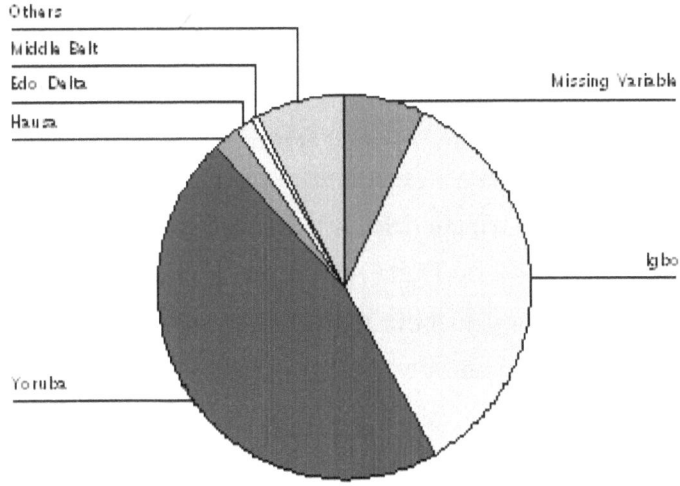

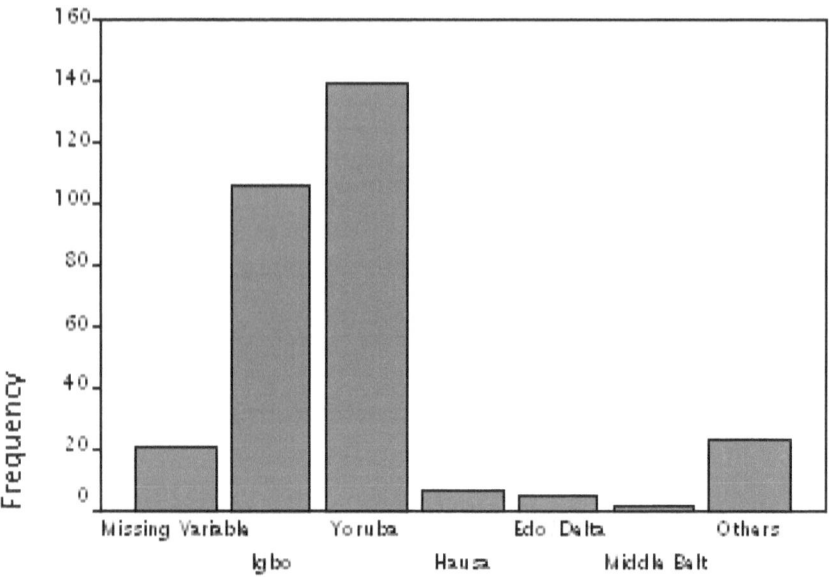

Tribe/Ethnic Group?

An objective analysis of the responses shows that those from the Yoruba tribe those who responded were 139, which represents 46%, while the Igbo tribe is 106, which stand for 35.1%. The Hausa and Middle Belt and Edo/Delta regions are 5, each which represent 4.3%. It is interesting to note that the others which make up the 7.6% of the respondents are not only from other parts of Nigeria but also includes tribes from East, Central and the West African sub regions. It is amazing that Seventh-day Adventists from all these parts of Africa practice and use African traditional medicine for so many reasons.

African Traditional Medicine

FIG. XXVII FREQUENCY TABLE ON THE NATIONALITIES OF RESPONDENTS

nationality?

		Frequency	Percent	Valid Percent	Cumulative Percent
Valid	Missing Variable	19	6.3	6.3	6.3
	Nigerian	263	87.1	87.1	93.4
	Others	20	6.6	6.6	100.0
	Total	302	100.0	100.0	

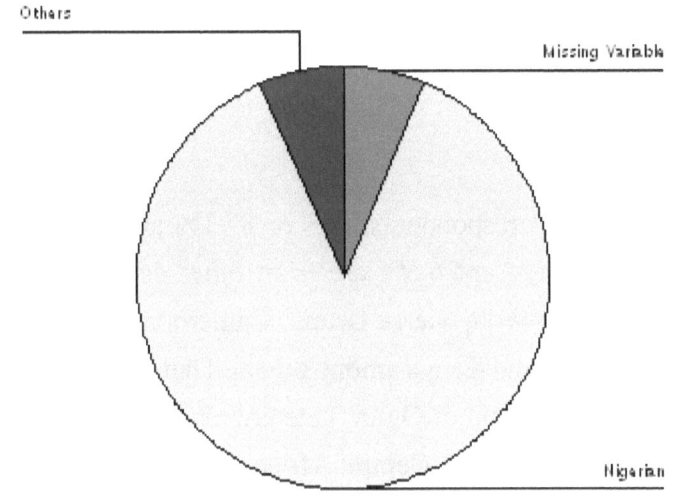

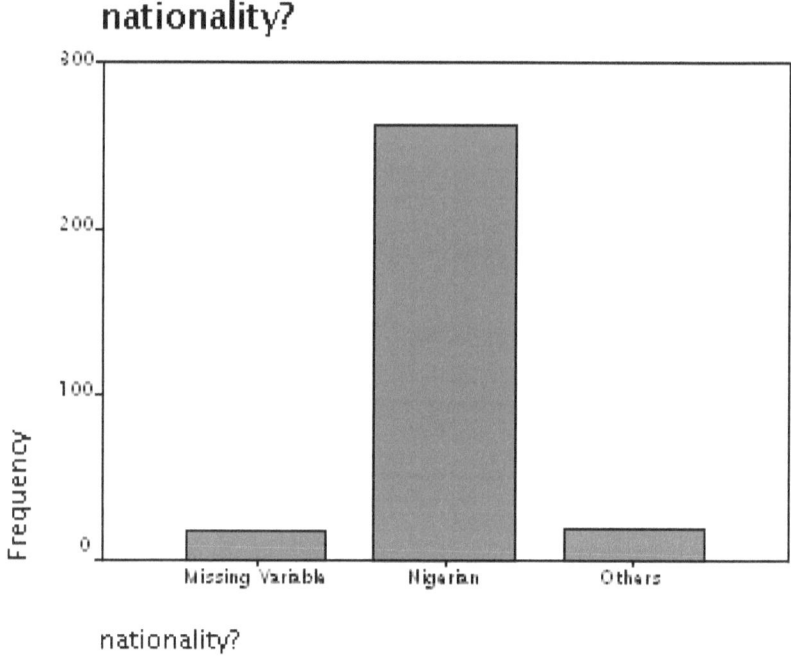

Out of the 302 respondents, 263 or 87.1% are Nigerians. The 20 others who represent 6.6% are from other countries in Africa such as Ghana, Liberia, Sierra Leone, Cameroon, Gambia, Niger, Burundi, Rwanda, and Kenya among others. Therefore, Seventh-day Adventists in Remoland of Ogun State are made up of people from different parts of West and Central Africa.

FIG. XXVIII FREQUENCY TABLE ON THE EDUCATIONAL STATUS OF RESPONDENTS

Educational Status?

		Frequency	Percent	Valid Percent	Cumulative Percent
Valid	Missing Variables	17	5.6	5.6	5.6
	Primary	19	6.3	6.3	11.9
	Secondary	53	17.5	17.5	29.5
	Post Secondary	139	46.0	46.0	75.5
	Others	71	23.5	23.5	99.0
	Do not Know	3	1.0	1.0	100.0
	Total	302	100.0	100.0	

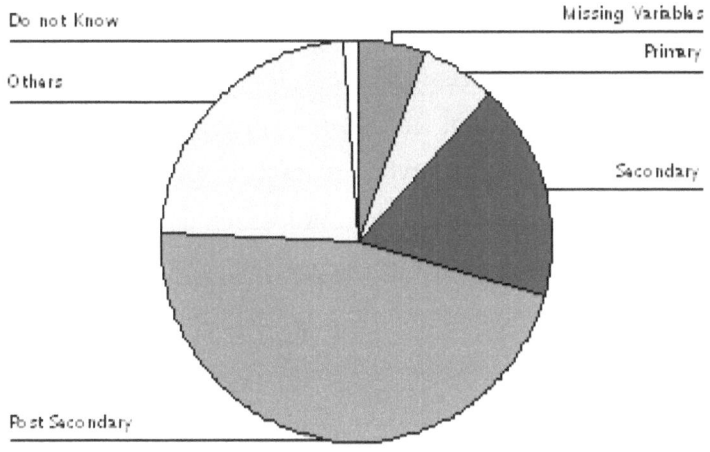

Educational Status?

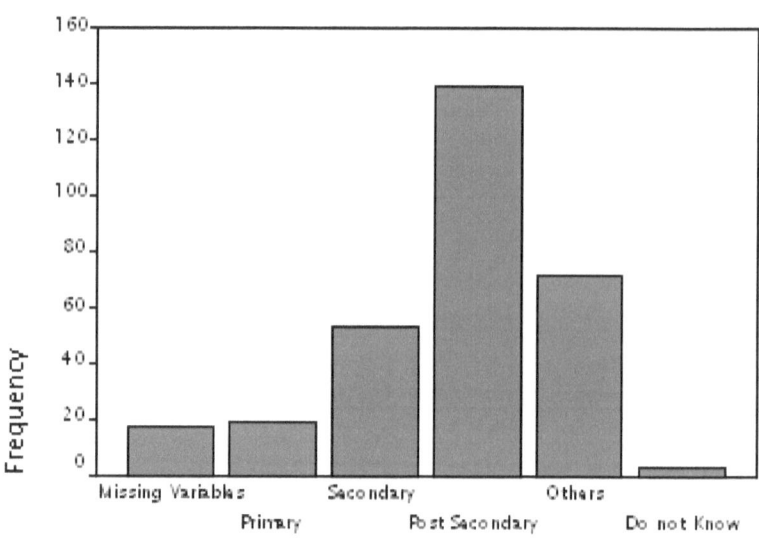

Educational Status?

People who are enlightened made the responses on the above question. For instance out of 302 respondents 139 have attained Post Secondary level, others who are up to 71 people are actually in Universities, colleges of education, Polytechnics and other Tertiary Institutions. 53 do have the Secondary School qualification while only 19 out of the whole lot are within the Primary school level.

FIG. XXIX MARITAL STATUS OF RESPONDENTS

Marital Status?

		Frequency	Percent	Valid Percent	Cumulative Percent
Valid	Missing Varibale	1	.3	.3	.3
	Single	173	57.3	57.3	57.6
	Married	121	40.1	40.1	97.7
	Widow	4	1.3	1.3	99.0
	Others	3	1.0	1.0	100.0
	Total	302	100.0	100.0	

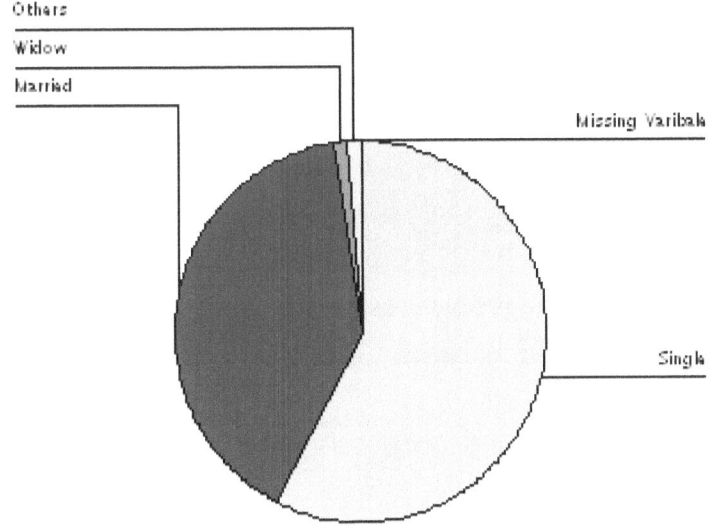

Marital Status?

Marital Status?

Bar chart showing frequency of marital status: Missing Variable, Single (~173), Married (~121), Widow, Others

According to the responses on this question, 173 people or 51.3% are single while 121 people or 40% are married. This large number of unmarried people is as a result of the fact that most of the respondents from the Babcock University community are students who are not yet married.

African Traditional Medicine

FIG. XXX FREQUENCY TABLE ON RELIGIOUS AFFILIATIONS OF RESPONDENTS BEFORE BECOMING SEVENTH-DAY ADVENTISTS

Religious Affiliation?

		Frequency	Percent	Valid Percent	Cumulative Percent
Valid	Missing Variable	10	3.3	3.3	3.3
	Christian	262	86.8	86.8	90.1
	Muslim	10	3.3	3.3	93.4
	African Traditional Religion	12	4.0	4.0	97.4
	Another Religion	4	1.3	1.3	98.7
	Do not Know	4	1.3	1.3	100.0
	Total	302	100.0	100.0	

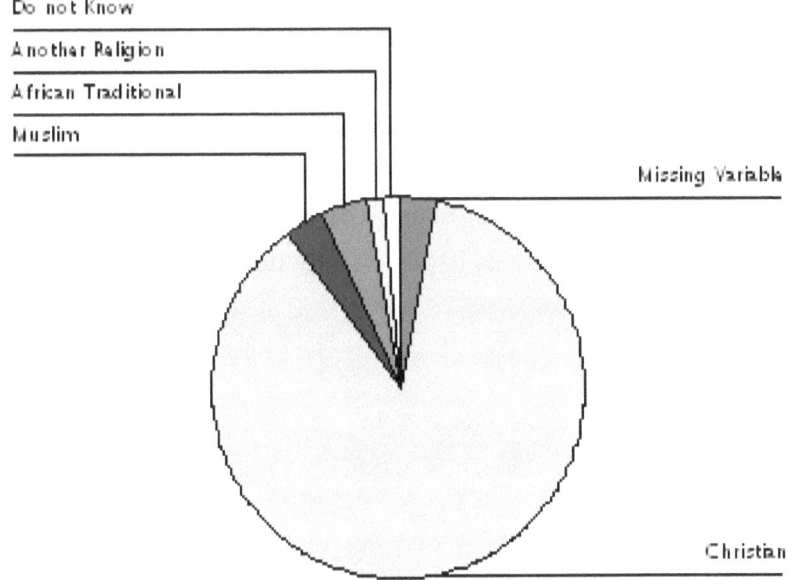

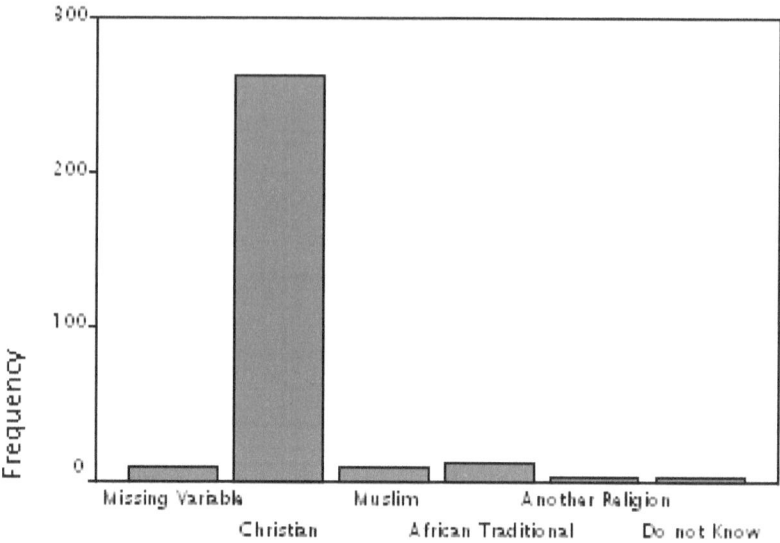

The responses show that most of the people have been Christians, which is 86.8%, while adherence of African Traditional Religion make up 4.0% and Muslims are 3.3% of the total respondents. Former members of the three major African Religions were however, represented in this study as had been ably demonstrated from these respondents.

African Traditional Medicine

FIG. XXXI LENGTH OF TIME OF BEING SDA CHURCH MEMBER

SDA Period?

		Frequency	Percent	Valid Percent	Cumulative Percent
Valid	Missing Variable	17	5.6	5.6	5.6
	0-12 months	56	18.5	18.5	24.2
	1-10 years	49	16.2	16.2	40.4
	11-20 years	60	19.9	19.9	60.3
	Above 20 years	120	39.7	39.7	100.0
	Total	302	100.0	100.0	

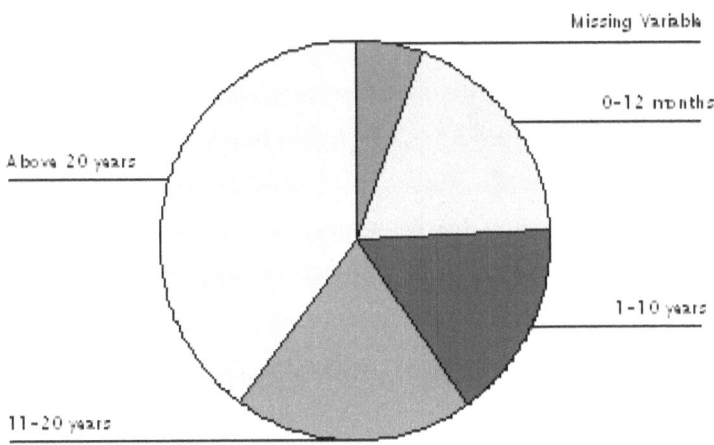

SDA Period?

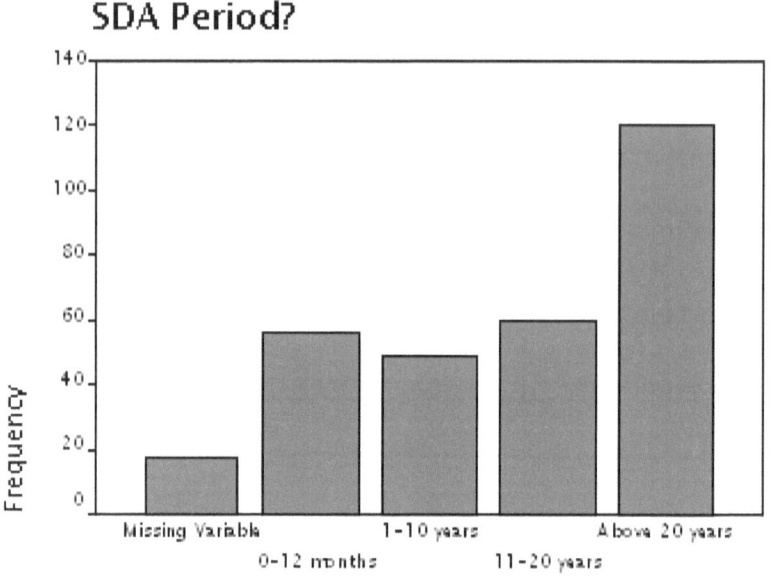

SDA Period?

The Table and charts above indicate that the respondents are not just new in the church. Those who had been in the SDA church for over 20 years are 120, which represent 39.7%. Those who have been in the church between 11-20 years are 60, representing 19.9%, follow this. While those who have been church members between 1-10 years represents 18.5% of the total respondents.

FIG. XXXII FREQUENCY TABLE SHOWING NO. OF SDA WHO USE ALTERNATIVE METHODS OF HEALING

Alternative Method?

		Frequency	Percent	Valid Percent	Cumulative Percent
Valid	Missing Variables	9	3.0	3.0	3.0
	Yes	163	54.0	54.0	57.0
	No	122	40.4	40.4	97.4
	Do not Know	8	2.6	2.6	100.0
	Total	302	100.0	100.0	

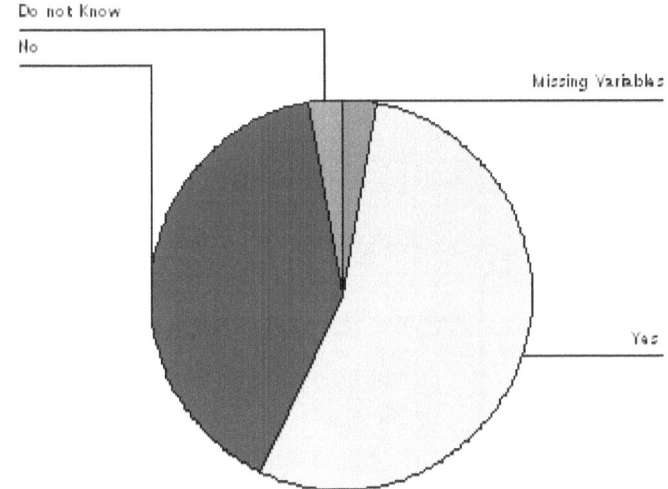

Alternative Method?

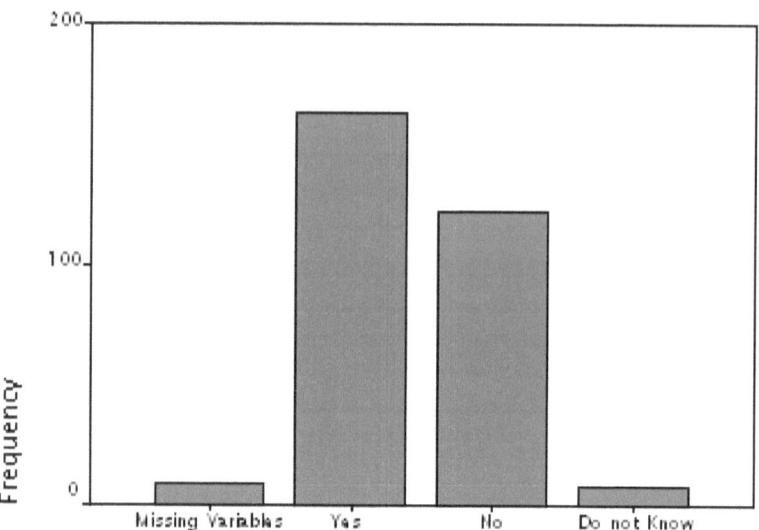

Source of Medication

		Frequency	Percent	Valid Percent	Cumulative Percent
Valid	Missing Variable	48	15.9	15.9	15.9
	Chemist Shop	62	20.5	20.5	36.4
	Traditional	83	27.5	27.5	63.9
	Self Help	54	17.9	17.9	81.8
	Another Method	29	9.6	9.6	91.4
	Do not Know	26	8.6	8.6	100.0
	Total	302	100.0	100.0	

African Traditional Medicine

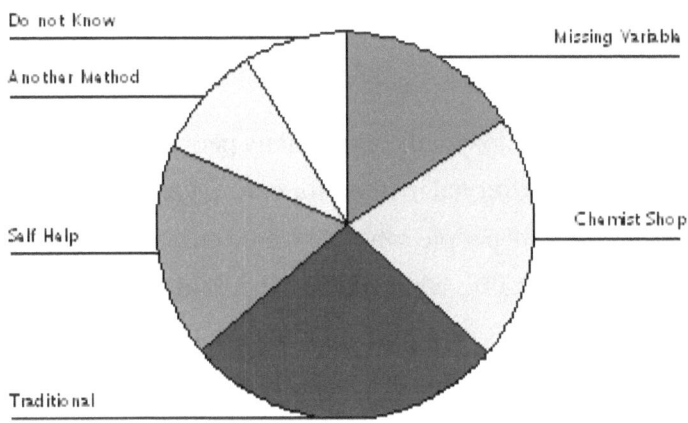

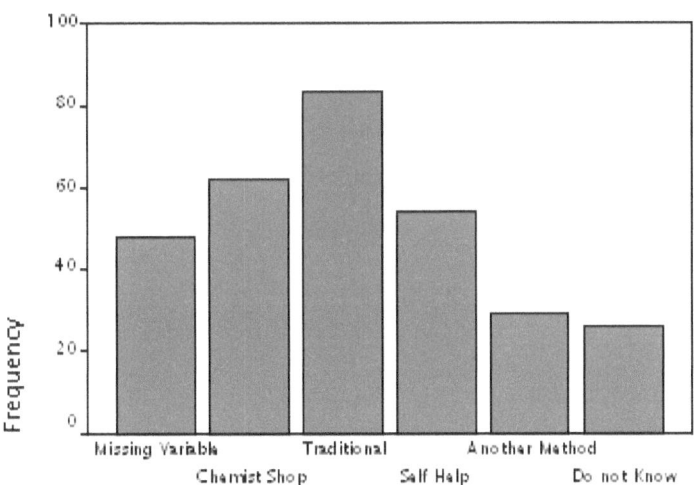

163 of the respondents representing 54% responded in the affirmative that they have used alternative methods of healing. Those who responded no were 122 which are 40.4% of the total respondents.

Apart from orthodox medication, many people have also received healing from the traditional method for curing various diseases in the past. The number of people who answered in the affirmative were 96, representing 59.8%, while those who said no represented the remaining 37.3%. This response is indicative that more people have used traditional medicine in the past. It is also interesting to note that 53 people who are actually 31.9% got their medication from the traditional medical personnel. The 45 people who are actually 27.1% of the total respondents got theirs from the Chemist Shop. The Chemist Shop here sells both modern and traditional medicine. The 26 people who represent 15.7% who are involved in getting the drug through self help are people who have knowledge of these drugs through training, experience or through personal reading. The good news is that many are aware of these traditional Medications and go for them.

FIG. XXXIII REASONS FOR TRADITIONAL MEDICINE

Reasons for Traditional Medication?

		Frequency	Percent	Valid Percent	Cumulative Percent
Valid	Missing Variable	98	32.5	32.5	32.5
	Affordable	22	7.3	7.3	39.7
	Available	22	7.3	7.3	47.0
	Effective	56	18.5	18.5	65.6
	Another Reason	22	7.3	7.3	72.8
	Do not Know	82	27.2	27.2	100.0
	Total	302	100.0	100.0	

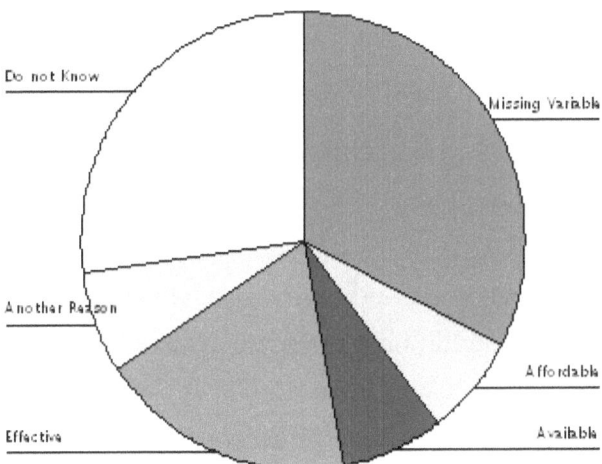

Reasons for Traditional Medication?

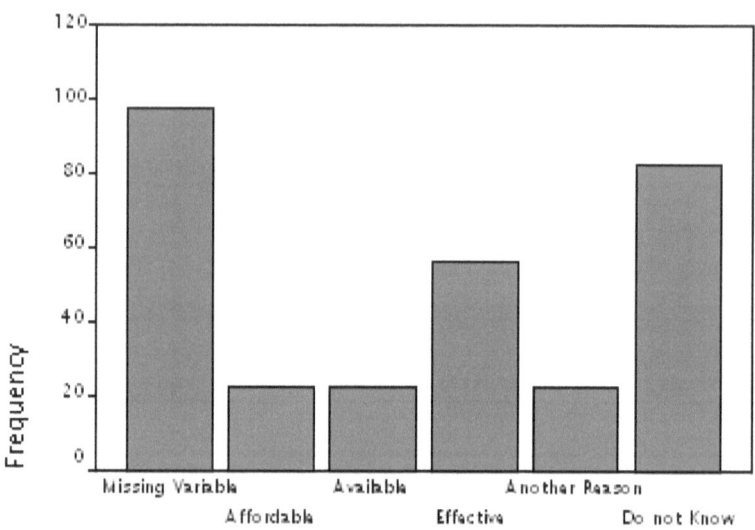

Reasons for Traditional Medication?

Many people go for traditional medicine simply because it is affordable, available and also effective. Another reason people have for patronizing traditional medicine is due to its prophylactic and preventive purposes. Many others might not have known the reasons for patronizing the traditional medicine dealers; this does not mean that they do not use it when needed. Others who are in this group might not want their identity to be known as people who patronize traditional medical healers.

African Traditional Medicine

FIG. XXXIV MOTIVATION FOR TRADITIONAL MEDICINE

Motivation?

		Frequency	Percent	Valid Percent	Cumulative Percent
Valid	Missing Variable	89	29.5	29.5	29.5
	Defied Orthodox	24	7.9	7.9	37.4
	Conviction	36	11.9	11.9	49.3
	Family Reasons	44	14.6	14.6	63.9
	Another Reason	38	12.6	12.6	76.5
	Do not Know	71	23.5	23.5	100.0
	Total	302	100.0	100.0	

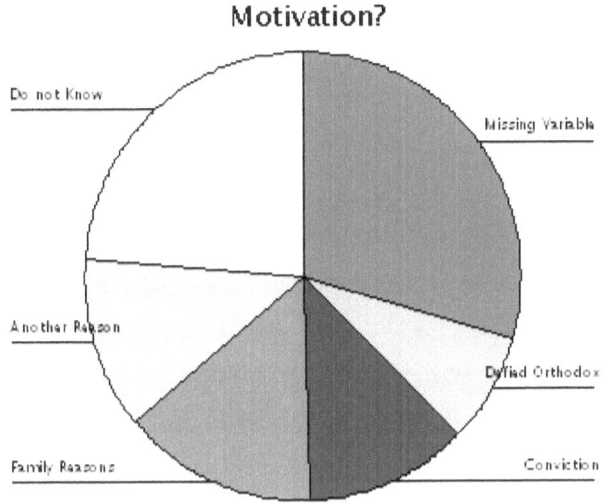

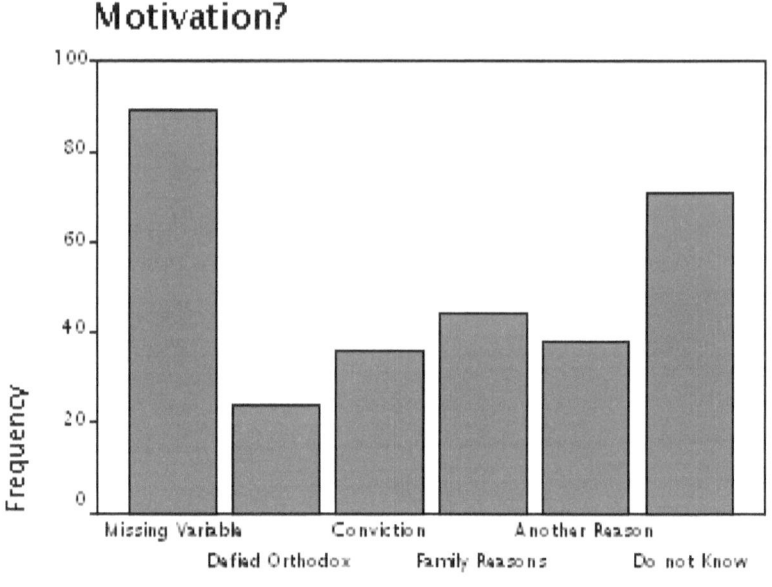

Many reasons have been given as the motivating factors for embracing traditional medication. For instance, a family that has found it beneficial will always recommend it, also when people are convinced as well as when the ill health has defied orthodox medication, the next objective option will be to embrace traditional medication.

FIG. XXXV PARTS OF THE BODY THAT NEEDED TO BE HEALED

Body Part?

		Frequency	Percent	Valid Percent	Cumulative Percent
Valid	Missing Variable	96	31.8	31.8	31.8
	Head	30	9.9	9.9	41.7
	Limbs	14	4.6	4.6	46.4
	Visceral Organ	27	8.9	8.9	55.3
	Others	62	20.5	20.5	75.8
	Do not Know	73	24.2	24.2	100.0
	Total	302	100.0	100.0	

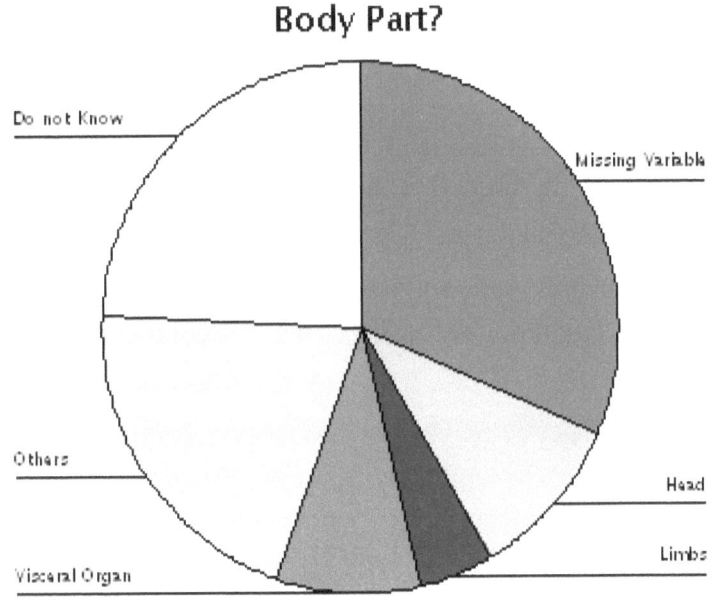

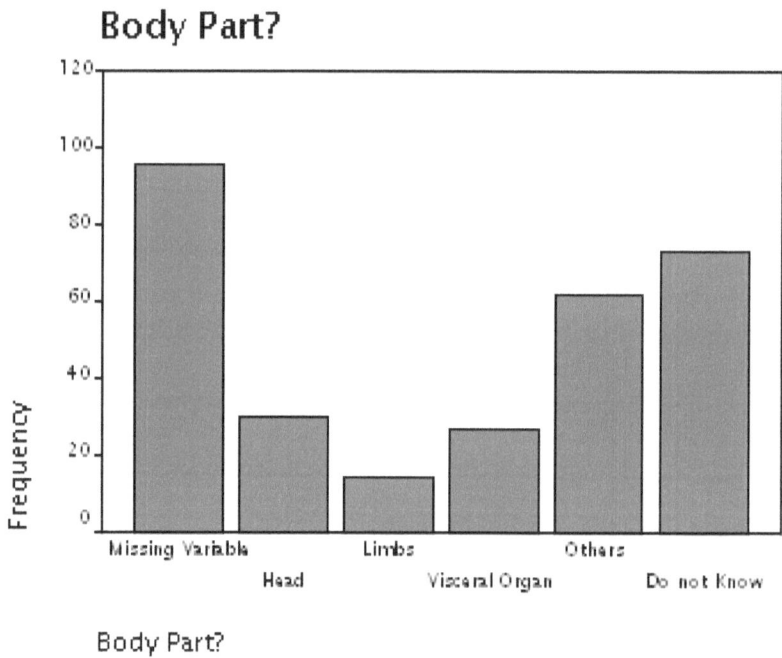

Body Part?

The parts of the body that the respondents indicated that were mostly affected included the visceral organs, the head, the hands and legs. Others include septicemia, malaria, typhoid fever and other ill health, which might not be localized in any section of the body.

FIG. XXXVI FORMS OF MEDICINE USED

Medicine Form?

		Frequency	Percent	Valid Percent	Cumulative Percent
Valid	Missing Variable	143	47.4	47.4	47.4
	Liquid	75	24.8	24.8	72.2
	Gaseous	5	1.7	1.7	73.8
	Powder	6	2.0	2.0	75.8
	Solid	8	2.6	2.6	78.5
	Poultice	6	2.0	2.0	80.5
	Roots	16	5.3	5.3	85.8
	Rhizomes	4	1.3	1.3	87.1
	Bark	11	3.6	3.6	90.7
	Leaves	28	9.3	9.3	100.0
	Total	302	100.0	100.0	

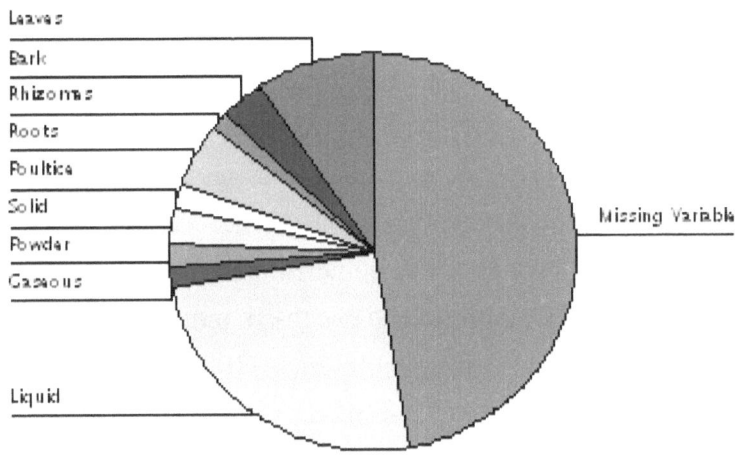

Medicine Form?

Medicine Form?

[Bar chart showing frequency of medicine forms: Missing Variable ~143, Liquid ~75, Gaseous ~2, Powder ~3, Solid ~5, Poultice ~3, Roots ~14, Rhizomes ~2, Bark ~8, Leaves ~25]

Medicine Form?

Respondents actually got their drugs in different forms which include liquid, leaves, roots, bark, powder, rhizomes, solid, gaseous and even poultice. These various forms indicate the varieties which are available when it comes to using traditional medicines. The frequency table for instance has demonstrated that 75 respondents, which represent 47.4%, prefer and use the liquid form of traditional medicine; 28 people which also represent 9.31% use their medication in the form of leaves while 16 respondents which represent 5.3% get their medication in the form of roots. A combination of the one, two or more of these materials was still another form in which some of the respondents receive their traditional medication.

FIG. XXXVII : LENGTH OF TIME MEDICINE WAS USED

Use Lenght?

		Frequency	Percent	Valid Percent	Cumulative Percent
Valid	Missing Variable	76	25.2	25.2	25.2
	1-12 months	60	19.9	19.9	45.0
	1-10 years	29	9.6	9.6	54.6
	11-20 years	18	6.0	6.0	60.6
	21 years and Above	49	16.2	16.2	76.8
	Do not Know	70	23.2	23.2	100.0
	Total	302	100.0	100.0	

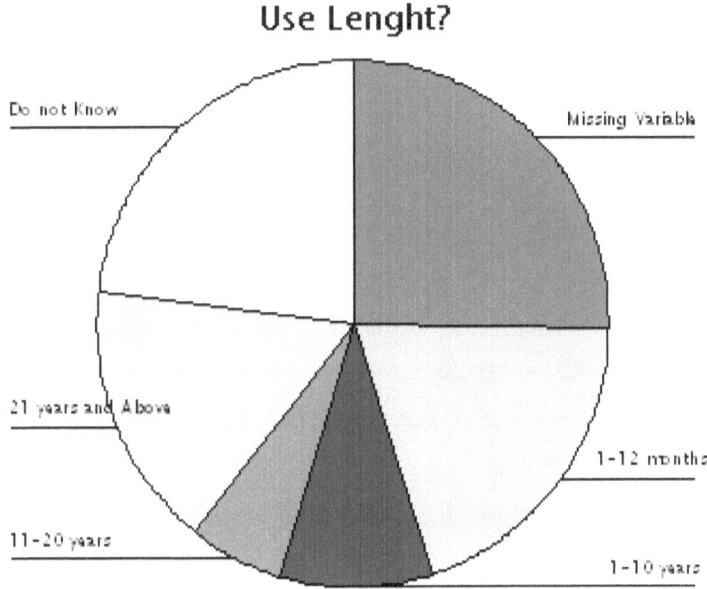

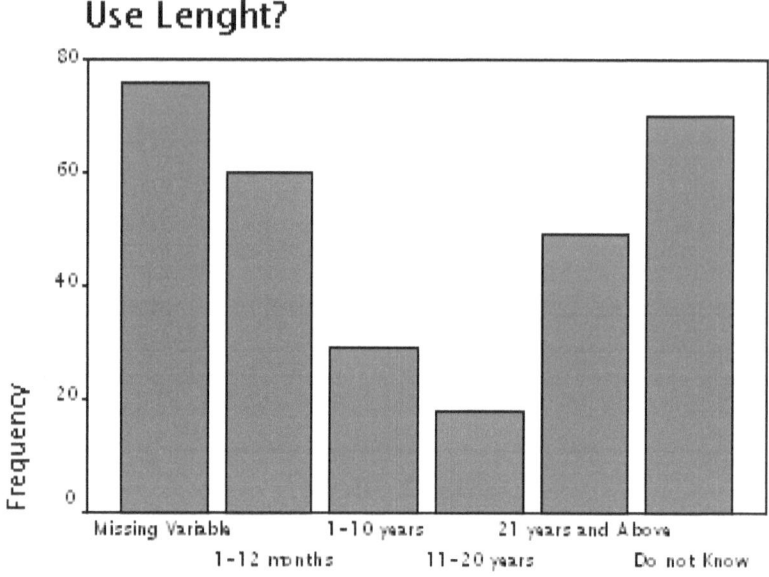

The figures above show that the length of the use of traditional medicine is on the increase. Some have used it between 1-12 months, representing 19.9%, while those who have used it between 1-10 years represent 9.6%. Those who have used it up to 21 years and above make up 16.2%. The fact still remains hat people have used traditional medicines for different lengths of time.

FIG. XXXVIII THE FREQUENCY OF USING TRADITIONAL MEDICINE

Frequency of Use?

		Frequency	Percent	Valid Percent	Cumulative Percent
Valid	Missing Variable	79	26.2	26.2	26.2
	Daily	9	3.0	3.0	29.1
	Weekly	7	2.3	2.3	31.5
	Monthly	2	.7	.7	32.1
	As needed	135	44.7	44.7	76.8
	Do not know	70	23.2	23.2	100.0
	Total	302	100.0	100.0	

The frequency of use of traditional medicine is determined by so many factors. The most outstanding is that people use it as the needs arise. The responses for the above question show that 135 people or 44.7% of the respondents use traditional medicine when there is need for it. 9 of the respondents use it on a daily basis while 7 use it weekly.

FIG. XXXIX NATURE OF THE SICKNESS

Nature of Sickness?

		Frequency	Percent	Valid Percent	Cumulative Percent
Valid	Missing Variable	111	36.8	36.8	36.8
	Pregnancy	5	1.7	1.7	38.4
	Accident	3	1.0	1.0	39.4
	headache	5	1.7	1.7	41.1
	Blood Related	6	2.0	2.0	43.0
	Do not Know	161	53.3	53.3	96.4
	Others	11	3.6	3.6	100.0
	Total	302	100.0	100.0	

Nature of Sickness?

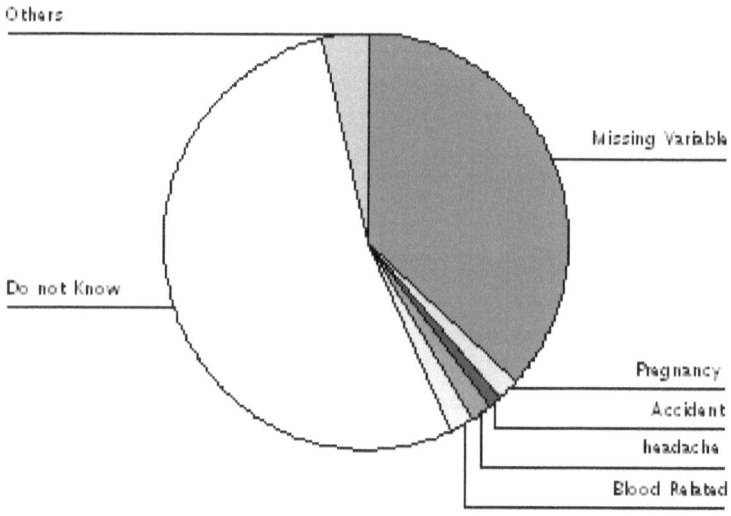

Nature of Sickness?

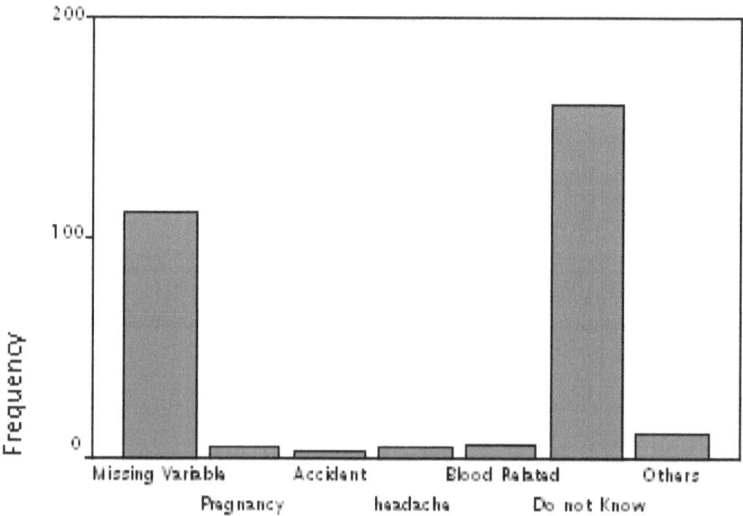

A lot of people, who have indicated that they do not know the nature of their sicknesses, still go to the Traditional healers for medication. Many people who are in this group do not know the nature of their sickness nor why they are ill. Other forms of ill health, which the respondents have indicated above, include headaches, blood/ pregnancy related sickness, accidents and others.

FIG. XL HOW DISEASES THAT DEFIED ORTHODOX MEDICATION WERE TREATED

Defy Orthodox Medicine?

		Frequency	Percent	Valid Percent	Cumulative Percent
Valid	Missing Variable	28	9.3	9.3	9.3
	Prayer/fasting	164	54.3	54.3	63.6
	Traditional	27	8.9	8.9	72.5
	Orthodox/Tradition	39	12.9	12.9	85.4
	Others	19	6.3	6.3	91.7
	Do not Know	25	8.3	8.3	100.0
	Total	302	100.0	100.0	

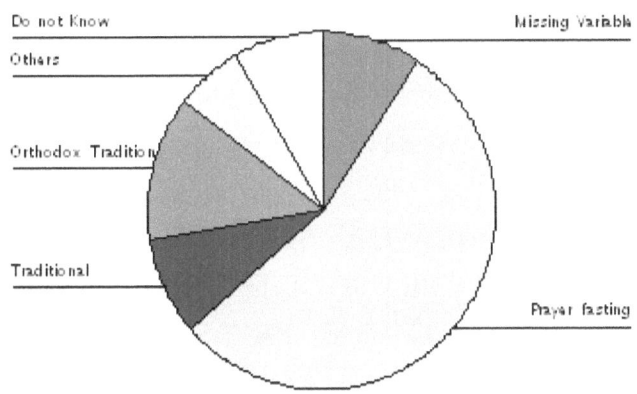

Defy Orthodox Medicine?

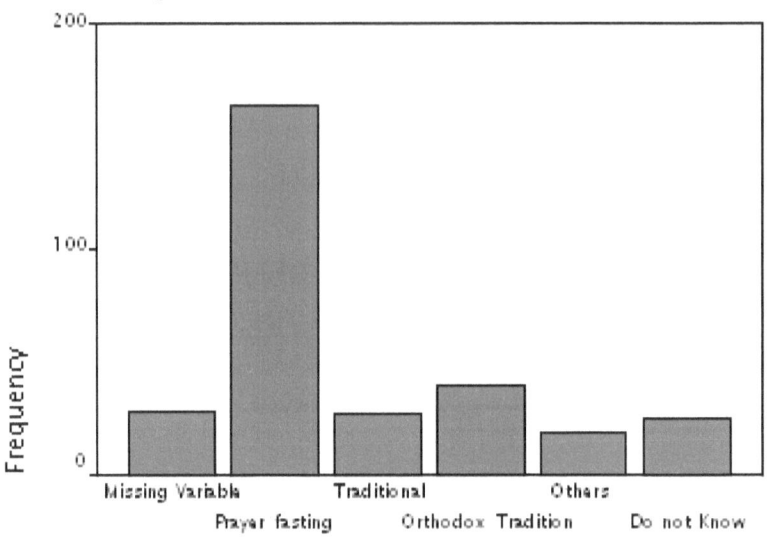

Defy Orthodox Medicine?

Apart from fasting and praying which traditional healers prescribe in exceptional cases, the combination of orthodox and traditional methods of healing has been suggested as a way to handle diseases which defy modern medication. 39 respondents which represent 12.9% suggested the above while only 27 respondents or 8.9% have suggested the application of only traditional medicine. It is not strange that 164 Christians who are used to prayer and fasting still resort to it to handle diseases that defy orthodox medication.

QUESTION 19: DOES THE SEVENTH-DAY ADVENTIST CHURCH SUPPORT THE USE OF TRADITIONAL MEDICINE AS A WAY OF HEALING ITS MEMBERS?

FIG. XLI SUPPORT OF TRADITIONAL MEDICATION BY THE SDA CHURCH

SDA Support?

		Frequency	Percent	Valid Percent	Cumulative Percent
Valid	Missing Variable	26	8.6	8.6	8.6
	yes	102	33.8	33.8	42.4
	No	77	25.5	25.5	67.9
	Do not Know	97	32.1	32.1	100.0
	Total	302	100.0	100.0	

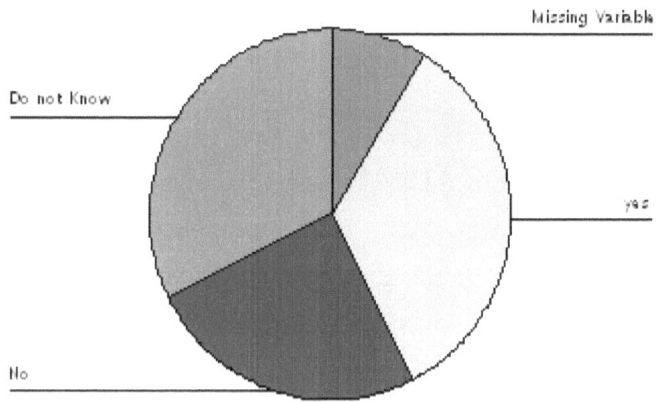

SDA Support?

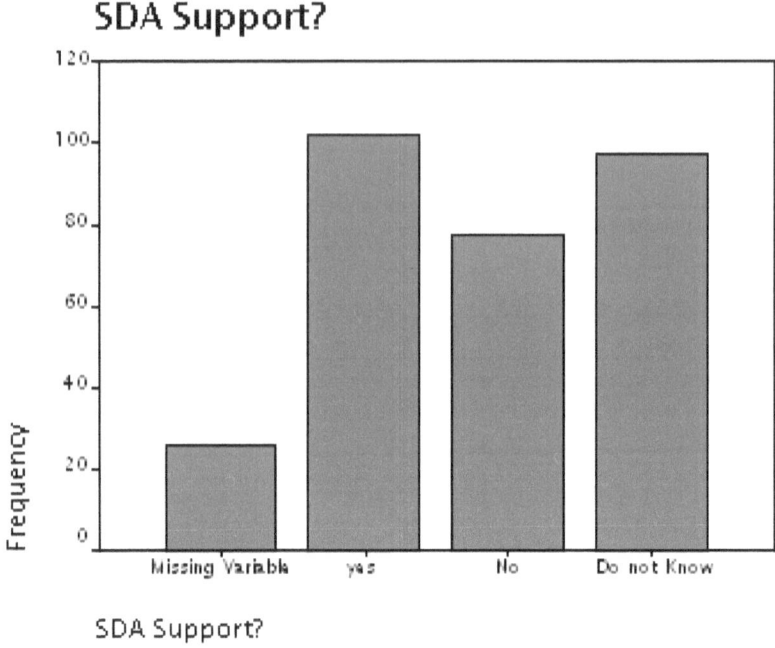

SDA Support?

102 respondents or 33.8% answered in the affirmative that the church supports the use of traditional medicine. The 97 respondents who indicated that they do not know if the SDA Church supports traditional medicine or not, suggests that there is need for awareness creation and education on the practice and use of traditional medicine among Seventh-day Adventist Church members in Remoland.

FIG. XLII WAYS THROUGH WHICH THE SDA CHURCH SUPPORTS THE USE OF TRADITIONAL MEDICINE

Ways of SDA Support?

		Frequency	Percent	Valid Percent	Cumulative Percent
Valid	Missing Variable	166	55.0	55.0	55.0
	Natural	45	14.9	14.9	69.9
	Leaves/herbs	26	8.6	8.6	78.5
	Feeding habits	20	6.6	6.6	85.1
	Economic	42	13.9	13.9	99.0
	Do not Know	3	1.0	1.0	100.0
	Total	302	100.0	100.0	

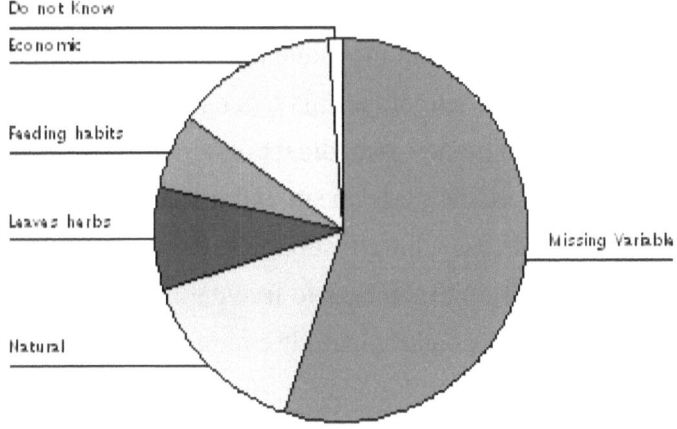

Ways of SDA Support?

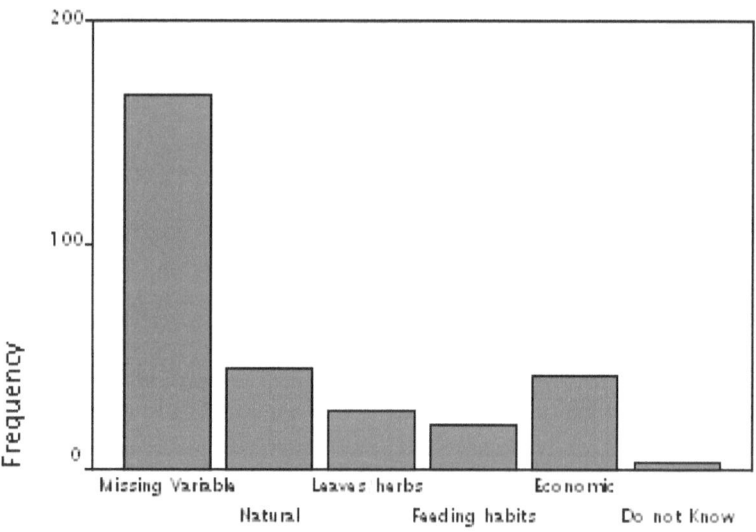

Ways of SDA Support?

The church encourages the members to embrace the practice and use of African traditional medicine due to the fact that it would positively impact their economy. This means that the members will spend little amount of money in medical bills since it is an established fact that traditional medicine is cheap and affordable. Respondents who indicated that the church supports the use of traditional medicine by encouraging members to live naturally were 45 which represent 14.9%. Living natural include eating original diet, drinking pure water instead of other beverages, exercising regularly among others. A total of 42 respondents which represent 24.7% are of the view that the economic advantage is one reason that has made the church support their use traditional medicine. 26 respondents which represent 8.6% are of the view that the church supports the use of traditional medicine by encouraging them to use appropriate leaves and herbs both for the prevention and healing of diseases. The third way in which the church supports this is by encouraging the members to embrace vegetarianism both in principle and practice. Members are equally counseled to refrain from using harmful substances such as alcohol, tea, coffee and flesh foods which adversely affect their health. 26 respondents that represent 6.6% are of the view that the church supports the use of traditional medicine by encouraging the members to embrace proper feeding habits which include eating the right quantity and quality of food devoid of flesh, and abstaining from alcoholic beverages among others.

FIG. XLIII WHY DO YOU THINK THE SDA CHURCH DOES NOT ENCOURAGE HER MEMBERS TO EMBRACE TRADITIONAL MEDICAL PRACTICE

Reasons Against?

		Frequency	Percent	Valid Percent	Cumulative Percent
Valid	Missing Variable	179	59.3	59.3	59.3
	Divine healing	10	3.3	3.3	62.6
	Idolatory	51	16.9	16.9	79.5
	Atheism	3	1.0	1.0	80.5
	Unrefined	4	1.3	1.3	81.8
	Alchohol Mix	4	1.3	1.3	83.1
	Do not know	49	16.2	16.2	99.3
	Ignorance	2	.7	.7	100.0
	Total	302	100.0	100.0	

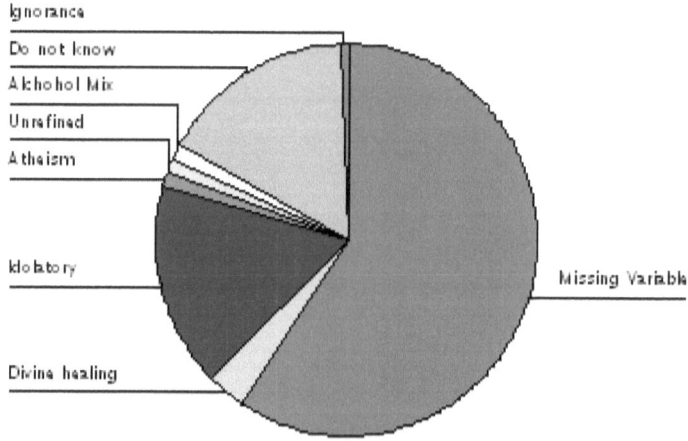

Reasons Against?

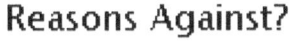

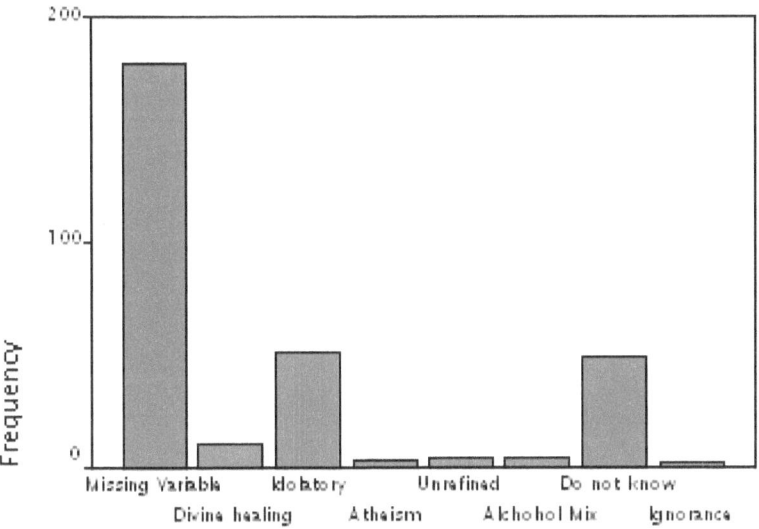

Some reasons were also proffered why the church seems to be reluctant in encouraging her members from embracing traditional medicine and they include the possibility of being involved in idolatry. 51 people who represent 16.9% of the total respondents are of this view. The unrefined nature of some traditional medicine products is another reason that had made the church to discourage her members from embracing this form of medication. The church also encourages her members to seek for divine healing directly from God and not through traditional medicine is another reason. Another reason includes the fear that the drugs are prepared with alcohol that might in the long run introduce the members to the use of alcohol in its various forms. Ignorance is another reason the members have given as a possible factor which prevents the church from encouraging her member from the use of traditional medicine. This is a very important factor because people tend to term anything traditional as being satanic. There is still the need to educate our people to differentiate between the explicable form of traditional medicine, which involves the use of herbs, sunshine, water, fruits, and other materials for healing and treating diseases just as *"Panadol"* might be used for analgesic purposes and the inexplicable form. In the inexplicable form we see in operation the unabated use of oracular diagnosis, incantations, ritual sacrifices and other cultic practices that might not be in consonance with the Christian belief, teaching and practice.

XLIV BIBLICAL SUPPORT FOR THE USE OF TRADITIONAL MEDICINE

Biblical?

		Frequency	Percent	Valid Percent	Cumulative Percent
Valid	Missing Variable	46	15.2	15.2	15.2
	Yes	123	40.7	40.7	56.0
	No	54	17.9	17.9	73.8
	Do not Know	79	26.2	26.2	100.0
	Total	302	100.0	100.0	

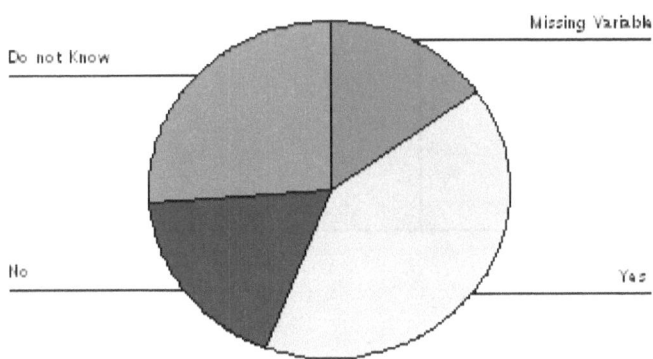

Biblical?

An objective analysis of the responses given to this question reveals that most Seventh-day Adventists are aware that the practice and use of traditional medicine has a biblical basis. Those who answered in the affirmative are 123 and this represents 40.7% of the total respondents. Those who indicated that traditional medicine was not biblical were 54 and that represented 17.9% of the total respondents. Those who do not know if the use and practice of traditional medicine is biblical or not are incidentally higher than those who responded in the negative since they were up to 79 representing 26.2% of the total respondents. Despite the fact that they do not know whether its practice was biblical or not, they still went ahead to use it when the needs arose.

FIG. XLV BIBLICAL EXAMPLES WHERE TRADITIONAL MEDICATIONS WERE USED

Examples?

		Frequency	Percent	Valid Percent	Cumulative Percent
Valid	Missing Variable	127	42.1	42.1	42.1
	Genesis (Reuben)	24	7.9	7.9	50.0
	2 Kings/Isaiah (Hezekiah)	31	10.3	10.3	60.3
	Timothy	8	2.6	2.6	62.9
	Exodus	10	3.3	3.3	66.2
	Revelation	6	2.0	2.0	68.2
	Do not know	87	28.8	28.8	97.0
	Luke	9	3.0	3.0	100.0
	Total	302	100.0	100.0	

African Traditional Medicine

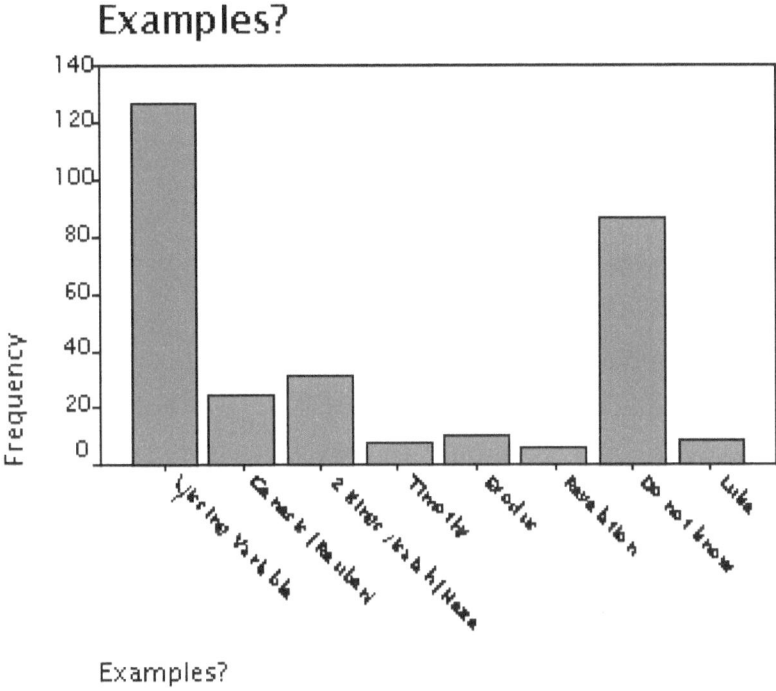

In responding to this question, a lot of examples were given from the Old and New Testaments of the Bible. The healing of king Hezekiah with the poultice of the fig tree as recorded in 2 Kings 20:1-7 was an example which many people remembered. 31 people or 10.3% of the total respondents gave this example. Others included the various healing activities of Jesus Christ such as spitting on the ground, making clay, anointing the eye and requesting the blind to go and wash which led the blind to see as recorded in John 9:1-7. Here we see the use of clay, soil and water for healing purposes, The story of the Good Samaritan who rendered medical assistance with oil and wine as recorded in Luke 10:25-34 was also cited. The use of mandrakes which are herbs with narcotic qualities as recorded in Genesis 30:14-16 and Songs of Solomon 7:13 were also cited. Finally, the healing to be received from the leaves of the tree of life in the New Jerusalem as recorded in Revelation 2:7, 22:2 was indicated.

The experience of the Israelites when they got to Marah where bitter water was made fit for human consumption when a tree was cast into it as contained in Exodus 15:23-25 was equally cited as another example of the practice and use of traditional medicine for the benefit of the people of God. In 1 Timothy 5:23 we have the record of Paul's counsel admonishing Timothy to take a little wine for the sake of his stomach and because of other recurring infirmities that the young minister of the gospel, Timothy was experiencing. This counsel was also cited as a good example of the use of traditional medicine in the scriptures. The respondents were aware of the numerous examples of the use of traditional medicine in the Bible and as indicated as a footnote on some copies of the questionnaire, some individuals who were using this alternative form of medication could not possibly remember any biblical example as at the time the questionnaire came to them.

FIG. XLVI WHO INTRODUCED YOU TO THE USE OF TRADITIONAL MEDICINE

Who Introduce you to Traditional Medicine?

		Frequency	Percent	Valid Percent	Cumulative Percent
Valid	Missing Variable	95	31.5	31.5	31.5
	Spouce	30	9.9	9.9	41.4
	Friend	45	14.9	14.9	56.3
	Church Member	27	8.9	8.9	65.2
	Medical Personel	20	6.6	6.6	71.9
	Do not Know	74	24.5	24.5	96.4
	Co-worker	5	1.7	1.7	98.0
	Co-resident	3	1.0	1.0	99.0
	Divine Inspiration	3	1.0	1.0	100.0
	Total	302	100.0	100.0	

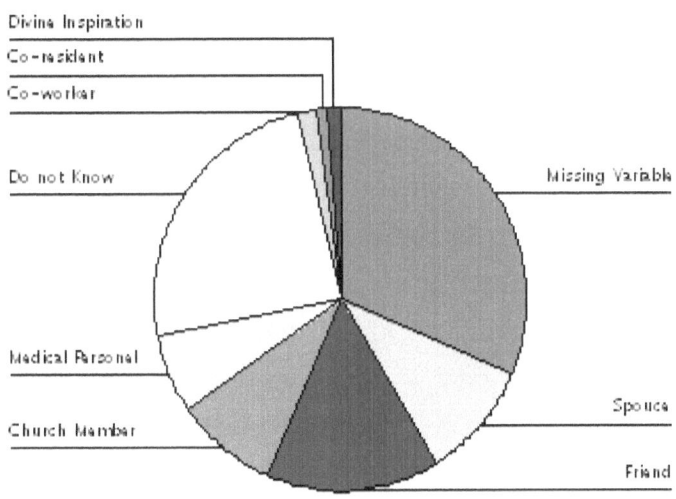

Who Introduce you to Traditional Medicine?

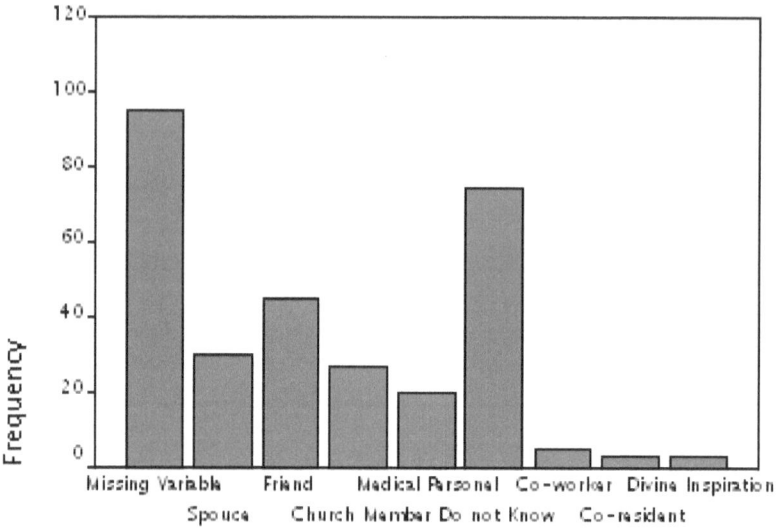

Who Introduce you to Traditional Medicine?

A lot of people were introduced into the use and practice of traditional medicine through those who are very close to them and also knew them very well. For instance, friends, fellow church members, medical personnel and spouses accounted for 14.9%, 8.9%, 6.6% and 9.9% respectively of people who were instrumental in introducing others to traditional medicine as indicated in the frequency, pie and other charts above. Two other groups who were instrumental in bringing the knowledge of traditional medicine to others included co-workers and co-residents. When people have tasted this form of healing, it becomes easier to share that good news with those around.

FIG. XLVII IS TRADITIONAL MEDICINE BETTER THAN THE MODERN ONE?

Traditional Supremacy?

		Frequency	Percent	Valid Percent	Cumulative Percent
Valid	Missing Variable	13	7.8	7.8	7.8
	Yes	81	48.8	48.8	56.6
	No	52	31.3	31.3	88.0
	Do not know	20	12.0	12.0	100.0
	Total	166	100.0	100.0	

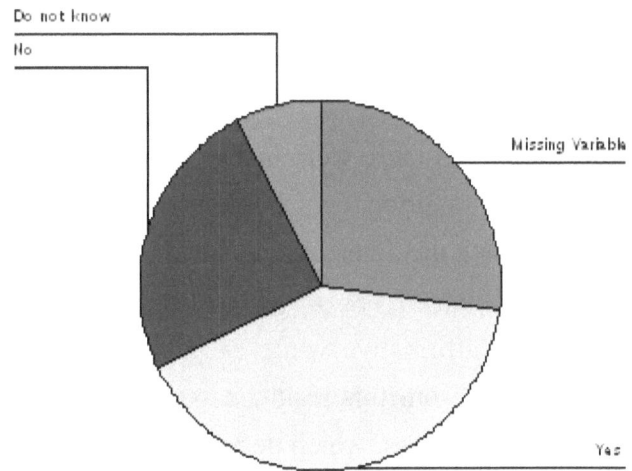

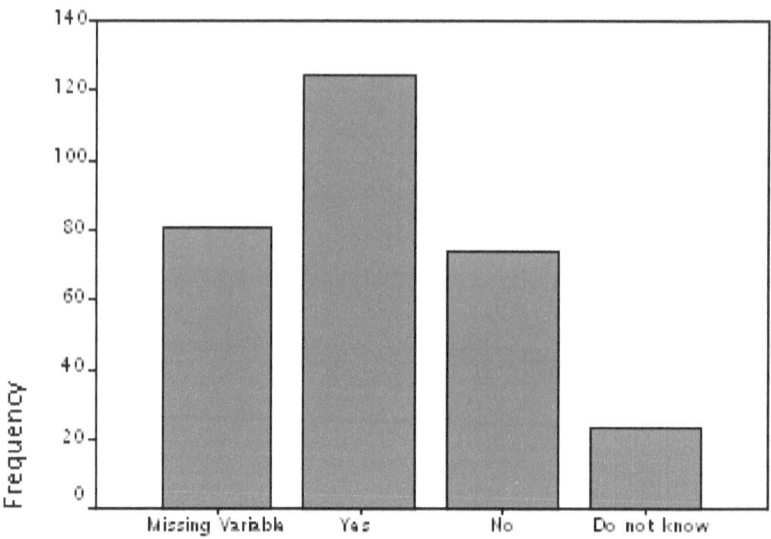

Traditional Supremacy?

This is to find out if there were instances and cases where the practice and use of traditional medicine were supreme or more effective than orthodox medicine. As indicated in the various charts, 124 people representing 41.1% of the total respondents answered this question in the affirmative while 74 people or 24.5% of the respondents said no. From this result, it is evident that there are health conditions or diseases, which defy orthodox medication, but the same cases were cured with traditional medicine.

African Traditional Medicine

FIG. XLVIII NATURE OF SICKNESS THAT LED TO THE USE OF TRADITIONAL MEDICINE

Nature?

		Frequency	Percent	Valid Percent	Cumulative Percent
Valid	Missing Variable	183	60.6	60.6	60.6
	Leprosy	12	4.0	4.0	64.6
	Hypertension	24	7.9	7.9	72.5
	Mystic	19	6.3	6.3	78.8
	Dibetes	21	7.0	7.0	85.8
	Jaundice	10	3.3	3.3	89.1
	Bone-setting	19	6.3	6.3	95.4
	Cancer	5	1.7	1.7	97.0
	Oedma	8	2.6	2.6	99.7
	Osteoporosis	1	.3	.3	100.0
	Total	302	100.0	100.0	

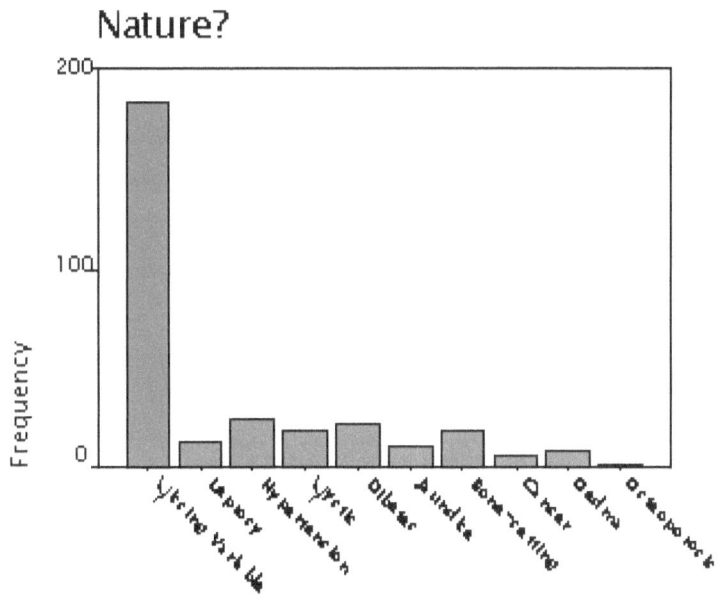

The nature of sickness which made people to seek the assistance of the traditional healers included leprosy, hypertension, mystic problems, diabetes, jaundice, bone-setting, cancer, oedema, and osteoporosis. These are just a few of the numerous health problems.

FIG. XLIX TIME FOR TRADITIONAL MEDICINE

Medical Time?

		Frequency	Percent	Valid Percent	Cumulative Percent
Valid	Missing Variable	105	34.8	34.8	34.8
	Before Dawn	12	4.0	4.0	38.7
	Before Night Fall	8	2.6	2.6	41.4
	Day Time	83	27.5	27.5	68.9
	At Night	16	5.3	5.3	74.2
	Do not know	78	25.8	25.8	100.0
	Total	302	100.0	100.0	

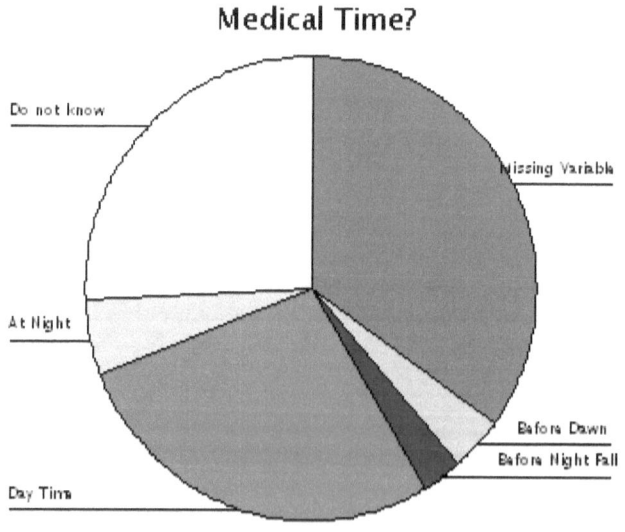

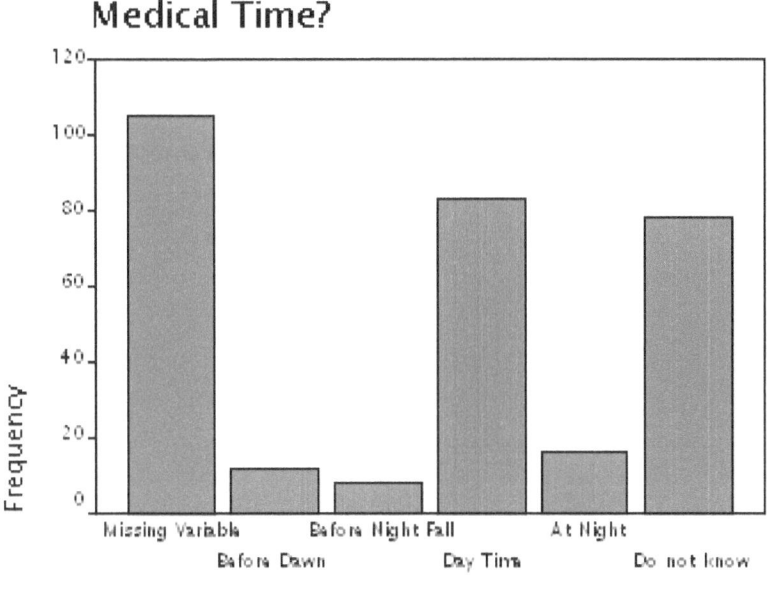

Medical Time?

From the responses to question 27, majority of the respondents indicated that they went for their medical treatment during the day. That was the time usually given by the traditional healer. The time for the medication may also depend on the nature of the treatment to be given. The nature of the sickness usually has a direct bearing on the timing of the treatment. For instance, someone who is infected with severe skin rashes and had to be treated with some drugs that might give the skin another color, will most likely apply that medication at night. This will enable such an individual to wash off the colored medicine early in the morning in order to attend to other duties of the day.

FIG.L REASONS FOR USING TRADITIONAL MEDICINE

Reasons?

		Frequency	Percent	Valid Percent	Cumulative Percent
Valid	Missing Variable	120	39.7	39.7	39.7
	None	21	7.0	7.0	46.7
	Believe	10	3.3	3.3	50.0
	Authentication	22	7.3	7.3	57.3
	Potency	10	3.3	3.3	60.6
	Invitation	17	5.6	5.6	66.2
	Identification	6	2.0	2.0	68.2
	Do not know	96	31.8	31.8	100.0
	Total	302	100.0	100.0	

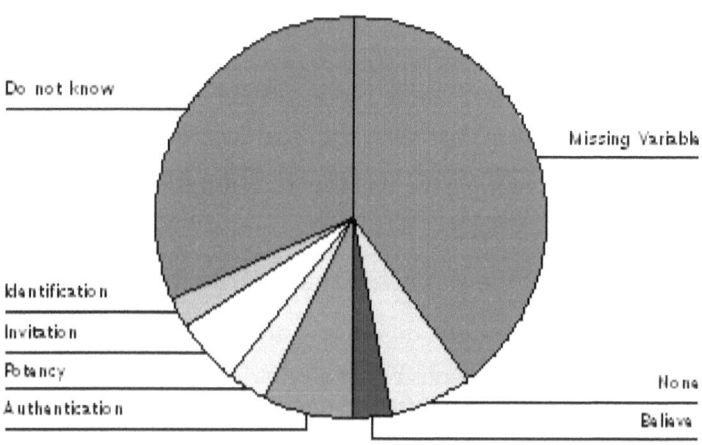

Reasons?

African Traditional Medicine

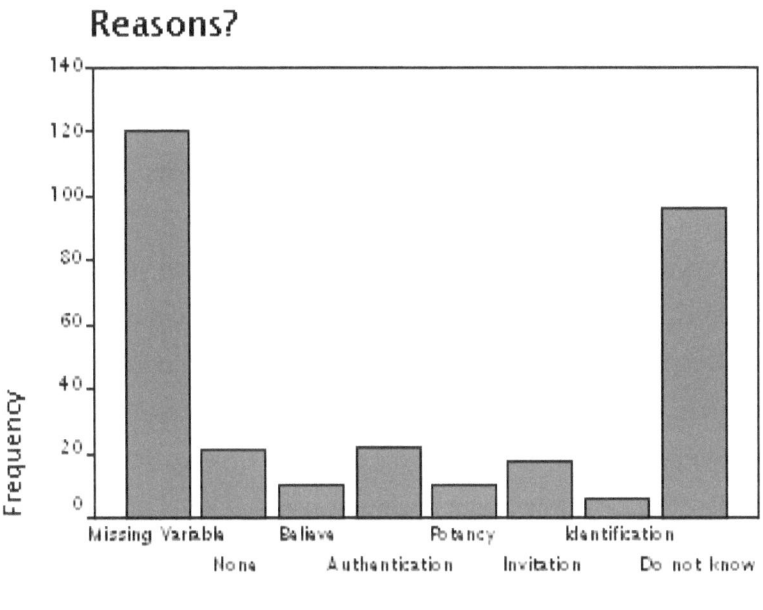

The reasons for going to the traditional healer's place for healing include invitation by the traditional healer, authentication and belief that the medicine will work best at that time, and due to the fact that the drug was potent. Concerning invitation, this was usually at the instance of the traditional healer. He informs the patients when they should come for counseling, treatment and what they should do before and after each visit to him. 10.2% of the respondents do visit the traditional healer at his own invitation. Next to that is the understanding and belief of some other people that traditional medicine works best at a particular time of the day or night. This time is usually the night when the body would be at rest and the drugs will have a conducive environment to function and achieve the desired results. 3.3% of the respondents were of this view. Authentication in this context means a time tried and proved to be the most effective. Those who have a long history of being cured of their diseases with traditional medications speak with certainty and confidence of the best time to apply the traditional medicine to enable them get the best result. 7.3% of the respondents are of this view.

The potency of the traditional medicine when used as and at when specified by the traditional healer always achieves it purpose of healing the sick of their diseases and that is another reason that had made compliance with time acceptable to the sick one. For instance, if a wound is to be treated with the poultice of a particular plant, the potency of that drug is highest when it was freshly administered. On the other hand, some decoctions become more potent as they stay longer and that is why they are usually taken after some stipulated number of days after its preparation. 3.3% of the respondents take their drugs at appointed times due to its high potency level at that period.

FIG. LI ARE MEMBERS AWARE YOU ARE USING TRADITIONAL MEDICINE

Awareness?

		Frequency	Percent	Valid Percent	Cumulative Percent
Valid	Missing Variable	95	31.5	31.5	31.5
	Yes	92	30.5	30.5	61.9
	No	46	15.2	15.2	77.2
	Do not Know	69	22.8	22.8	100.0
	Total	302	100.0	100.0	

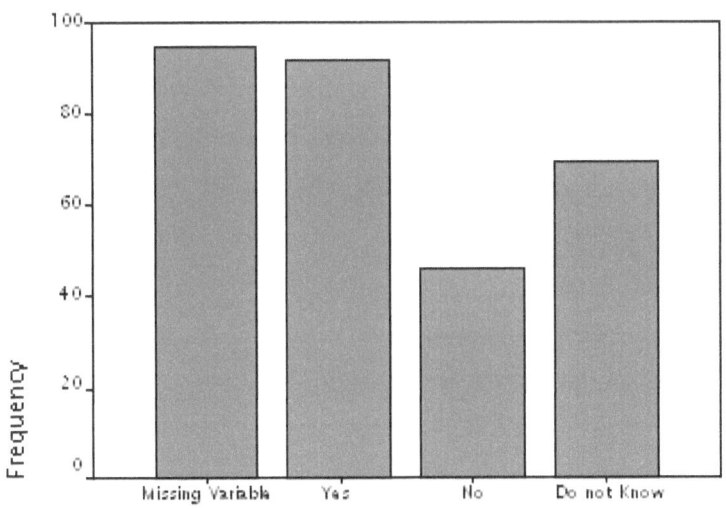

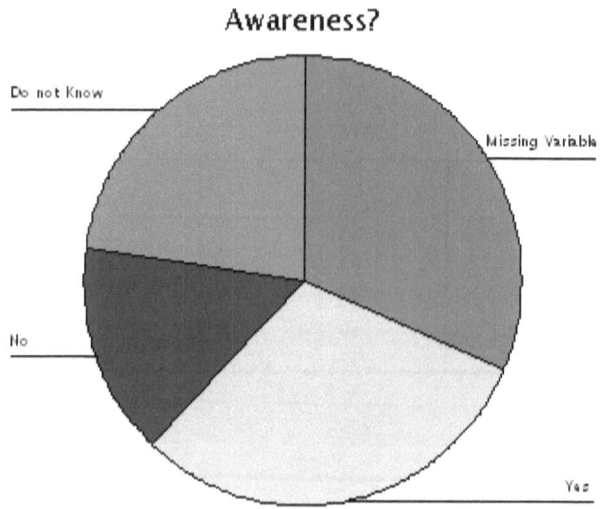

The use of traditional medicine among Seventh-day Adventists in Remoland of Ogun State for both preventive and prophylactic purposes is not done in secrecy. The church members who use traditional medicine are aware that other believers within the church know how and where they get their medications. 92 of the respondents which represent 30.5% of the those who responded answered in the affirmative that other members are aware of their use of traditional medicine. 46 people who represent 15.2% of the total respondents indicated that other members were not aware that they were patronizing the traditional medicine personnel.

FIG. LII ATTITUDE OF THE CHURCH TOWOARDS TRADITIONAL MEDICATION

Church Attitude?

		Frequency	Percent	Valid Percent	Cumulative Percent
Valid	Missing Value	105	34.8	34.8	34.8
	Suprised	27	8.9	8.9	43.7
	Apprehension	28	9.3	9.3	53.0
	Negative Comment	11	3.6	3.6	56.6
	Another	50	16.6	16.6	73.2
	Do not Know	81	26.8	26.8	100.0
	Total	302	100.0	100.0	

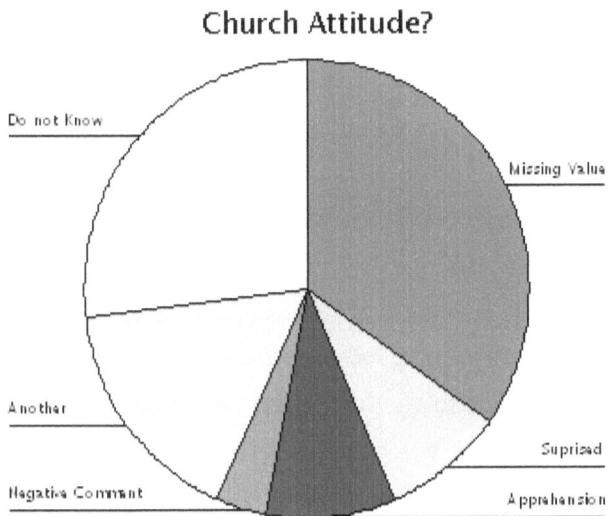

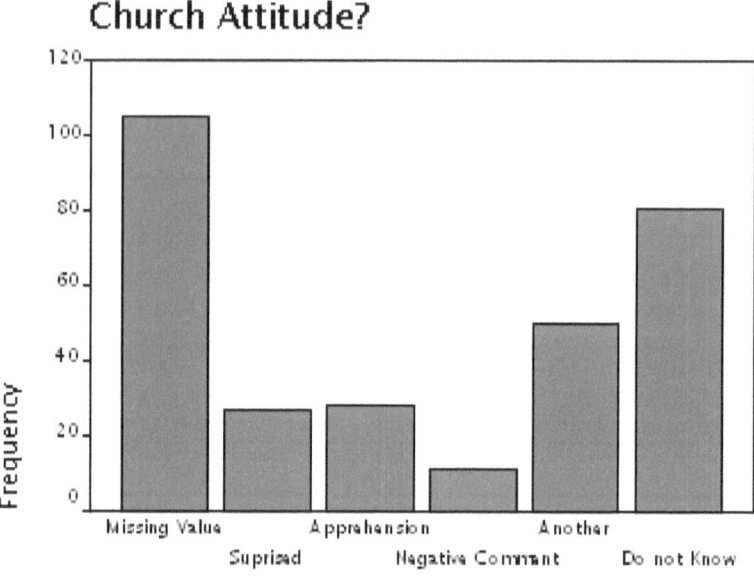

A lot of reactions were expressed by the Seventh-day Adventist Church members and these included being apprehensive, 28 respondent which is also 9.3% of the total respondents displayed this attitude. Others expressed surprises when this knowledge was known to them. Those in this group make up 8.9% of the total respondents. 50 people who represent 16.6% of the total respondents had different attitudes which were expressed in various other ways such as "let him do what he knows is the best for his recovery", "he is old enough let him take of himself." These statements and others like them were used by the members of the Seventh-day Adventist Church to show their attitude and reactions on making this recovery. 3.6% of the total number of those who sent in their questionnaire also made negative comments.

FIG.LIII PASTOR'S ATTITUDE TOWARDS THE USE OF TRADITIONAL MEDICINE

Pastor's Attitude?

		Frequency	Percent	Valid Percent	Cumulative Percent
Valid	Missing Value	104	34.4	34.4	34.4
	Suprised	19	6.3	6.3	40.7
	Apprehension	28	9.3	9.3	50.0
	Negative Comment	12	4.0	4.0	54.0
	Another	42	13.9	13.9	67.9
	Do not Know	97	32.1	32.1	100.0
	Total	302	100.0	100.0	

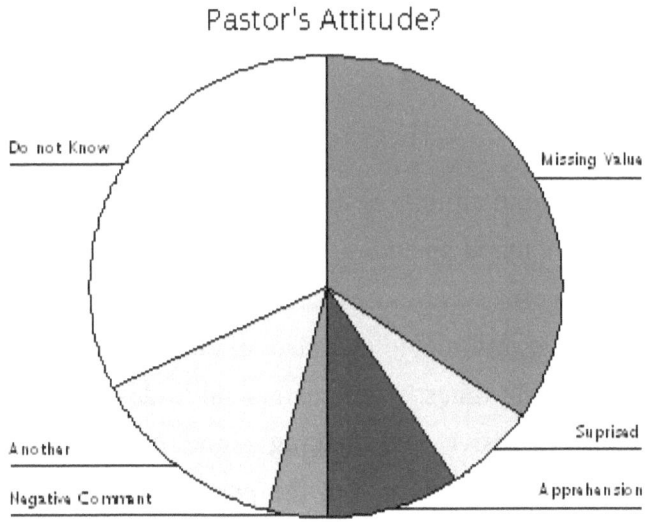

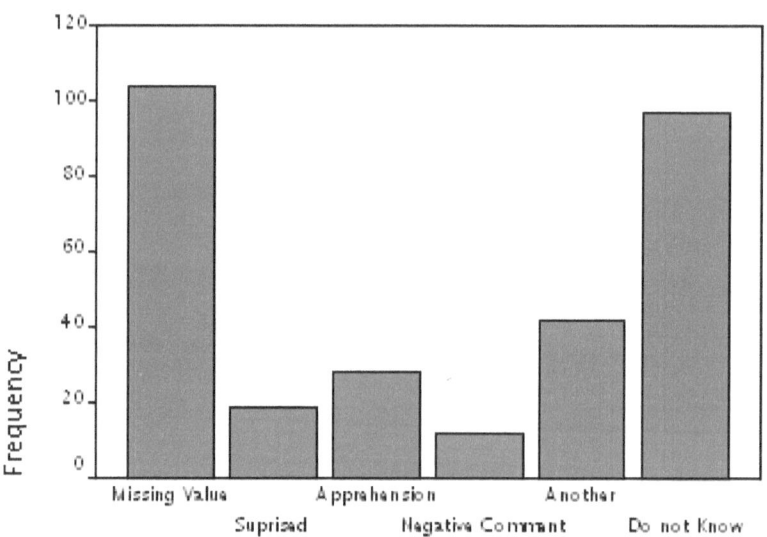

The reaction and attitude of the pastor depended on a number of factors which included his understanding of traditional medicine as a way of healing, his acceptance that traditional medicine is biblical, reliable, effective, affordable and also an effective method to keep one healthy at all times. The pastors' attitudes included being surprised, apprehensive and making some negative comments. These indeed are indications that the pastors need enlightenment and further education on the importance of traditional medicine. On the other hand the 97 which represent 32.1% of the total respondents whose responses were 'do not know' could be a way of keeping silent, or not making their views and attitudes known to any one due to fear or insecurity.

FIG.LIV ANY EDUCATION ON THE IMPORTANCE OF TRADITIONAL MEDICATION?

Importance?

		Frequency	Percent	Valid Percent	Cumulative Percent
Valid	Missing Variable	75	24.8	24.8	24.8
	Yes	63	20.9	20.9	45.7
	No	123	40.7	40.7	86.4
	Do not Know	41	13.6	13.6	100.0
	Total	302	100.0	100.0	

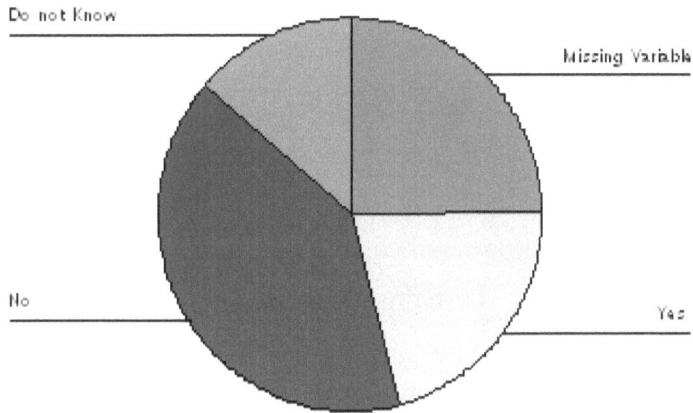

Importance?

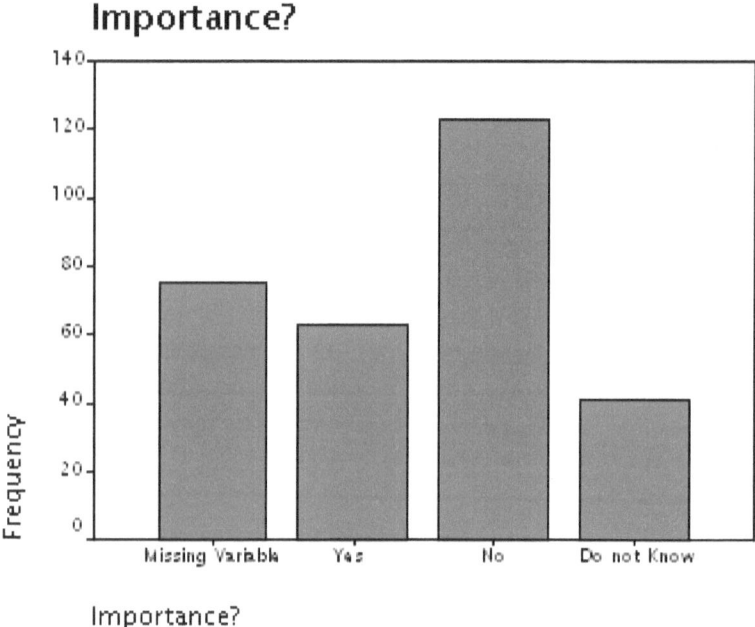

Concerning appropriate education on the importance of traditional medicine, 63 people who represented 20.9% of the total respondents indicated that there has been enlightenment and education on this important subject in the past. On the other hand, 123 of the members who represent 43.4% of the total respondents denied seeing any education being given on this important subject. Another 13.6%, or 41 members claimed that they were not aware if such an education had ever been given to them by the church leadership. The two groups that claimed they do not know and those who answered negatively are clear indicators that the church members need a balanced education on the importance of using traditional medicine to meet the health needs of man. This might also need some specialized training on the part of the church leadership to know what to do and how best to accomplish them.

FIG. LV HAS THE CHURCH DISCIPLINED ANY ONE WHO PRACTICED OR USED TRADITIONAL MEDICINE?

Any Discipline?

		Frequency	Percent	Valid Percent	Cumulative Percent
Valid	Missing Variable	68	22.5	22.5	22.5
	Yes	36	11.9	11.9	34.4
	nO	143	47.4	47.4	81.8
	Do not Know	55	18.2	18.2	100.0
	Total	302	100.0	100.0	

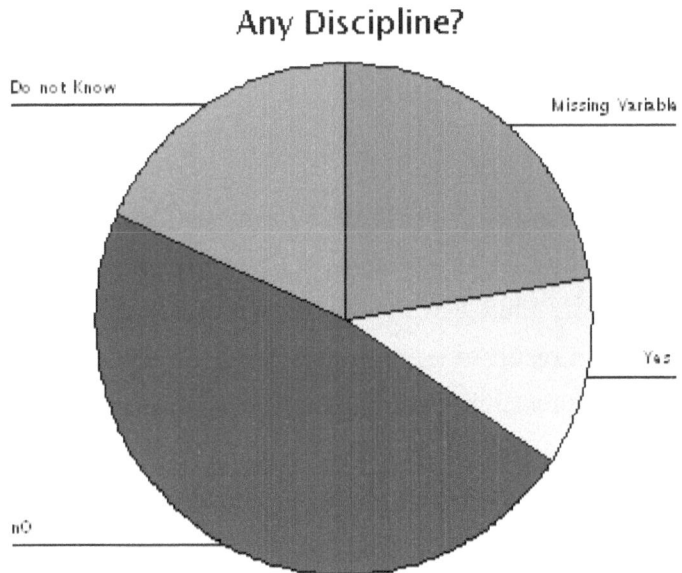

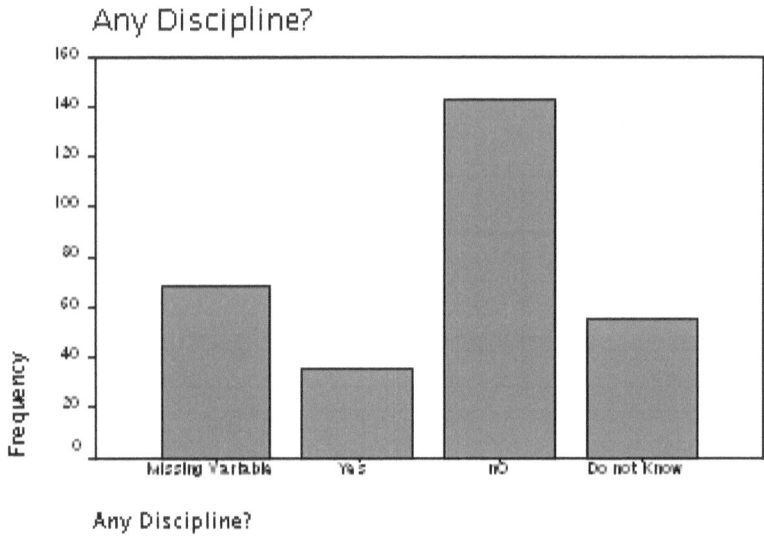

This question is to help us have an objective analysis of the view of the church leadership on the practice and use of this type of alternative way of healing by the members. 36 people who represent 11.9% of the total number of those who responded through the questionnaire indicated that some church members have been disciplined as a result of using traditional medicine. 143 members representing 47.4% of the total respondents indicated that to the best of their knowledge no one had ever been disciplined as a result of practicing or using traditional medicine. Those who do not know of any discipline are 55 representing 18.2% of the total respondents.

FIG. LVI HAS TRADITIONAL MEDICINE MADE ANY OBSERVABLE IMPACT IN YOUR LIFE?

Any Impact?

		Frequency	Percent	Valid Percent	Cumulative Percent
Valid	Missing Variable	67	22.2	22.2	22.2
	Yes	95	31.5	31.5	53.6
	No	92	30.5	30.5	84.1
	Do not Know	48	15.9	15.9	100.0
	Total	302	100.0	100.0	

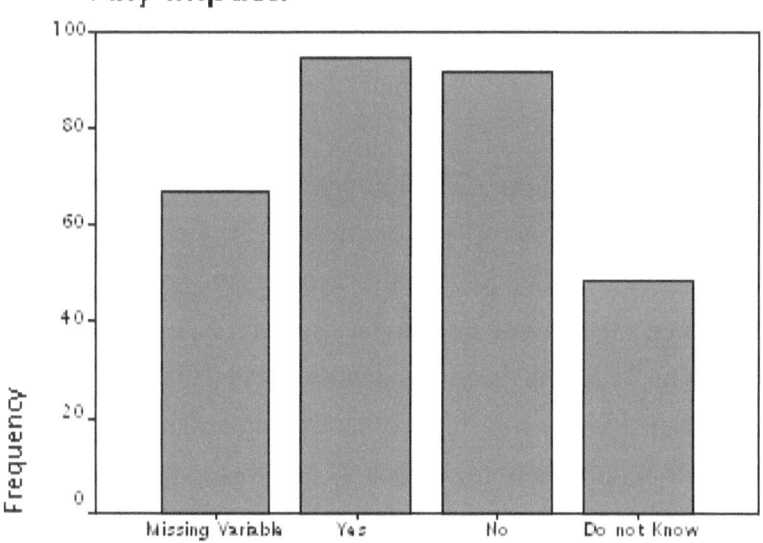

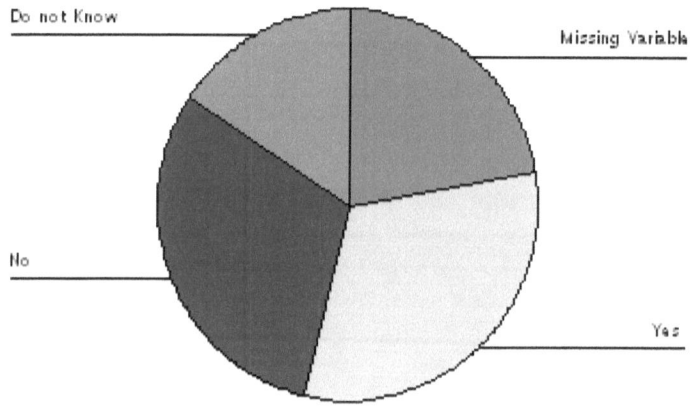

Any Impact?

The practice and use of traditional medicine should have some impacts on the users in one way or the other. If there is no impact at all, it might be an indication that the members are not being involved with this type of alternative medicine. In their response, 95 members representing 31.5 of all the respondents indicated that their lives have been impacted in one way or the other by using traditional medicine. Those who reported no impact are 92 and this represents 30.5% of the total respondents. 48 members representing 15.9% of the total respondents indicated that they do not know.

FIG LVII HAS TRADITIOANL MEDICINE MADE ANY IMPACT IN YOUR LIFE?

Impact In Life?

		Frequency	Percent	Valid Percent	Cumulative Percent
Valid	Missing Variable	112	37.1	37.1	37.1
	Recovery	82	27.2	27.2	64.2
	No side effects	15	5.0	5.0	69.2
	Recommendation	2	.7	.7	69.9
	Do not know	88	29.1	29.1	99.0
	Economic	3	1.0	1.0	100.0
	Total	302	100.0	100.0	

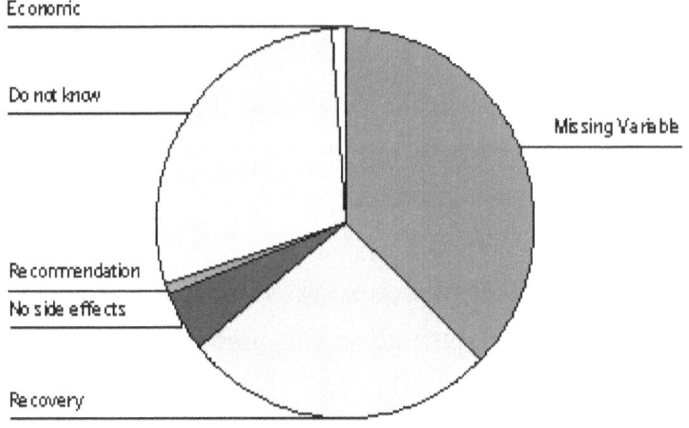

Impact In Life?

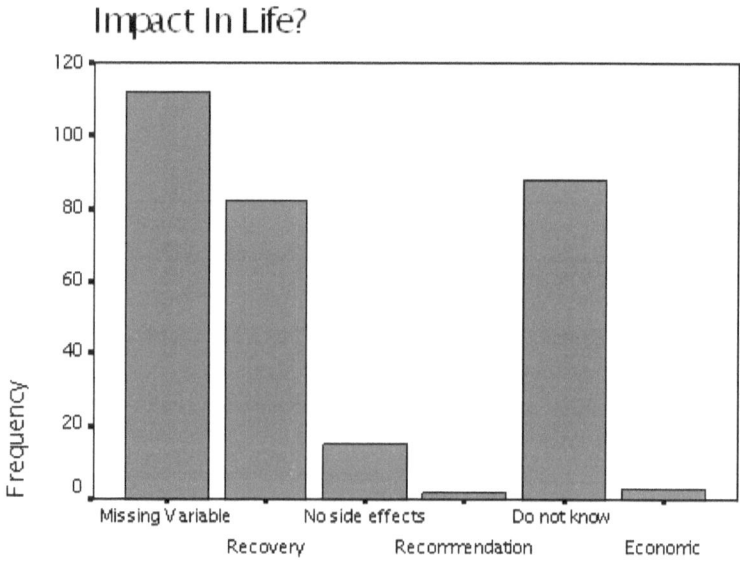

Impact In Life?

The purpose of this further question on impact is to know the specific ways and areas in which traditional medicine has impacted the lives of the Seventh-day Adventists in Remoland of Ogun State. Some of the areas that were pointed out included recovery from sickness, no side effects experienced after using traditional medicine and the economic factor indicating that it was affordable. Specifically, 82 members representing 27.2% of the total respondents indicated that traditional medicine was used to cure one disease or the other which ultimately led to their recovery from their sickness. Those who had no side effects after using traditional medicine were 15 and this represents 5.% of the total respondents. Those whose impacts were observed through the economic factor were 3 and that represented 1.0% of the total respondents.

FIG LVIII HAS TRADITIONAL MEDICINE MADE ANY IMPACT ON THE FAMILY?

Impact on Family?

		Frequency	Percent	Valid Percent	Cumulative Percent
Valid	Missing Variable	118	39.1	39.1	39.1
	Healing	48	15.9	15.9	55.0
	Economic	10	3.3	3.3	58.3
	Prevention	11	3.6	3.6	61.9
	None	115	38.1	38.1	100.0
	Total	302	100.0	100.0	

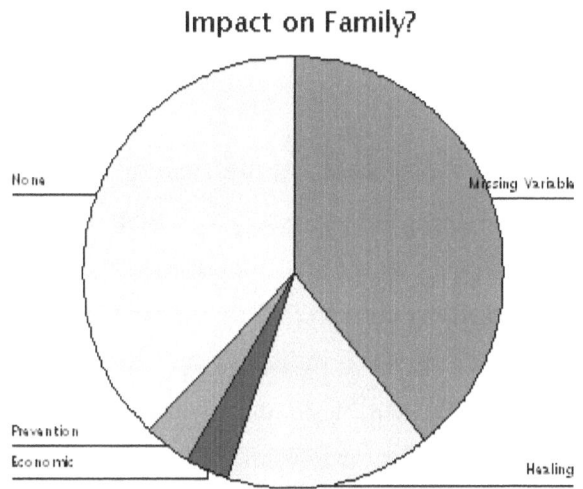

Impact on Family?

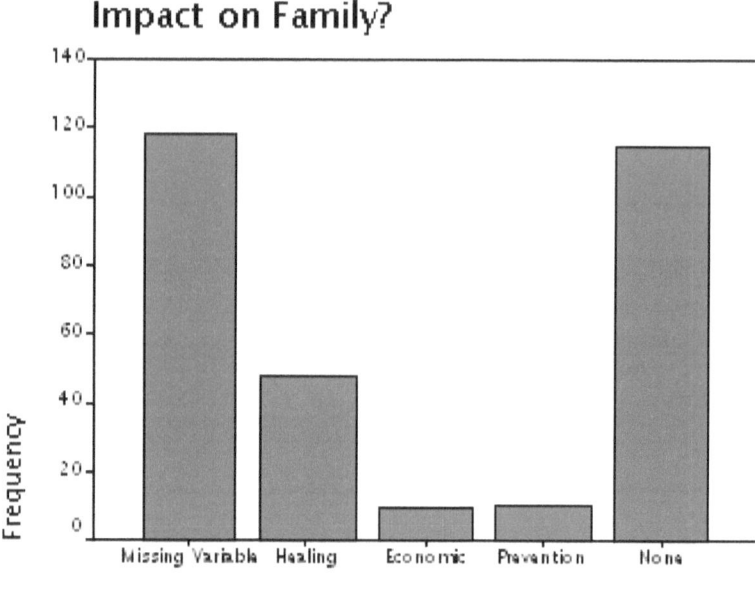

This question is to further elicit information to buttress the fact that some members of the Seventh-day Adventist Church are actually using traditional medicine and that this use is positively impacting them and their family members. 48 members representing 15.9% of the total respondents have indicated that the use of traditional medicine has brought healing to their various families. Another group of 11 members which represents exactly 3.6% of those who responded to the questionnaire pointed out that traditional medicine was used to protect their families and also prevent them from the attack of many diseases. The third group indicated that the use of traditional medicine had economic impacts on their families. A total of 115 members which represents 38.1% of the total respondents seem to be neutral on the impacts of the use of traditional medicine had made on their families. Since many had equated the use of traditional medicine with idolatry, it is not surprising that some members would deny its positive impacts on their families. The solution is to give a balanced education to the members of the church by emphasizing that using what God had created for the benefit of man is neither a denial of faith nor an idolatrous practice.

FIG LVIX HAS TRADITIONAL MEDICINE MADE ANY IMPACT ON THE CHURCH

Impact on Church?

		Frequency	Percent	Valid Percent	Cumulative Percent
Valid	Missing Variable	125	41.4	41.4	41.4
	1.00	1	.3	.3	41.7
	None	9	3.0	3.0	44.7
	Backsliding	15	5.0	5.0	49.7
	Reorientation	8	2.6	2.6	52.3
	Awareness	6	2.0	2.0	54.3
	Healing	24	7.9	7.9	62.3
	Do not Know	114	37.7	37.7	100.0
	Total	302	100.0	100.0	

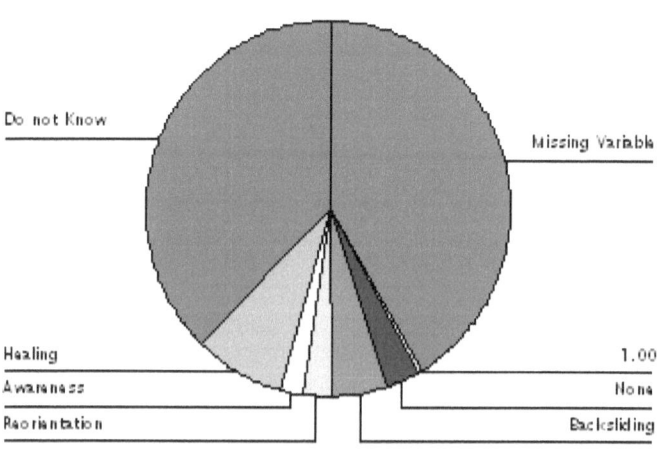

Impact on Church?

African Traditional Medicine

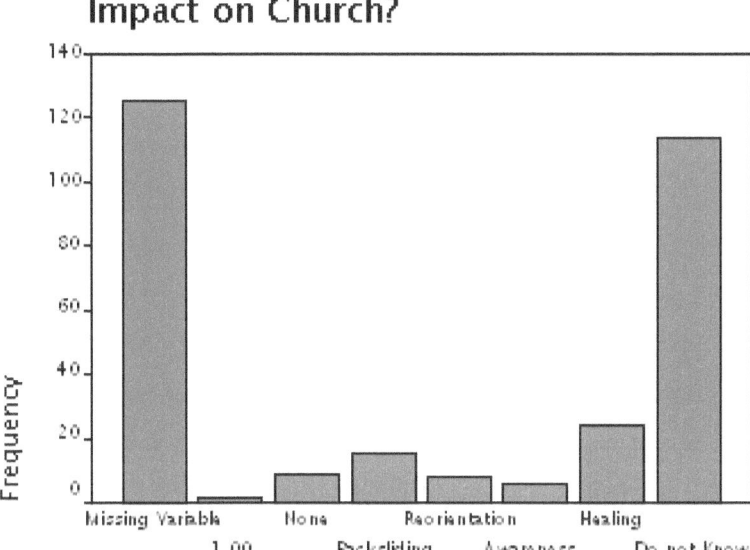

Impact on Church?

The use and practice of traditional medicine have both negative and positive impacts on the members of the Seventh-day Adventist Church in Remoland. Among the positive impacts are the healings that members receive by using traditional medicine. 24 members representing 7.9% noted this as a positive impact on their families. The use of these alternative methods of healing was seen as a way of creating awareness that something better than the orthodox form of medication is available. 6 people representing 2.0% of all the respondents indicated this as an important impact in their church. Another 2.0% of the people indicated that the use of traditional medicine has created for them a new awareness on the efficacy and effectiveness of this means of healing. For 8 of those who responded, the impact was in the form of reorientation into what they never knew before. Their earlier views of traditional medicine that was negative had now been changed. They now see the use of traditional medicine in a new dimension.

All the members who responded did not give the impression that there were no negative impacts, which the use of traditional medicine had on the church members. The use of traditional medicine by the Seventh-day Adventists in Remoland of Ogun State also had some negative impacts as it led to the backsliding of 15 members, which represents 5% of the total respondents. This negative impact could also be traced to the fact that some people cannot differentiate between the explicable from the inexplicable forms of traditional medicine. The solution for this problem of misunderstanding lies in educating the members of the church.

FIG LX WHAT IS THE EXTENT OF USING TRADITIONAL MEDCINE?

Extent of Traditional Usage?

		Frequency	Percent	Valid Percent	Cumulative Percent
Valid	Missing Variable	110	36.4	36.4	36.4
	Until Healed	11	3.6	3.6	40.1
	Use Prayerfully	6	2.0	2.0	42.1
	Work in Groups	2	.7	.7	42.7
	Do not Know	173	57.3	57.3	100.0
	Total	302	100.0	100.0	

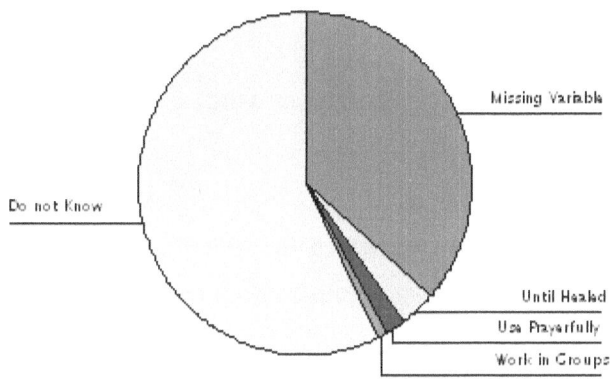

Extent of Traditional Usage?

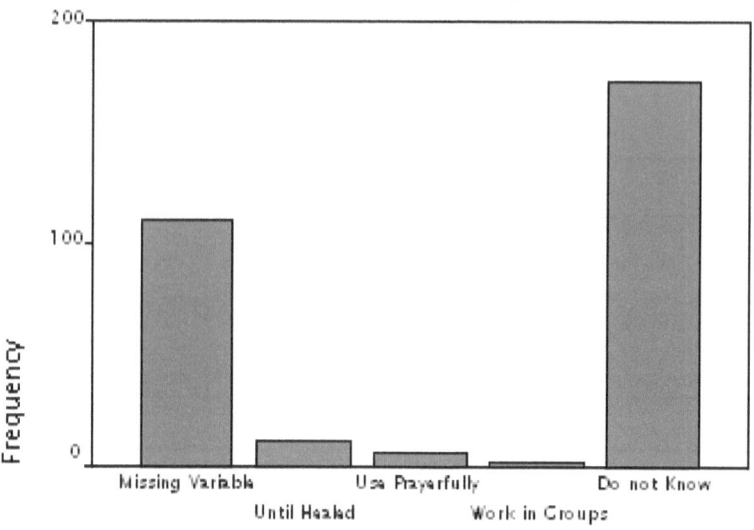

Extent of Traditional Usage?

Some of the responses, which were given by the members, indicate their willingness to use traditional medicine until they were healed, 3.6% of those interviewed were of this view while in order to be on a safer ground others would like to work in groups. 5 members or 2.0% of those who responded to the questionnaire would like to use traditional medicine prayerfully. Still, 173 members representing 57.3% of the total respondents did not know to what extent they could go in their use and practice of traditional medicine.

FIG LXI DO YOU SEE ANY DANGERS IN THE USE OF TRADITIONAL MEDICINE?

Any Dangers?

		Frequency	Percent	Valid Percent	Cumulative Percent
Valid	Missing Variables	88	29.1	29.1	29.1
	Yes	41	13.6	13.6	42.7
	No	17	5.6	5.6	48.3
	Do not Know	156	51.7	51.7	100.0
	Total	302	100.0	100.0	

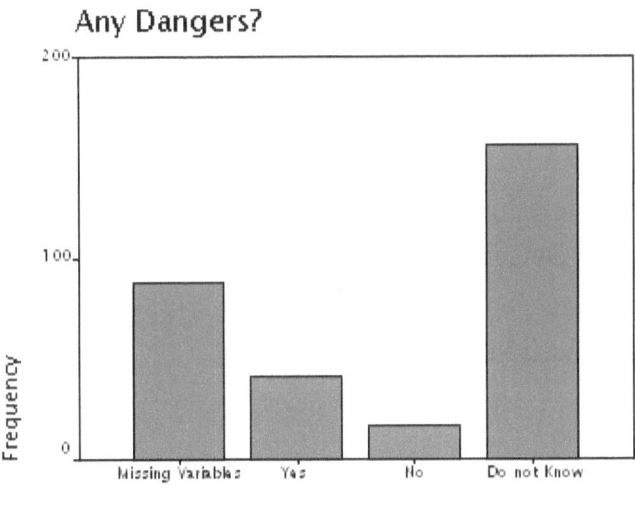

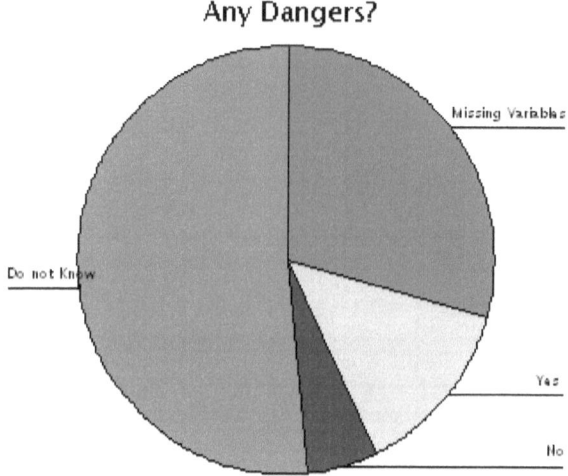

Any Dangers?

Some members are of the view that the use of traditional medicine is laden with a lot of dangers for the church members. 41 of the members were of the view that the use of traditional medicine had some evil or dangers associated with it. Only one respondent said no evil or dangers are associated with it. 156 people that represent 51.7% responded that they do not know.

FIG LXII LIST DANGERS ASSOCIATED WITH TRADITIONAL MEDICINE

List Dangers?

		Frequency	Percent	Valid Percent	Cumulative Percent
Valid	Missing Variable	101	33.4	33.4	33.4
	Idolatry	16	5.3	5.3	38.7
	Witch haunting	4	1.3	1.3	40.1
	No Dosage	9	3.0	3.0	43.0
	Unhygienic	16	5.3	5.3	48.3
	No Date	1	.3	.3	48.7
	Do not Know	155	51.3	51.3	100.0
	Total	302	100.0	100.0	

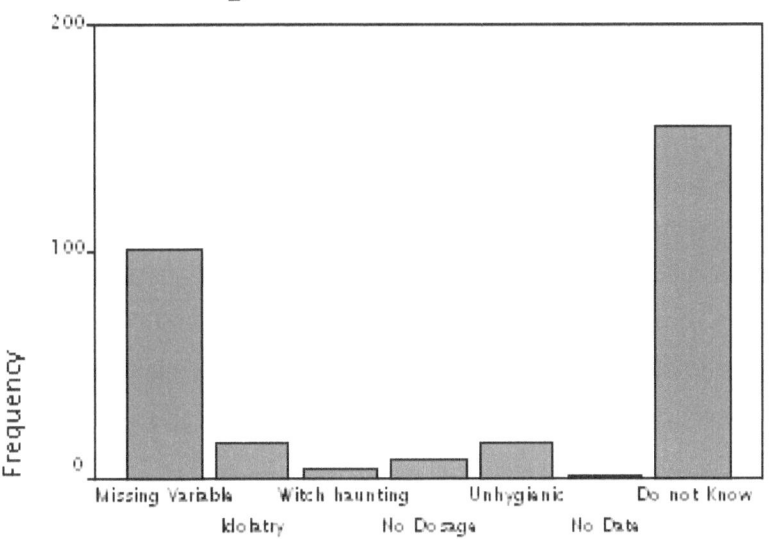

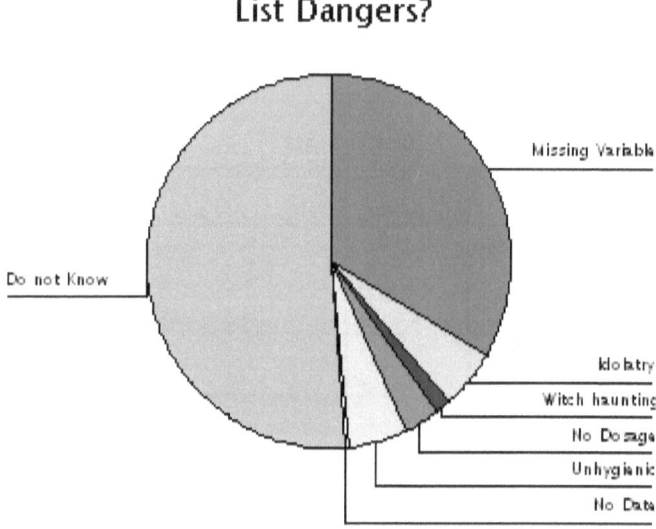

Some of the dangers which could be associated with the use and practice of traditional medicine as seen by the members of the church are that it could lead to idolatry; some are prepared in unhygienic conditions which could become avenues for the transmission of other diseases. Next is that most of the preparations do not contain both the date of manufacture and the date of the expiry. Another danger indicated by the members is on the absence of dosage specifications clearly provided for the various preparations. A majority of those who responded equally chose to be neutral by responding that they do not know.

FIG LXIII WHY SOME SDA CHURCH MEMBERS ABHOR TRADITIONAL MEDICINE?

Reasons for Abhorrence?

		Frequency	Percent	Valid Percent	Cumulative Percent
Valid	Missing Variable	102	33.8	33.8	33.8
	Unbiblical	13	4.3	4.3	38.1
	Ignorance	2	.7	.7	38.7
	Idolatry	11	3.6	3.6	42.4
	Do not Know	174	57.6	57.6	100.0
	Total	302	100.0	100.0	

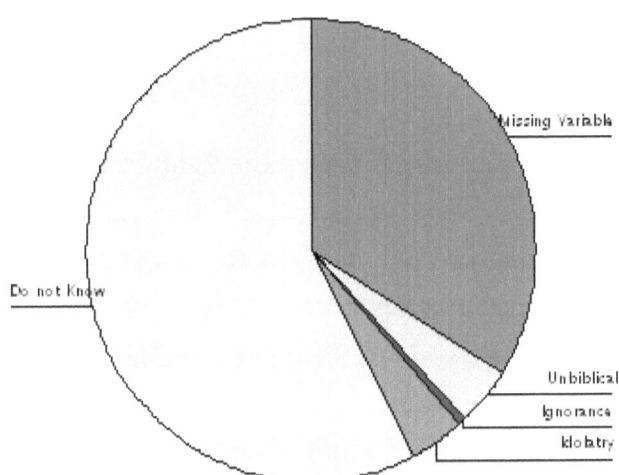

Reasons for Abhorrence?

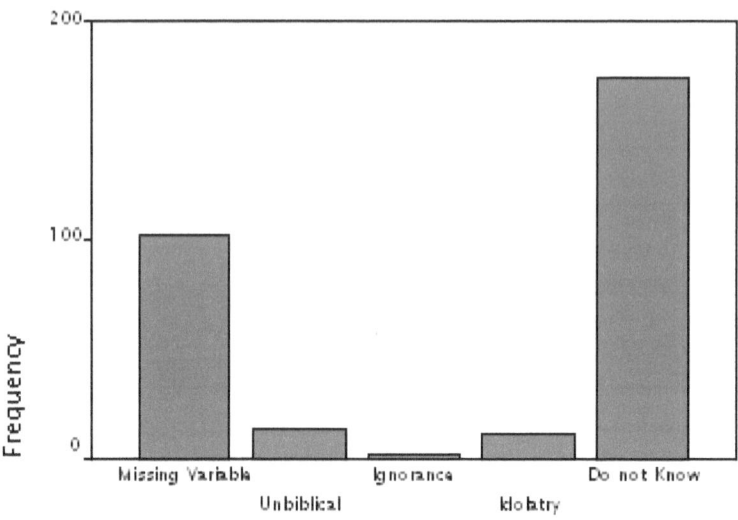

This last question was to shed more light on why Seventh-day Adventists abhor the use and practice of traditional medicine among them. It is amazing that a majority of those who responded to the questionnaire did not even know why they abhor the use of traditional medicine among them. 174 of them representing 57.6% of the total respondents are in this category. If members do not have any reasons for abhorring the use of traditional medicine, then enlightening and disabusing their minds of preconceived ideas about traditional medicine will greatly help them to appreciate the importance and usefulness of this alternative method of health and healing. Eleven members abhor the use of traditional medicine due to the fact that it might lead them to idolatry while two did so out of ignorance. Those who abhorred it because it is deemed unbiblical are 13.

6.6 THE PRACTICE AND USE OF AFRICAN TRADITIONAL MEDICINE AMONG SEVENTH-DAY ADVENTISTS IN REMOLAND OF OGUN STATE AND SOME STUDY VARIABLES.

Cross tabulation of the number of women who used African traditional medicine as well as the length of time it was used compared with the men who used and practiced it among Seventh-day Adventists in Remoland of Ogun State.

	Use Length					
	1-12 months	1-10 years	11-20 years	21 years and above	Do not know	Total
Gender? Male	40	23	13	39	38	153
Female	18	4	5	10	32	69
Total	58	27	18	49	70	222

A total of 153 men were involved in using this alternative means of treatment as compared with 69 women. A critical analysis of this reveals that 25.5% of men have used African traditional medicine for various purposes for 21 years and above while only 14.5% of women have done so within period of time. In the same manner, 8.5% of the male have used African traditional medicine from 11-20 years as compared with only 7.23% of the female counterpart. The same trend is equally observed among those who have used it between 1-10 years. The men in this category were 15% while the women were 5.8% of the total number of male and female respondents respectively. Even those who have used this form of medication between one and 12 months the males were 26.1 % and the females 26.1%. Within all the age groups, the male counterpart seems to have used African traditional medications more than the females except those who have used it between one and twelve months. During the fieldwork it was discovered that most male traditional healers who were interviewed were handling both male and female health issues. For instance, the male healers were also handling pregnancy matters, pre-natal as well as post-natal medical issues. On the other hand, almost all the female traditional healers were primarily traditional birth attendants.

Cross tabulations of Seventh-day Adventists in Remoland of Ogun State who are from different tribes/ethnic groups that used African traditional medicine compared with the length of time it was used.

	Use Length?					Total
	1-12 months	1-10 years	11-20 years	21 years and above	Do not know	
Tribe/Ethnic Group						
Igbo	18	16	2	6	52	94
Yoruba	25	4	13	29	14	85
Hausa	3	1	1		1	6
Edo/Delta	1	2		1	1	5
Middle Belt	1		1			1
Others	6	2	17	9	68	18
Total	54	25		45		209

A look at the figures above reveal that 85, 94 and 6 people responded from the Yoruba, Igbo and Hausa tribes respectively. Seventh-day Adventists who have used African traditional medication between 1-12 months were 29.4%, 19.1% and 50% among the Yoruba, Igbo and Hausa tribes respectively. Still in the same order those who have used as well as practiced African medicine from 11-20 years were 15.3%, 2.1% and 16.6% respectively. Those who have used this alternative method of health and healing for 21 years and above among the Yoruba and Igbo tribes as outlined above are 34.1% and 6.4% respectively. From the above information, it is evident that neither the tribe nor ethnic group which one belongs is a hindrance to the use and practice of African traditional medicine especially among Seventh-day Adventists in Remoland of Ogun State. Seventh-day Adventists in Remoland irrespective of their place of origin recognize and utilize African medicine for their health and healing. By putting all the tribes and ethnic groups together it is revealed that 25.8% and 22% have used traditional medicine from 1-12 months and above 21 years respectively.

Cross Tabulation Of The Length Of Time Members Have Been Seventh-day Adventists Compared With The Length Of Time They Had Used African Traditional Medication.

	Use Length?					Total
	1-12 months	1-10 years	11-20 years	21 years and above	Do not know	
SDA Period						
0-12 months	7	5	4	7	8	31
1-10 years	18	6	2	4	12	42
11-20 years	9	7	4	6	18	44
Above 20 years	26	11	8	25	32	102
Total	60	29	18	42	70	219

It was also discovered that those who have been members of the Seventh-day Adventist Church for over 21 years also used this alternative form of healing more than others. Out of the 42 members who have used African traditional medicine for 21 years and above 60% of them have been Seventh-day Adventists for over 20 years. In the same way, those who have used African traditional medication between one and twelve months are 60. Out of this, 43.3% have been members of the Seventh-day Adventist Church for over 20 years. One can equally conclude that the longer members stay in the SDA Church, the more they use this alternative form of medication for health and healing purposes. This is also as a result of the Seventh-day Adventist Church's orthodoxy and orthopraxy, which are Bible based as expressed in the AH-NEWSTART principle. Indeed, the longer people stayed in the Seventh-day Adventist Church, the more they learn and practice these natural health principles espoused by the Adventist Church.

Cross Tabulation On Comparing The Former Religious Affiliation Of Seventh-Day Adventist With Their Frequency And Length Of Using Traditional Medication After They Had Become Members Of The SDA Church.

Use Length?	Frequency of Use?						
	Daily	Weekly	Monthly	As needed	Do not know	7.00	Total
Missing Variable							
Religious Affiliation							
Christian				2			2
Muslim							
Another Religion				1			1
Total				3			3
1-12 months							
Religious Affiliation							
Christian	3	6		39	4		54
African Traditional Religion				3			3
Total	3	6		44	4		57
1-10 years							
Religious Affiliation							
Christian				1	24		25
African Traditional Religion					3		3
Total				1	27		28
11-20 years							
Religious Affiliation							
Christian				14			14
Muslim				1			1
African Traditional Religion	2						2
Total	2			15			17

21 years and above							
Religious Affiliation							
Christian	2	1		36	1	1	41
Muslim				2			2
African Traditional Religion				1			1
Another Religion				2			2
Do not Know					1		1
Total	2	1		41	2	1	47
Do not Know							
Religious Affiliation							
Christian	2			3	54		59
Muslim					2		2
African Traditional Religion				1	2		3
Another Religion					1		1
Do not Know					3		3
Total	2			4	62		68

One factor which was common among Seventh-day Adventists who were former members of other religious groups was their consistent use of African traditional medications after they had become SDA Church members. It was discovered that they consistently continued to use this alternative form of medication for health and healing purposes as the needs arose. This also meant that their becoming Seventh-day Adventists did not nullify their uses of these traditional medications; it was rather enhanced through their interaction with other church members. This is an indication too that the Seventh-day Adventist Church in Remoland both in principle and practice uses African traditional medicine.

Cross Tabulation Of The Attitude Of Church Members Toward The Users Of African Medication Compared With The Attitude Of The Pastor.

	Pastor's Attitude?					
	Surprised	Apprehension	Negative Comment	Another	Do not know	Total
Church Attitude						
Surprised	12	3	4	2	5	26
Apprehension	1	19	4	2	2	28
Negative Comment	4	4	2		1	11
Another		2	1	38	8	49
Do not Know	1		1		79	80
Total	18	28	12	42	95	194

It was quite a revelation that the attitude of both the pastor and members of the SDA Church was that of surprise, apprehension and some even made some negative comments. This is an indication that a lot of enlightenment needs to be made in the form of creating more awareness on the importance of African traditional medicine.

Cross Tabulations Of The Various Ways Seventh-day Adventists Support The Use Of Traditional Medication.

	Ways of SDA Support?					
	Natural	Leaves/ herbs	Feeding Habits	Economic	Do not Know	Total
SDA Support						
Yes	39	3	17	13		91
No	2	19		15	1	20
Do not Know	1	4	2	14	2	21
Total	42	26	19	42	3	132

It was discovered that Seventh-day Adventists support the use of traditional medication by applying natural remedies, using leaves and herbs, and through their eating habits. That fact that traditional medication is cheap also motivates them to its usage. A total of 91 respondents which represent 69% of the total number who responded to the questionnaire demonstrated that they use traditional medicine in the above mentioned ways for their healing and well-being. Concerning the eating habits, most people in this group are vegetarians. The members are either lacto-ovarian vegetarians or complete vegans. Out of the 91 respondents who apply various forms of traditional medication, 39% use it in the form of natural remedies; 24.2% use it in the form of leaves and herbs; 18.7% use it through their eating habits while 14.3% use it due to its economic advantage.

African Traditional Medicine

Impact on Family	Religious Affiliation?					
	Christian	Muslim	African Traditional Religion	Another Religion	Do not know	Total
Missing Variable						
Impact In Life						
Recovery		11				11
Total		11				
Healing						
Impact In Life						
Recovery	32	1				33
No side effects	4	2				6
Recommendation	1					1
Do not Know	3					3
Total	40	3				43
Economic						
Impact In Life						
Recovery	3	2				5
No side effects	2					2
Do not Know	1					1
Economic	2					2
Total	8	2				10
Prevention						
Impact In Life						
Recovery	8		1			9
No side effects	2					2
Total	10		1			11
None						
Impact In Life						
Recovery	17		2		1	20
No side effects	5					5
Recommendation	1					1
Do not Know	76		2	1	3	82
Economic	1					1
Total	100		4	1	4	109

Cross tabulations of the former religious affiliations compared with impacts in life and family

As indicated above, the former religious affiliation of Seventh-day Adventists did not prevent them from enjoying the benefits of traditional medication. Their use of traditional medication actually had impact on their lives and families. The use of this alternative form of medication led to the health and recovery of Muslims, adherents of African Traditional Religion as well as Christians from others faiths.

6.7: REPORT OF PERSONAL INTERVIEWS

In the course of this research, one hundred people were interviewed on their practice and use of Africa Traditional Medicine. This was done on a ratio of 50 percent Seventh-day Adventists and 50 percent non-Seventh-day Adventists. The Seventh-day Adventists in this group were ten selected Pastors, fifteen men leaders, fifteen women leaders, and ten medical personnel. The other who were not Seventh-day Adventists included fifteen traditional birth attendants, two bone setters, and thirty three herbal and other traditional medical practitioners.

The report of personal interviews has been broken down into four different sub-sections which include the responses of Seventh-day Adventist pastors; responses of Seventh-day Adventist men and women leaders; responses of Seventh-day Adventists medical personnel and responses of non-Seventh-day Adventists are presented and discussed below:

6.7.1: **RESPONDENTS' UNDERSTANDING OF AFRICAN TRADITIONAL MEDICINE**

RESPONSES BY SEVENTH-DAY ADVENTIST PASTORS:

One of the Pastors understands African Traditional Medicine as using natural things around us for health and healing. Another minister revealed that for the past ten years, he has never taken any tablet or injection for any reason. For him traditional medicine is what "we are born with, grow with, and cured with from our immediate environment." Other ministers see it as "unrefined medicine to the orthodox medication."

RESPONSES BY SEVENTH-DAY ADVENTIST MEN AND WOMEN LEADERS:

The current women's ministries leader and a retired educationist understood African traditional medicine as "the medicine derived from trees and herbs." But to another member, it means "the use of medicinal herbs for health and healing." A youth leader at the Babcock University District understands African traditional medicine to be "native medicine used for curing diseases." For another, it means "the use of herbs to cure ailments." Others understand it to be the "way of healing which has been handed to us from our forefathers".

RESPONSES BY SEVENTH-DAY ADVENTISTS MEDICAL PERSONNEL:

A medical practitioner at the Babcock University Medical Centre understands African traditional medicine to be "the use of natural remedies." A former Medical Director, understands it as "natural food therapy." A midwife for the past twenty years, sees African traditional medicine as, "using herbs for the treatment of some diseases." Still on various understanding of African traditional medicine by Seventh-day Adventist medical personnel, a male nurse understands the subject under consideration as "the use of herbs in the treatment of diseases which may sometimes include spiritual invocation in the form of incantation." Others understand it as "another way of treating diseases," and "the use of plant for medicine."

RESPONSES FROM NON-SEVENTH-DAY ADVENTISTS:

A medical practitioner on private practice understands African traditional medicine as "natural remedies used to cure sickness and to keep healthy," but to another it is "using various plant products, sacrifices and incantations to achieve physical well being." It is "local herbs mixed very well for the care of pregnant women and new born babies" says a traditional birth attendant at Ilishan-Remo. Another traditional birth attendant at Sagamu understands it as the use of natural materials plus sacrifices to bring health and happiness to humanity."

Others understand African traditional medicine as "using natural drugs/herbs and "Ifá" consultation to achieve health and healing." (Among the adherents of African Traditional Religion in the Western part of Nigeria, it is believed that Ifá is what God sent before the advent of Christianity, Islam and other imported religions. Ifá refers to the system of divination and the verses of the literary corpus known as the Odú Ifá. Orunmila had been identified as the Grand Priest of this religious organization[504]). One traditional healer on the other hand understands African traditional medicine as "using mystic power and natural materials both for healing and success in life's business." He explained further that herbal medications are used for medicinal purposes while oracles are consulted when the needs arise. He was also quick to point out that magical powers are not used for healing but to help those who are cheated to reclaim what rightly belongs to them. It is also used for good luck, safe journeys, business prosperity as well as protection against ones enemies. This corroborated with the information of other older traditional healers who maintained that their services which involve consultation with the ifa are to bring good luck to people and freedom to those who are oppressed.

6.7.2: **RESPONSES ON MATERIALS USED IN TRADITIONAL MEDICAL PRACTICE**

The responses given by the Seventh-day Adventist Pastors, male and female leaders and the medical personnel revealed that the following material are used for African traditional medicine: leaves of appropriate trees, herbs, roots, clay, charcoal, water, honey,

---

[504] http://en.wikipedia.org/wiki/If%C3%A1

rhizomes, trunk of trees, seeds, stone, fire and calabash. However one, a Seventh-day Adventist male nurse added "blood" to be one of the materials used in this form of medical practice. Responses from non-Seventh-day Adventists included all the above mentioned materials plus olive oil, bones, black soap, pepper, saps of plants and powder.

6.7.3: **WHO INTRODUCED YOU TO AFRICAN TRADITIONAL MEDICINE?**

The response from the other three groups of Seventh-day Adventists show that they were introduced to this medicine by their fathers, mothers, grandfather, grandmother, father-in-law, mother-in-law, friends, and through personal discovery. A lady said that God introduced her to it. One medical doctor indicated that he learnt about it from the media and by reading medical books. A gospel minister revealed that he knew of this form of medication through the writings of Ellen G. White. Another Pastor said God introduced him to it through Ezekiel 47: 12 and Revelation 22: 2 which say:

> And by the river upon the bank thereof, on this side and on that side, shall grow all trees for meat, whose leaf shall not fade, neither shall the fruit thereof be consumed: it shall bring forth new fruit according to his months, because their waters they issued out of the sanctuary: and the fruit thereof shall be for meat, and the leaf thereof for medicine. In the midst of the street of it, and on either side of the river, [was there] the tree of life, which bare

twelve [manner of] fruits, [and] yielded her fruit every month: and the leaves of the tree [were] for the healing of the nations.

The responses from non-Seventh-day Adventists are similar since they learnt it from fathers, mothers, aunt, uncle or grandparents. It is interesting to note that they were introduced to traditional medicine by inheritance. Some traditional healers specifically said "they inherited African traditional medical practice" from their fathers. A medical practitioner who combines the two methods of healing under discussion revealed the he studied African traditional medicine in medical school at the University of Ibadan.

6.7.4: **BENEFITS ONE CAN DERIVE FROM THE USE OF AFRICAN TRADITIONAL MEDICINE?**

The responses were all in the affirmative. Everyone agreed that there were numerous benefits which could be derived from the use of this medicine. Some of the benefits which were mentioned included: restoration of health, prevention of ill health, provision of employment, it is cheap to procure and it is readily available. In addition to the above benefits one respondents' said "you also become very popular both far and near." And according to another respondent "you become a good neighbour because you heal those around you almost free of charge."

6.7.5 DANGERS THAT YOU HAVE DISCOVERED IN THE PRACTICE AND USE OF THIS MEDICINE?

All the people who were interviewed responded that there are dangers associated with the use of traditional medicine. These dangers become more glaring when instructions concerning the usage of the medicine are not followed. Both modern medical practitioners and the traditional healers pointed out that mixing the two forms of medication and using same at once could endanger the user's life.

6.7.6 LIST OF SOME DANGERS

RESPONSES BY SDA MEDICAL PERSONNEL:

The medical personnel who were interviewed mentioned the following dangers which are associated with the use of African traditional medicine:

1. Overdose and death
2. Infection and death
3. No dosage regimen
4. Use of toxic substances e.g. alcohol
5. Not hygienic
6. Cause liver damage and peptic ulcer

RESPONSES BY SDA PASTORS:

All the pastors who responded indicated that the measurement of the medicine or the dosage is not known, it could cause more harm than good. Another identified danger was 'fainting and stomach pain when the medicine has not been taken as prescribed by the healer'. It is important to point out that no single pastor associated the practice and use of African traditional medicine with the danger of idolatry or demon worship.

RESPONSES BY SDA MEMBERS:

The members of the church considered overdose, under dose, dirty environment, associating the production and dispensing traditional medicine with incantations, magic and other mystical powers as some of the dangers seen in traditional medication.

RESPONSES BY NON SEVENTH-DAY ADVENTISTS:

According to one respondent 'mixing modern medicine with traditional one can cause a lot of danger and could lead to death'. Another respondent maintained that "wrong usage, wrong dosage and telling lies to a traditional healer concerning a disease are all dangerous". It is therefore important to follow the rules or instructions on the drug usage. A male respondent sees a danger in "using the wrong medicine for the wrong disease as a result of misinformation by the patient". Other dangers include combining the use of traditional with that of the orthodox; disobeying the instruction of "Ifa" could bring evil consequences; and using the medicine at the wrong time could also be dangerous.

6.7.7 COMPARISON OF TRADITIONAL WITH THE MODERN WAYS OF MEDICATION

Most of the SDA church pastors supported the fact that the traditional way of treating diseases is better than the orthodox method, while a majority of those who were interviewed said traditional is better, a few others were of the opinion that the orthodox method of medication is better. The response of the members for the above question was most interesting as more than 75% of them indicated that the modern way of medication is better than the traditional method.

In the same vein, none of the various traditional medical practitioner indicated that the modern way of medication is better than the traditional. About 95 percent of them said that African traditional medicine is the better way of treating diseases that plague humanity. The other 5 percent are of the opinion that both should be combined.

6.7.8 REFERRAL OF PATIENTS TO A TRADITIONAL MEDICAL HEALER? (QUESTION FOR MODERN MEDICAL WORKERS).

All the responses from the Seventh-day Adventist medical personnel were negative. No nurse, midwife or modern physician ever admitted referring any patient to any traditional healer at any time in their medical practice.

6.7.9 **REFERRAL OF PATIENTS BY OTHER MEDICAL WORKERS OR HOSPITALS? (QUESTION FOR TRADITIONAL HERBALIST).**

Many of the traditional healers responded that patients have actually been referred to them from the modern medical workers as well as from hospitals. About 80% of the traditional healers responded in the affirmation to this question.

6.7.10 **NATURE OF THE SICKNESS REFERRED TO YOU?**

According to one respondent "sickness associated with spiritual powers which the modern medicine cannot handle" is usually referred to him. Sickness associated with child birth which could have led to caesarean operations are also handled by the traditional healers. A woman traditional birth attendant said that "instead of giving birth by surgical operation—it is handled in a few minutes here and the baby is delivered normally".

Another respondent was emphatic in saying "there has been many birth related cases that had been referred to him both from the health centers and other modern medical institutions." He also added that "he had referred many cases which he could not handle to modern hospitals." Still on birth related cases, both male and female traditional healers from Ikenne, Ilishan, Irolu, Ilara and Sagamu among others all confirmed that they had handled several birth cases which were referred to them by modern or orthodox medical personnel.

One respondent confirmed that many bone cases had been referred to him after the orthopedic medical institutions could not provide a complete solution to the patients. Even cases that have received attentions at modern hospitals were later sent to him for corrections and amendments.

6.7.11 OPINIONS ON THE COMBINATION OF AFRICAN TRADITIONAL MEDICINE AND MODERN WAYS OF HEALING

RESPONSES FROM SDA PASTORS:

Almost all the Seventh-day Adventist Pastors who were interviewed were of the opinion that the two ways of healing should be combined to achieve complete health for man. One Pastor said "my best opinion is to counsel the federal government to encourage and support traditional healers to operate in better ways to enable them compliment what the modern medical workers are doing. When both are enlightened, then better health will be the result". In a similar statement, another Pastor asserted that "African traditional medicine and modern ways of healing are good to man. There are some diseases that modern medicine cannot heal which the traditional medicine can cure".

It was one senior Pastor, who had not taken any modern medical treatment for the past ten years as earlier mentioned that differed from others. He said "there should not be any combination of the two ways of healing except in a situation where the traditional method fails". In spite this minister's position, a higher percentage of the pastors were of the opinion that the two should be combined to meet the health needs of humanity.

RESPONSES FROM SEVENTH-DAY ADVENTIST MEN AND WOMEN'S LEADERS:

The responses of the members differ from one another. Some are of the opinion that to combine the two methods of healing is dangerous while others think that complete health can only be achieved by using modern medicine in combination of African traditional one. In the opinion of one respondent, "the combination is aright because two good heads are better than one. The modern medicine personnel should bury their pride and learn something good or new from the traditional medical workers". In the same way, a women's ministries leader opined that "the two should be adequately combined for better and complete health for humanity". Another woman contended that if the two methods of healing must be combined, it should be administered one after the other". On the other hand are members of the Seventh-day Adventist church who said that modern medicine should not be combined with African traditional medicine because it could lead to complications and even death.

RESPONSES FROM SEVENTH-DAY ADVENTIST MEDICAL PERSONNELS:

One medical doctor is of the opinion that before any combination could be embarked upon traditional medicine should be 'subjected to scientific test to show its efficacy and this should be followed by formulating dosage regimen for it". However, other medical personnel have different opinions. For instance, one respondent is of the opinion that "this is one of the means of finding solution and improvement in the care of patients because the use of African traditional medicine would consider the socio-cultural beliefs of Africans in the treatment of patients. Modern medicine would also be of advantage in case there is any health problem which is difficult to be handled by the use of the former".

In the opinion of others, the combination should be encouraged because some bacteria are not easily destroyed except with modern drugs. A higher percentage of our medical personnel have seen the need and are also of the opinion that the two methods of healing should compliment one another in the health care delivery system of man. A male nurse said that "in a nutshell, I believe that combination is only in some certain (few) areas of medicine and we need experts to handle it carefully."

In a similar reaction, another female respondent was of the view that, "there are some benefits from traditional medicine which have been developed to suit the present medical practice. If both methods are combined, many diseases that do not respond to modern medicine will be cured by a combination of both." Still on combining the two methods of healing, a medical doctor said it will "help harness the traditional properties in naturally occurring substance in the environment which modern medical practice will help standardize."

RESPONSES FROM NON SEVENTH-DAY ADVENTISTS:

The responses from traditional medical practitioners who are not Seventh-day Adventists fall into two groups. The first group consists of those who are of the opinion that the two types of medication should not be combined. According to one respondent, "If you know what you are doing, traditional medicine cannot and should not be mixed with modern medicine. For over twenty years, I have never used modern medicine myself or prescribed it for anyone". Another traditional healer shares the same opinion that both methods of healing should not be combined. Many others, however, were of the opinion that combining the two methods of healing is good for man. In the words of a male respondent, "the two can be used at different times or one after the other. But the two should not be used at the same time". The point being made is that a lot of wisdom is needed when the need to combine the two methods of healing arises.

The NARL Specialist Clinic-The modern Center of Natural Remedies-Center for Research and Development of Phyto-medicines located at Ibadan, Oyo State of Nigeria is a place where modern and traditional medications are combined with much success. According to a respondent there, "herbs are used effectively without incantations, rituals, or sacrifices." He further said, "the coming of the Whites led to a shift from herbal medications to synthetic medicine. However, people are now realizing the side effects of synthetic drugs and they are now yearning for the original and natural." Indeed NARL Clinic which has a total of 47 workers has been meeting the health needs of numerous individuals for the past 19 years of its existence. The personal interviews have revealed a lot of things which included the following among others;

1. All the people who were interviewed supported the practice and use of African traditional medicine in meeting the health needs of Seventh-day Adventists in Remoland as well as in other parts of the world.
2. It is remarkable to note that none of the Seventh-day Adventist Church pastors who were interviewed ever associated African traditional medicine with idolatry or demon worship.
3. Among all those who were interviewed, there was just one individual who was introduced to traditional medication through the message and writings of Ellen G. white. This is an indication that the pastors of Seventh-day Adventist Church in Remoland and beyond, need to spend quality time in studying the writings of Ellen G. White, especially on health matters.

CHAPTER SEVEN

7.0 SUMMARY, RECOMMENDATION AND CONCLUSIONS

7.1 Summary Of Findings

The purpose of this study has been to undertake a contextual study of the practice and use of African traditional medicine among the Seventh-day Adventists in Remoland of Ogun State. To achieve this purpose, I undertook 9-month intensive fieldwork spread over the summers of 2002, 2003 and 2005 to enable me research into the social, economic, political, cultural and religious practices of Remo people with emphasis on the use and practice of African traditional medicine among the Seventh-day Adventists. Apart from numerous literature review, and oral interviews that were held with many people, materials for this study were also collected with an open-ended, semi-structured questionnaire and the data collected was analyzed using simple frequency tables. In carrying out this research, a multi-dimensional methodology was adopted which included the phenomenological, religious leaders, descriptive and participant observation approaches among others.

This chapter further provides a brief summary of the materials presented in this study. Then some conclusions are provided that demonstrate the effective use and practice of African traditional medicine among Seventh-day Adventists in Remoland of Ogun State. Following that are some suggestions that have been given for further studies. Finally, the contribution of this study to existing knowledge was highlighted.

This section also presents an over view of the first six chapters of this study. Focus is given to the role of Ellen G. White and her impact on the health and medical philosophy of the Seventh-day Adventist church. Chapter one provides information on the methodology used in this work. Starting with the statement of the problem, through the objectives of the study, delimitation, limitation, definition of terms, review of relevant literature and the instrumentation used in this work were all discussed. The organization of the thesis was also handled in this section.

Chapter two examines the identification of the Seventh-day Adventist Church and its location within Remoland of Ogun State in Nigeria. The historical and ethnographic backgrounds of the people were considered. This was followed by the culture and the socio-economic activities of the people in Remoland. Then the three major religions in Africa, namely African Traditional Religion, Christianity and Islam that are also located within Remoland were considered.

Chapter three examines the history of the practice of traditional medicine from biblical times to contemporary period. The earliest information concerning the use of herbs and food therapy is recorded in the cosmogenic account of Genesis where the instruction for the use of herbs, which is an integral aspect of traditional medicine, was given to man.

Apart from its use after creation in the Garden of Eden, the Old Testament is replete with information on various forms of natural and traditional medical practices. It is true that Yahweh Himself is the Healer of His people, when the needs arose; Yahweh gave specific instructions on what should be done to effect the healing of His people with *materia medica*. This was seen when a tree was cast into bitter water of Marah to make it pure and safe for human consumption. It was also the case in healing King Hezekiah with the poultice of figs. The situation was not altered when Naaman, the Syrian army commander was healed by washing seven times in the flowing water of River Jordan. Prophet Jeremiah, Ezekiel and others made appropriate references to the healing powers of the famous balm of Gilead.

During the New Testament era, the use and practice of traditional medicine was also in vogue. This was evident in the humanitarian first-aid service of the Good Samaritan who used oil and wine to assist someone in need. The use of clay and soil were not just for creation but they are also symbols of healing, deliverance and restoration to life. This was amply demonstrated in the life and ministry of Jesus Christ in healing different types of diseases.

In our modern society, whenever an average person hears the word "oil" he or she would think of petroleum oil. During Bible times, however, oil means "Olive oil." It was considered the most versatile, useful and essential oil put in place by the all Wise God.

Apart from its use as a prophylactic agent, it also serves as oil for lamplight, lubricator for squeaking hinges, agent for anointing kings and priests, preserver of fish and meat products, tonic for hair as well as an integral part of sacrifices.

Another important section within chapter three, deals with the use and practice of traditional medicine in contemporary time. In our contemporary time, the use of traditional medicine is on the increase as it has been estimated that some 80% of Africans patronize the traditional healers for their health needs. In view of its availability, affordability and its effectiveness in handling the health needs of people, the WHO has urged various nations to give traditional systems of medicine adequate support as well as for the formulation of policies to regulate its use at the national level. Some medicinal plants are used both as food and medicine. The bitter leaf, paw paw, coconut, aloe vera, lemon, garlic among others are in this group. The various ways in which they are used both as food and medicine were also explored within this chapter.

Chapter four considered the practice of traditional medicine among Seventh-day Adventists and also traced the history of the church's health and medical philosophy. The background of the Seventh-day Adventist health message could be traced back to the vision God gave to Ellen G. White at Otsego in May 21, 1863. It was also called the comprehensive health vision. That health vision was concerned with the physical well being of Seventh-day Adventists and others around them, preventive medicine, causes of diseases, care for the sick, and the use of remedial agencies for taking care of the sick. This philosophy of health has been simplified for applications among Seventh-day Adventists and for all God's children through the acronym, AH-NEWSTART.

AH-NEWSTART means:

A—Attitudes
H—Hygiene
N—Nutrition
E—Exercises
W—Water
S—Sunlight
T—Temperance
A—Air
R—Rest
T—Trust in God

In order to put these principles into practice, the Seventh-day Adventist church from her earliest days embraced the publications of these truths for all to read. Some of the health publications include: The Health Reformers (1866); The Pacific Health Journal (1904); Health (1932); Christian Temperance and Bible Hygiene (1890); Healthful Living (1896); The Ministry of Healing (1905); Counsels on Health (1923); Medical Missionary (1932); Counsels on Diet and Foods (1938); and many others.

Health care institutions were also established to cater for the sick the way it should be done. The first of such institutions was the Western Health Reform Institute that was opened on September 5, 1866. Soon other medical institutions were established in many parts of North America. As time progressed, Nigeria in Africa was blessed with such institutions. In Nigeria for instance, we have the following health and medical institutions: Seventh-day Adventist Hospital, Ile-Ife, Osun State; Babcock University Medical Centre, Ilishan-Remo, Ogun State; Seventh-day Adventist Hospital and Motherless Babies Home, Aba, Abia State; Jengre Seventh-day Adventist Hospital, Plateau State and many others. All these medical institutions have contributed in advancing the philosophy of health as espoused by the church.

Chapter five deals with the impact of the use and practice of African traditional medicine among Seventh-day Adventists in Remoland of Ogun State. This section demonstrated that Seventh-day Adventists use and practice the explicable form of African traditional medicine. In this traditional healing, there are no rituals involved. The use of chickens, eggs, cola nuts, white or red cloth is not required by the herbalist. This is the traditional medicine, which is devoid of incantations, sacrifices, use of psychic phenomena, magic and the use of mystic powers for the purposes of healing and the prevention of diseases. It is true that a majority of the people uses and practices the inexplicable type of traditional medicine, which involves incantations, sacrificing animals, the pouring of libations, the use of magic, and the free use of other psychic phenomena. On the other hand, Seventh-day Adventists who use and are involved in the traditional healing profession, use the explicable form of traditional medicine. Seventh-day Adventists practice and use this type of traditional medicine due to its availability, affordability, effectiveness, economic benefits and the general well being the users derive from it as well as a result of their religious convictions based on the Bible and the writings of Ellen Gould White.

Chapter six contains the data analysis and presentation of findings on the practice and use of African traditional medicine among Seventh-day Adventist in Remoland of Ogun State. The data which had been collected with the questionnaires were analyzed with simple frequency table which was electronically processed on the statistical package for social sciences (SPSS, Inc. USA).

7.2 Suggestions/Recommendations

Having undertaken a contextual study of the practice and use of African traditional medicine among Seventh-day Adventists in Remoland of Ogun State, a lot of other issues have been raised and they have given rise to the following suggestions:

A. The information, which, have been presented in this thesis, constitutes an information base that could be used by other researchers in the future to carry out further investigation on the use and practice of African traditional medicine among Seventh-day Adventists in other parts of Yorubaland. It is therefore suggested that the information could also be used to compare and contrast the perception of other religious groups within Remoland on their use and practice of African traditional medicine.

B. It is also suggested that further research could be carried out to find out what had led Seventh-day Adventists in Remoland of Ogun State to use and practice only the explicable form of African traditional medicine. Is this action due to their orthodoxy, orthopraxy, or their peculiar understanding of the Bible and the Spirit of Prophecy among them?

C. Next, a comparative research could also be carried out between Seventh-day Adventists in Remoland where the members embrace the explicable form of traditional medicine and another group who depends on the modern system of medication for the health care delivery system to ascertain the state of health of the two groups.

D. Our educational institutions from the post primary to the tertiary should include the study of the practice of traditional medicine in their curriculum. When competent teachers teach students, the students in turn will positively have an impact upon the members of the church.

E. Seventh-day Adventists in Remoland should be educated to differentiate between utilizing what God has created and put in place for the benefit of humanity from any devilish practice. This education, apart from citing contemporary break through in the use and practice of traditional medicine, should also be Bible based and Spirit of Prophecy centered. The Scripture itself is replete with incidents of herbal medicinal practices. It is interesting to note that herbal medicine is an integral part of traditional medicine and the instruction to use herbal medicine has been noted as been direct instructions from the God of the whole universe Himself. For example, when King Hezekiah was sick, the prophet Isaiah brought him news that he was going to die. That was a painful message to the sick monarch. He there and then cried bitterly to the Lord, the Lord heard his cry and came to the rescue of the king. He was cured with the poultice of figs. Indeed one word or touch of God would have been enough to cure the sick king instantly. Instead, he was instructed to apply a bunch of figs to his sore. That natural remedy which was blessed by God healed the king. It is fascinating to note here that the God of nature who directed human beings to use natural remedies then still wants us to use that prescription now.

F. The study of agricultural science both in principle and practice should be revitalized and reactivated within our schools with full students and staff participation. The focus would be on growing medicinal plants, herbs, shrubs, and mushrooms among other conventional agricultural activities. The department of Agriculture and Industrial Technology in cooperation with the Health Sciences Department of our universities, as well as medical schools where they are available should work as a team to have this dream translated into reality. A further work could be taken to liaise with the Department of Pharmacy, where it is also available to get this achieved. The production, packing, and the preservation of these medicinal plants cannot be overemphasized.

G. It is clear from the above that right from the beginning of man's life, God has put the herbs in place for our benefits. If we would come back to God's original design for all humanity, disease would be rare while abundant health would be very common. Herbal medication, which is an integral part of traditional medicine, should be restored to its rightful position in this era of science and technology. In Seventh-day

Adventist hospitals, traditional medications that are both effective and efficacious should be provided and dispensed with other modern medications as the needs arise.

The call for further study and improvement in the dosage and other aspects of traditional medicine should be further emphasized. This will lead to a wider acceptability of this alternative health care system. The important roles, which present religious leaders should play in educating their members on the importance of traditional medicine, should be pointed out to these leaders.

A comprehensive look at this research has actually revealed that Seventh-day Adventists also use and practice this alternative form of medicine for prophylactic and preventive purposes. This study has therefore provided us with a better understanding of the educational, medical and health programmes of the Seventh-day Adventist Church, not only in Remoland but also across the world since the Seventh-day Adventists operate over five hundred hospitals, sanitariums, dispensaries and medical institutions in more than two hundred countries of the world. Following that, this research has also highlighted the various important roles, which the use and practice of African traditional medicine have played and will continue to play in the church in particular and to the society in general.

BIBLIOGRAPHY

UNPUBLISHED MATERIALS

This Section describes the principal Libraries, Archives, and Collections, research Centers and Unpublished Sources, which have been used in this dissertation. Published sources as well as oral Interviews will be treated in appropriate and designated sections of the Bibliography

Adventist Historical Village
Battle Creek, Michigan,
USA.

The Historic Adventist Village, located in the West-end of Battle Creek, Michigan, is indeed a village which has been preserved to share the history of a people who lived to honour God. Some significant historic sites in this village include the restored and replicated Review and Herald Publishing House, the Western Health Reform Institute, the Home of James and Ellen White, the homes of other pioneers and The Welcome Center. The Welcome Center houses the various health equipments, which were discovered by our church pioneers. Materials on evangelism, education, health and medical operations are also located at the Welcome Centre. This Adventist Historic village was the source of some rare information on Ellen White and H. J. Kellog who were pioneers in the health ministry of the Seventh-day Adventist Church.

Center for Adventist Research,
James White Library,
Andrews University,
Berrien Spring, Michigan,
USA.

The Adventist Heritage center and Ellen G. White Branch office located within the James White Library on the main campus of Andrews University is known as the Center for Adventist Research. This center has a large collection of manuscripts on every phase of the Seventh-day Adventist work. In addition, there are monographs, photographs, artifacts and research papers. Specific information on J. N. Andrews, the first foreign missionary the Seventh-day Adventists sent to Europe was gathered from this center.

Ellen G. White Estate, Main Office,
General Conference of Seventh-day Adventists,
Silver Spring, Maryland,
USA.

The Ellen G. White Estate is one of the most important archives that provided valuable information for this research. The White Estate is rich with important letters, manuscripts, books, and other original collections from Ellen White. Her original writings on natural health, God's original plan for man's health, longevity and natural remedies are all located here. These materials were used while writing this thesis.

Ellen G. White-SDA Research Center
Babcock University
Ilishan-Remo, Ogun State
Nigeria.

The center was established in 1990 for a comprehensive study of the Bible, Seventh-day Adventist Church history and mission. The centre enables researchers to discover the biblical foundation for the gift of prophecy, the life, ministry and the writings of Ellen G. White. The collection includes Ellen G. White letters and manuscripts, Ellen G. White published works, 21 volumes of manuscript releases, Adventist periodicals, General Conference Bulletins. Ellen G. White Biographical index, and other research aids. These were consulted for information in the course of this research.

Hezekiah Oluwaseanmi Library
Obafemi Awolowo University
Ile-Ife, Osun State
Nigeria

The Hezekiah Oluwasanmi Library contains a large assemblage of information on African Traditional Medicine from the Yorubaland and other African perspectives. These were helpful since the work under consideration was carried out in Remoland, which is located within Yorubaland in Nigeria.

Private Library of Elisha O. Babalola
Obafemi Awolowo University
Ile-Ife, Osun State
Nigeria.

Certain information that were helpful in this research were found in the Private Library of Dr. Elisha O. Babalola. These included his personal works on various aspects of African Traditional Medicine. His works on the combination of orthodox medicine with that of African Traditional Medicine to achieve complete health for humanity were very useful.

PRIMARY ORAL SOURCES

LIST OF THOSE INTERVIEWED

Aborishade, Daniel S. has been a pastor at the No.1 Seventh-day Adventist church Ilisan Remo for the past 4 years. These 4 years were equally used to do an undergraduate study in Theology Babcock University.

Aborishade, Yetunde (Mrs.) is the Shepherdess of the No.1 Seventh-day Adventist Church, Ilisan Remo. She is the Sabbath School Superintendent. According to her she uses the alternative form of medication because it is very cheap and could be located easily. She learnt the use of African medicine from her grand mother, but she uses it now to take care of her family.

Adebayo Oladele, lives at No 4 Ajegunle Street, Ilishan-Remo of Ogun State. He is a professional traditional medical practitioner for the past 20 years. He handles all cases. The effectiveness of the treatment depends on the nature of the sickness. Even modern hospitals refer cases to him and for the past 20 years he has never referred any medical case to any other source. He however, specializes in fertility cases. He was interviewed on November 4, 2005 from 5.oo pm to 5.30 pm. The best way to achieve complete health for humanity is through a combination of the traditional and modern systems of medication.

Adeyemi, Sarah M. A. is a youth promoter of the No. 1 SDA church, Ilisan Remo. She also claimed that God introduced her to traditional medication through Bible studies. She further opined that it was dangerous to combine both traditional and modern way of treatment.

Akande, David resides at No. 7 Iworu Street, Ilisan Remo. He works in the Choir section of the No.1 SDA Church, Ilisan Remo. He gained knowledge of traditional healing from his father who was a traditional medical practitioner.

Akinlabi O. (Mrs.) is a teacher, who also serves as the Clerk of SDA Church, Ilisan Remo. According to her, God introduced her to African traditional medicine.

Akintoye Onamade A. lives at Odunlami Close, Iperu Remo. He is a teacher by profession. He serves as the clerk of the Seventh-day Adventist Church, Iperu Remo.

Asiyanbola, John A. resides at No.59 Imosimi, Ilisan Remo. He is an electronic-electronical engineer. Using the right mixture of leaves and herbs is the only way to get complete cure for malaria or fever. His parents introduced him to this form of medication.

Ashamba, Bidimba is a Pastor from Congo. He is also studying for an M.A degree in pastoral ministry at Babcock University, Ilisan Remo Ogun State, Nigeria.

Awodele, I. O. (Mrs.) is a Medical Practitioner at the Babcock University Medical Centre, Ilisan Remo Ogun State. She has served in that capacity for the past 2 years.

Awoniyi, James Ayodeji is a student of Babcock University. He is a 200 level Theology student as well as the Adventist Youth Leader. According to him African traditional medicine is using native medicine to cure diseases and to keep healthy. The dangers he has discovered are lack of hygiene in preparing the drugs as well as in not observing adequate dosages for it.

Awoniyi, Olatunde is also a student at Babcock University who serves as a deacon in the SDA Church. The medicine which our fore-fathers handed to us through our fathers which is effective in handling diseases is African traditional medicine. Since two heads are better than one, the modern medical worker has a lot to learn from African traditional healers for a balanced health for mankind.

Awuloha, Festus, N is the current youth Director of the Eastern Nigeria Union Mission with headquarters at Aba, Abia State. He is currently an M. A. degree student at Babcock University, Ilisan Remo, Ogun State.

Babs Tunde Olubajo, Traditional Doctor in charge of Banke Traditional Orthorpaedic Center is a specialist in treating fractures, polio, sprain, dislocation, etc. He was interviewed at No. 19 Obada Market Street, Idode-Oke-Sopen, Ijebu-Igbo, Ogun State from 1.00 p.m. to 1.45 p.m. on Monday, February 23, 2004. He is in support of the combination of the knowledge of the traditional healers with that of orthodox medication to achieve Optimum result in the health care delivery system.

Bamidele, Tobi is a teacher by profession. He lives at No.5 Obori Basin Valley—Araroun, Ilisan Remo. He serves the No.1 Seventh-day Adventist Church as Associate Treasurer.

Bello, Shakirat resides at No. 4 Ajegunle Street. He is a teacher and serves as an Usher at the No. 1 SDA Church, Ilisan Remo. He said African traditional medicine is the first aid one takes before going to the hospital.

Binuyo, Biodun is a nurse and works at the Babcock University Medical Centre, Ilisan Remo, Ogun State. He is a Seventh-day Adventist.

Biobakun, C. A is the resident minister at the Seventh-day Adventist church, Iperu-Remo, Ogun State. As a result of his use and practice of African traditional medicine, he has never gone to any modern hospital for the past ten years. He has a big herbarium at his Iperu residence.

Blessing, N. has worked as a nurse for the past 24 years. She is currently working at The Babcock University Medical Centre. She serves the No.2 Seventh-day Adventist church, Ilisan Remo as the Health and Temperance Director.

Chiabuotu, Chidinma has been a nurse for the past 7 years. She is serving at the Babcock University Medical Centre, Ilisan Remo, Ogun State.

Chief Adelaja—Taran Lafia of Irolu—Ilisan road, opposite the Irolu Health Centre has been a traditional healer for 14 years. He handles sleep disorders; mystic attacks and promotes business prosperity for people. He was trained at Cotonuo where he also got his healing powers.

Chief Dr. Wole Ogunsanya, the Obaisegun of Irolu Remo, Ogun State. He works as a traditional birth attendant as well a general traditional healer. He is the current Chairman of the traditional healers association in Ikenne Local government area. He is also the Chairman of Irolu Health Centre Committee. He is of the opinion that modern and traditional medicine should be used to meet the needs of humanity.

Chief (Mrs.) A. O. Orisagbemi Olomo-Wewe, is the Director of the Orisagbemi Iya Olomo-Wewe Maternity Home, which is located at No.107 Akarigbo Street, Shagamu, Ogun State, and she is also a member of Nigeria Association of Native Doctors. An internationally acclaimed Traditional Birth Attendant since 1990. She uses only herbs, leaves, roots, barks and other natural materials in bringing solution to any problem associated with pregnancy. She is a specialist in native drugs and herbs. She was interviewed on Wednesday, February 4, 2004 between 2.00p.m. and 3.00p.m

Chief (Dr) O. P. Somefun is currently the treasurer of the Ogun State Traditional Healers Association. He is an herbalist native doctor who combines Ifa with herbal medication. Before he embraces any healing exercise, he must get information from Ifa. He was interviewed between 6.45-7.00PM on August 28, 2005.

Chief Saloko Sabowade, is living at No. 15 Araroma Street, Ilishan-Remo, Ogun State. He was interviewed on Sunday, 27th August 2005 by 4.00 p.m. He has been a traditional healer for more than thirty-five years.

Dina, Peace is a Nurse Assistant at the Babcock University Medical Centre. She is an adult who has served in her present position for 12 years.

Djata, Francis is a Seventh-day Adventist member from Iperu. For him herbs are gifts from God for the benefit of man.

Djata Juliana, is the leader of the Women's Ministries Department of the Seventh- day Adventist Church, Iperu Remo.

Ebedi, Ibrahim is a traditional healer who also sells the drug from place to place. He comes from Olomi Academy, Ibadan three times a week to sell his medicine in Shagamu. He has been doing this for the past 20 years. His father introduced him to the traditional medical work. He is of the opinion that both ways of treating the sick should be combined for greater success.

Ebenezer O. Olapade, Medical Director, NARL Specialist Clinic, Ibadan—The Modern Centre of Natural Remedies—Center for Research and Development of Phytomedicines. He was interviewed at NARL Specialist Clinic, Ibadan on Friday, March 14th, 2003 from 12.00 noon to 2.00 p.m. He is currently using known and tested orthodox medicine in conjunction with traditional remedies (without incantations) to treat and heal various diseases and he is of the view that the orthodox medical workers and traditional healers should work together for greater success.

Ekpendu, Ikechi C. is a clergyman from Aba who has been in pastoral ministry for 8 years. He is currently the Director of Evangelism and Family Life at the Eastern Nigeria Union Mission, Aba, Abia State. He is currently at Babcock University for the M.A pastoral ministry studies.

Jacques Mansaly, is a Pastor from Dakar, Senegal, who has been in the ministry for 7 years. He is studying towards an M.A degree in Theology at Babcock University, Ilisan Remo, Ogun State.

Kara, S.B has been a gospel minister for the past 29 years in Rivers Conference Port Harcourt. He is currently an M.A student in Babcock University, Ilisan Remo, Ogun State.

Kwarbai, Ishaya Iliya has been a gospel minister for the past 23 years. He is currently the president of the North West Nigeria Conference and headquarters in Kaduna. He is currently an M.A. student at Babcock University.

Kassoule, Lukan is a pastor form Niamey, Niger Republic. He has worked as a publishing Director for many years, but he is currently studying for an M.A degree in pastoral ministry at Babcock University.

Lasisi, Israel is a mason from Ilishan Remo, Ogun State who works with the Babcock University building department in the construction of new buildings. He was interviewed on May 18, 2003

Leopold Agbossassa M. is a Pastor from Cotonou, Benin Republic who has been in the ministry for the past 16 years. He is an M.A Theology student at Babcock University. His parents and friends introduced him to African traditional medicine and according to Him; combing modern medication with African traditional one is the best way to maintain health.

Mark Beatrice is a medical worker who for the past 20 years has been a midwife at the Babcock University Medical Center. She is a deaconess as well as a health instructor for the No. 1 Seventh-day Adventist Church, Ilisan Remo.

Mbaegbu, Priscilla U. is a hall administrator for the past 5 years at Babcock University. She sees African traditional medicine as using natural remedies for the health of humanity. The only danger she has observed in the use of this form of treatment is the absence of dosage in most cases.

Miss Esther Boluwaju Sholaru is a nurse who works at the Opemiro Eleweobiwere Traditional Maternity Home. She had done her general nursing coupled with the midwifery training in another modern hospital. She finds her former training very useful in the traditional maternity home. She emphasized the unity of both the traditional and modern forms of medicine to achieve complete healing for man. She plans to deliver her children in this maternity home when she marries. She was interviewed on December 22, 2005 from 3.00 pm to 3.25 pm.

Mr. Adeyemi Soyemi is living at No. 7 Ajegunle Adeyemi Street, Ilishan-Remo, Ogun State, was interviewed on August 27th, 2005 by 4.30 p.m. He is a traditional healer.

Mr. Odubanwo Olusola, is from the Itunmuleruwa compound of Ilishan Remo. He is a Seventh-day Adventist Church member, who was interviewed on Sunday, 27th August, 2005 between 1.00pm-2.00p.m

Mr. Sikiru Sumaila, lives at No. 030 Ago Ilara Street, Ilishan-Remo, Ogun State. He is a Seventh-day Adventist Christian who was interviewed on Sunday, August 27, 2005 between 2.30 p.m.-3.00 p.m

Mrs. Toyin Jinadu is a Traditional Birth Attendant who owns and manages Opemiro Eleweobiwere Traditional Maternity Home. She has been running this traditional maternity home for the past 15 years. All her three children were delivered there. She said that this type of maternity for delivering babies is very cheap as well as being close to the people. According to her, a normal delivery will cost only N2, 500.00 while a difficult one will cost N3, 000.00. She was interviewed on December 22, 2005 from 2.30 pm to 3.00 pm.

Mustapha, Alli, is a Medical Laboratory Technician at the Babcock University Medical Center. He has served in this capacity for the past 13 years.

Nkwazema, Roseline is a teacher and Evangelist at the Seventh-day Adventist Church, Iperu Remo, Ogun State.

Odiase, J. O. is a Medical Doctor. He is a Seventh-day Adventist serving at the Babcock University Medical Center as a physician.

Odubanjo Falabake, is a Native Doctor in Ilishan-Remo of Ogun State. He works with herbs, roots, rhizomes, barks of medicinal plants and leaves for various treatments. According to him, before he embarks on the treatment of major diseases, he consults "IFA" for permission and blessings on his work. He further commented that what IFA is to him in his herbal medical profession is what JESUS CHRIST is to Christians. He was interviewed from 5.00-5.45 p.m. on Wednesday, February 11, 2004 in the company of Mr. Oduojukan who translated for me.

O. Olaifa, Consultant of Olayode Native Doctor has been working for the past 20 years. His home located at No. 2 Igido Street, Ilishan-Remo, Ogun State also serves as the native hospital. There are no in-patients. People come there to collect their drugs and then go back to their different homes. If a patient comes and his Ifa tells him not to render any services to the individual, he would then refer that person to another native doctor.

Olanipekun Rafiu is, the Director of Ilesanmi Traditional Clinic—Traditional Maternity. He has been in this work since 1991 and has attended several government-organized seminars and has the following licenses and certificates;
  1. License from the Ministry of Health, Ogun State of Nigeria—Certificate of participation—(Dec. 2005).
  2. Ogun State Traditional Healers Association—Ikenne Local government branch—Issued 27-3-2002

3. Certificate of the Ogun State Traditional Healers Association (2001)
4. Remo North—South Medical Herbalists Association of Nigeria—Issued 11-3-1991

He showed these certificates to us to demonstrate the fact that the traditional healers and modern medical practitioners are working together.

Oluremi Olatunji has been a traditional healer for the past 6 years. He resides and practices at No. 7 Ajedunle Street, Ilishan Remo, Ogun state. He has no formal education but he inherited the gift of healing from his father who was a successful traditional healer for many years before his death. He specializes in caring for children and in treating various forms of diabetes with herbal preparations. Incantations and oracular consultations are used for good luck, safe journeys, success in business, the retrieval of bad debts as well as to regain friends. He was interviewed on December 22, 2005 from 4.30 pm to 5.00 pm.

Olusola, Oluwatoyin Ogbudu is a teacher. She teaches Sabbath School lessons at the Seventh-day Adventist Church, Ilisan Remo, Ogun State.

Onyenweaku, Nnamdi E. is a pastor from East Nigeria Conference, Aba, Abia State who has been working for the past 9 years. He is currently an M.A pastoral ministry student at Babcock University.

Ogunbiyi, R.B. (Mrs.) is a retired teacher after serving for 35 years. She currently resides at No.1 C.A.C Road, Ilisan Remo. She is the Women's Ministries leader of No.1 SDA Church, Ilisan

Remo. She is gifted in treating all forms of stomach ache with herbs.

Ogundene Janet is a nurse who has worked at the Babcock University Medical Center for the past 3 years. She is a Seventh-day Adventist.

Ogunsanya, S.O has been a pastor with the Southwest Nigeria Conference, Akure for the past twelve years. He is currently studying for an M.A degree in Religion at Babcock University, Ilisan Remo, Ogun State.

Ogunyelu, Samuel Sunday is the Personal Ministry leader as well as Elder of the Seventh-day Adventist Church living at 4 Oyegunle Street, Ilisan Remo, Ogun State.

Oyerinde, Israel M.A has been a minister of the gospel in the Southwest Nigerian Conference of the Seventh-day Adventist Church for the past Seventeen years. He is currently the director in charge of Youth, Education, Chaplaincy and Children's Ministries. He is also an M.A Religion degree student at Babcock University, Ilisan Remo, Ogun State.

Oyerinde 'Yemisi is a teacher who leads out in the Children's Department of the Seventh-day Adventist Church, Iperu Remo Ogun State.

Paul Ibire of No. 17 Itunde-Itunlisi Street, Irolu Remo, has been treating bone related problems for 35 years. He inherited this form of healing from his father. He is not willing to disclose what he uses in handling problems associated with bones

Saheeb, Owodunni Oreoluwa lives at No.15 Awolowo Avenue, Town planning, Ilisan Remo. He has been in the teaching profession for 23 years. He is the Personal Ministry Leader at the No.2 Seventh-day Adventist Church, Ilisan Remo. He grew up with herbs. And since there are some diseases which modern medicine cannot cure, such as asthma, traditional medicine should then be used to treat and cure them completely.

Saibu Gbadamosi resides at No. 14 Jigboye Street, Iperu—Remo. For the past 21 years, he has been practicing as a traditional birth attendant and doing general traditional healing. He handles all cases related to child bearing and advocates for a combination of the two forms of healing.

Sarah Bola Taiwo is a native of Ilishan Remo in Ogun State. She has practiced the art of healing with roots, leaves and other natural means for the past 13 years. As far as she is concerned, the natural way of healing is better than the orthodox means. The natural way is more permanent. She moves from place to place administering her drugs to people in their homes, shops, working places, etc. She was interviewed on November 4th, 2005 at 3.00-4.00 p.m.

Sonola, Olaniyi Faniyi, has been managing the Fannel Herbal Maternity Home for the past 13 years. The herbal aspect of the medical work inherited while he learnt the traditional birth attendant for three years. He refers patients when the need arises and he plans to expand his hospital soon.

Sotunsa, John O. is currently the acting Medical Director of the Babcock University Medical Center. He has been serving the Medical Center for the past 4 years. He is also the health leader of the Town Planning Seventh-day Adventist Church. According to him, African traditional medicine involves the use of plant and animal parts for the health of humanity.

Sunday Onasanya, started practicing traditional healing in 1972. He both learnt and inherited the art of healing from his father who was a known healer. He produces medications for *jedi-jedi* which people from places like Lagos, Abeokuta, and Ibadan patronize. His drugs take care of malaria, stomachache, pile and diabetes. He was interviewed between 6.00pm-6.30 pm on the 28th day of August 2005.

Tajudeen, Alonje (TJ Osonyintola) is a general herbal practitioner as well as a traditional birth attendant. He has been working in these capacities for the past 23 years at Ajegunle Street, Ilara—Ilisan Road, Ilara—Remo, Ogun State.

Temitayo, Adeyemi Omoba is the Medical Director of Temitayo Natural Clinic with Head Office at Alfa-Nla Street, Capital Road, Agege Lagos State. He has 22 different natural clinics around the country where people are receiving treatment and cure with 100% herbal products for the past 30 years. He was interviewed on Monday, January 5, 2004 at his Head Office.

Tigue, Thio is a Pastor from Abidjan, Cote d'Ivoire. He is an M.A Theology student at Babcock University. He has been a minister of the gospel for the past 9 years. He learnt of traditional medication from his parents, and he supports that both the traditional and modern ways of medication should be combined to achieve complete health for Humanity.

Tshimanga, Mbwebwe has worked as a teacher, pastor, Director and President respectively at the Seventh-day Adventist church, Congo in the last 33 years. He is an M.A student now at Babcock University, Ilisan Remo, Ogun State.

Yusuf, Bako, lives at 14 Egbami Street Ogere, but worships at the Seventh-day Adventist Church Iperu—Remo, Ogun State.

SECONDARY SOURCES

A. BOOKS

Abogunrim, G. O. ed., (et al). Christian Presence and West African Responses Though the Years: Being the Proceeding of the August, 1982, Nigeria Zonal WAATI Conference and the August, 1983 West Africa Conference, WAATI

Adodo, Anselm, Nature Power, Akure: Don Bosco Training Centre, 2000.

Adegbola, F. A. Ade, Traditional Religion in West Africa, Ibadan: Oluseyi Press, 1998.

Adelowo, Dada E, Methods and Theories of Religion, Ado-Ekiti: Olugbenga Press and Publishers, 2001.

Adeniyi, M. O. & Babalola, E. O. ed., Yoruba Muslim-Christian Understanding in Nigeria, Lagos: Eternal Communications, 2001.

Africa-Indian Ocean Division, Working Policy, Accra: Advent Press, 1998.

Agboola, David T., A History of Christianity in Nigeria: The Seventh-day Adventists in Yorubaland. Ibadan: Day Star Press, 1988.

Araoye, Margaret Olabisi, Research Methodology with Statistics for Research and Social Sciences. Ilorin: Nathadex Publishers, 2004.

Asika, Nnamdi, <u>Research Methodology and the Behavioural Sciences,</u> Lagos: Longman Nigeria PLC, 2002.

Austin, Phylis, <u>More Natural Remedies</u>, Michigan: Family Health Publications, nd.

Ayeni, S. F., <u>You Can Be Healthier</u>, Lagos: Ebun-Ayeni (Nigeria) Ent., 2001.

Babalola, E. O., <u>Theology and Sociology of Yoruba Indigenous Religion</u>, Lagos: Concept Publications (Nig.) 2002.

_____ <u>African Traditional Religions. A Phenomenological and Comparative Analysis</u>, Ile-Ife: 2001.

_____ <u>Interaction of Religions in Yorubaland: A Theological and Social Analysis,</u> Ile-Ife: Babs-Adedeji and Sons Press, 2001.

_____ <u>Traditional Religion, Islam and Christianity: Patterns of Interaction</u>, Ile-Ife: Olajide Printing Works, 1992.

Billington, Ray, <u>Religion Without God</u>, London: Routledge, 2002.

Blide, Richard Rylander, <u>7 Steps to Heart and Lung Fitness</u>, Florida: Anna Publishing, Inc., 1978.

Boots, S., <u>African Religion: A Symposium,</u> New York: Nok Publishers, 1977.

Borg, W. R. and M. D. Gall, <u>Educational Research : An Introduction,</u> 4th ed., New York: Longman, 1983.

Bouquet, A. C., <u>Comparative Religion</u>. New York: Pengiun Books, 1941.

Brieger Gert H and Jerome J. Bylebyl, eds.,<u> Bulletin of the History of Medicine</u>. Baltimore: The John Hopkins University Press, 1993.

Bryant, John, <u>Health and The Developing World</u>, London: Cornell University Press, 1969.

Caman, Joan, Who's Who in the Old Testament: Together with the Apocrypha, London: Routledge, 2002.

Clements, William M., ed., Religion, Aging and Health: A Global Perspective, New York: The Haworth Press, 1988.

Clerke, T. C., Nature's Big Beautiful Bountiful Feel-good Book, Connecticut: Keats Publishing Inc., 1977.

Damsteegt, Gerrard, Foundations of the Seventh-day Adventists Message and Mission, Michigan: Andrews University Press, 1990.

Daodu, Tunde, Aloe Vera: The Miracle Healing Plant, Lagos: Healthfield Coperation, 2000.

Dawson, B., Religion and Culture, London: Sheed and Ward, 1948.

Dickson, Kwesi A. and Paul Ellingworth, eds., Biblical Revelation and African Beliefs, New York: Orbis Books, 1963.

Donnellan, Craig, Food for thought, vol. 36, Cambridge: Independent Educational Publishers, 1998.

Dopamu, P. Ade, Esu: The Invisible Foe of Man, Ijebu-Ode: Shebiotimo Publications, 2000.

Douglass, Herbert E., Messenger of the Lord, Ontario: Pacific Press Publishing Association, 1998.

Dysinger, William, Heaven's Lifestyle Today, Hagerstown MD: Review and Herald Graphics, 1997.

Eddy, Mary Baker, Science and Health with Key to the Scriptures, Boston: The First Church of Christ, 1994.

Eliade, Mireca, The Sacred and the Profane, New York: Harper and Row, 1961.

_____ What is Religion? An Inquiry for Christian Theology, New York: The Seaburn Press, 1980.

_____ Rites and Symbols of Initiation, New York: Harper and Row Publishers, 1964.

_____ Images and Symbols: Studies in Cosmology, Translated by P. Mairet. New York: Sheed and Ward, 1969.

Elujoba, A. A., Pharmacognosy for Health and Culture—The PHC Jungle Connection. Ile-Ife: Obafemi Awolowo University Press, 1999.

Fayemi, P. O., Nigerian Vegetables, Ibadan: Heinnamann Educational Books (Nigeria) PLC, 1999.

Felhaber, Tary, ed., South African Traditional Healers' Primary Health Care Handbook, Cape town: Kagiso Publishers, 1997.

Fellows, Ward J., Religions East and West, New York: Holt, Rineholt and Winston, 1979.

Fisher, Mary Pat, Religion Today: An Introduction, London: Routledge Curzor, 2002.

_____ Religion in the Twenty-First Century, London: Routledge Curzor, 1999.

Gehman, Richard, African Traditional Religion in Biblical Perspective, Kijabe: Kesho Publications, 1989.

General Conference Corporation of Seventh-day Adventists. Seventh-day Adventist Church—Yearbook 2010—Proclaiming God's Grace. Washington DC: Review and Herald Publishing Association, 2010.

Greenberg, Katherine Hayes, Versatile Vegetables, California: Owlswood Productions, Inc., 1980.

Guzman-Ladion, Herminiade, Healing Wonders of Herbs: Guide to the Effective Use of Medicinal Plants, Florida: Inter-American Division Publishing Association, 1988.

Hardinge, Marvyn G., A Physician Explains Ellen White's Counsel on Drugs, Herbs and Natural Remedies, Hagerstown, MD: Review and Herald Publishing Association, 2001.

Hawley, Don, Come Alife, Washington D.C.: Review and Herald Publishing Association, 1975.

Heirnaux, Jean, The People of Africa, New York: Charles Scribners Sons, 1975.

Hollist, Nestor Olayimika, A Collection of Traditional Yoruba Oral and Dental Medicaments, Ibadan: Book Builders, 2004.

Idowu, Bolaji, Olodumare-God in Yoruba Belief, London: Longmans, 1962.

_____ African Traditional Religion: A Definition, Ibadan: Fountain Publications, 1991.

_____ African Traditional Religion, MarylKnoll: Oriba Books, 1973.

Insoll, Timothy, Archaeology and World Religion, New York: Taylor and Francis Group, 2001.

Jones, Jeanne, The Fabulous High-Fibre Diet, California: 101 Productions, 1985.

Johns, Edward B., Health for Effective Living, Toronto: McGraw-Hill Book Company, Inc., 1958.

James, George Wharton. The Indians' Secrets of Health, California: The Radiant Life Press, 1917.

Janvier, George E., How to Write A Theological Research Thesis, Kaduna: Baraka Press and Publishers, 2001.

Kayode, J. O., Understanding African Traditional Religion, Ile-Ife: University of Ife Press, 1984.

Klaaren, Eugene M., Religious Origins of Modern Science, Michigan: William B. Eerdmans Publishing Company, 1977.

Kloss, Jethro <u>Back to Eden</u>, California: Woodbridge Press Publishing Company, 1975.

Knight, George R., <u>Meeting Ellen White,</u> Hagerstown, MD: Review and Herald Publishing Association, 2000.

Lau, Benjamin, <u>Garlic for Health</u>, Wilmot: Lotus Light Publications, 1988.

Lonergan, L. H., <u>The Wheel of Health</u>, California: Loma Linda University School Health, 1976.

Lessa, William A., <u>Reader In Comparative Religion</u>, New York: Row Peterso Company, 1958.

Lucas, J., <u>The Religion of the Yorubas</u>, Hull, England: A Brown and Sons, 1942.

Ludington, Ailean, <u>Health Power: Health By Choice Not Chance</u>, Hagerstown, MD:

Review and Herald Publishing Association, 2000.

Lust, John, <u>Drink Your Troubles Away</u>, New York: Benedict Lust Publications, 1967.

McClintode, Robert, <u>God's Healing Leaves: A User's Guide to Herbology</u>, Michigan: Remnant Publications, Inc., 1998.

Maquet, Jacques, <u>Africanity: The Cultural Unity of Black Africa</u>, London: Oxford University Press, 1972.

Mary, Midglen <u>Evolution as a Religion Strange Hopes and Strange Fears</u>, London: Routledge, 1994.

Maxwell, C. Mervyn, <u>Magnificent Disappointment</u>, Ontario: Pacific Press Publishing Association, 1994.

Mbiti, John S., <u>The Prayer of African Religion</u>, New York: Orbis Book, 1975.

_____ <u>Introduction to African Religion,</u> Second Edition, Nairaobi: Heinennman International, 1990.

_____ African Religion and Philosophy, Nariobi: Heinemann Educational Books, 1985.

_____ New Testament Eschatology in an African Background, London: Oxford University Press, 1971.

Moore, George Foot, The Birth and Growth of Religion, New York: Charles Scribner's Sons, 1923.

Nicholson, I. F., The Administration of Nigeria 1900-1960: Men Methods and Myths, Oxford: Clarendon Press, 1966.

Noss, David and John B. Noss, ed., Man's Religions, New York: Macmillan Publishing Company, 1984.

Numbers, Ronald L., Prophet of Health, Knoxville: The University of Tennessee, 1992.

Odumuyiwa, E. Ade, God: The Contemporary Discussion, Ilorin: Decency Printers and Stationaries Ltd., 2005.

Ojo, J. O., Understanding West African Traditional Religion, Ile-Ife: S. C. Popoola Printers, 1999.

Ojo, Afolabi G. J., Yoruba Culture: A Geographical Analysis, London: University of London Press. 1966.

Okezie, Goodluck N., My Terminal Project Work, Lagos: Emaphine Reprographics Ltd., 2002.

Olaniyan, Richard, Nigerian History and Culture, London: Longman, 1988.

Olapade, Ebenezer O., ed., Traditional Medicine in Nigeria, Toyin Okebunmi Printers, 1998.

Oluikpe, Benson, Thesis Writing: Its Form and Style, Onitsha: Africana Publishing Limited, 1982.

Omoyajowo, Akinyele, Religion, Society and Religion, Ijebu-Ide: Vicoo International Press, 2001.

Onasanya, S. A. and A. T. Oduyale, Historical Foundation of Ilishan Town, Shagamu: Ojoko-Biri-Kale Press, nd.

Osuala, E. C., Introduction to Research Methodology, Ibadan: Africana-Fep Publishers, 1993.

Owoeye, Jide, ed., Research Design and Methodology, Ibadan: College Press and Publishers, 1999.

Pamplona-Roger, George, New Lifestyle: Enjoy It: Food for Healing and Prevention, Madrid: Editorial Safeliz, 1998.

_____ Encyclopedia of Medicinal Plants, Spain: Editorial Safeliz, 1999.

Parrinder, Geoffery, Religion in an African City, Westport, Connecticult: Negro University Press, 1953.

_____ West African Religion, London: Epworth Press, 1949.

_____ African Traditional Religion, London: Sheldon Press, 1954.

_____ Africa's Three Religions, London: Sheldon Press, 1969.

Platvoet, Jan James Cox and Jacob Olupona, (eds.), The Study of Religions on Africa Past, Present and Prospects, Cambridge: Roots and Branches, 1996

Ray, Benjamin C., African Religion, New Jersey: Prentice-Hall, Inc., 1976.

Rebok, Deuton Edward, Our Firm Foundation, vol. 11, Washinton, DC: Review and Herald Publishing Association, 1953.

Ridgeon, Lyoyd, Major World Religion-From Their Origins to the Present, London: Routledge Curzor, 2003.

Robinson, D. E., The Story of Our Health Message, Nashville, Tennessee: Southern Publishing Association, 1965.

Simpson, E. George, Yoruba Religion and Medicine in Ibadan, Ibadan University Press, 1980.

Sofowora, Abayomi, ed., Medicinal Plants and Traditional Medicine in Africa, Ibadan: Spectrum Books, 1993.

Soriyan, John Olubanjo, A Comprehensive History of Saint Saviour's (Angelican) Church Ikenne Remo (1898-1986): A Short History of Remoland-Earliest time to Present Day, Ibadan: African Press Limited, 1986.

_____ ed., Antihypertensive Agents from Natural Sources, Ile-Ife: University of Ife Press, 1979.

Salau, T. I., Introduction to Research Methodology, Ilaro: Limbs Press, 1998.

Sawyer, Harry, God, Ancestor or Creator?, London: Longmans Group, 1970.

Scade, John, Cereals, London: Oxford University Press, 1975.

Schuller, Robert, Tough Times Never Last—Tough People Do, Ibadan: Oluseyi Press, 1983.

Schwarz, Richard W., Light Bearers to the Remnant, Ontario: Pacific Press Publishing Association, 1953.

Shryock, Harold, Highways to Health, Washington DC: Review and Herald Publishing Association, 1954.

Smith, Edwin W., African Ideas of God, London: Edinburg House Press, 1966.

Spalding, Arthur W., Origin and the History of the Seventh-day Adventists, vol. 1, Washington DC: Review and Herald Publishing Association, 1960.

Stein, Daine, All Women Are Healers: A Comprehensive Guide to Natural Healing, California: The Crossing Press, 1990.

Sutherland, Stewart, Leslie Houldon, Peter Clarke and Friendhe Hardy, The World's Religions, Boston: G. K. Hall and Co., 1988.

Taryor, Nya Kwainon St., Impact of African Tradition on African Christianity, Chicago: The Strugglers Community Press, 1984.

Tilden, J. H., Food: Its Influences as a Factor in Disease and Health, Connecticut: Keats Publishing, Inc., 1976.

Timmreck, Thomas C., Dictionary of Health Services Management, MD: FrRynd Communications, 1987.

Tkai, Debora, ed., The Doctors Book of Home Remedies: Thousands of Tips And Techniques, Pennsylvania: Rodale Press, 1998.

Turaki, Yusufu, Foundation of African Traditional Religions and Worldview, Enugu: International Bible Society, 2001.

Turner, H. W., History of an African Independent Church: Church of the Lord Aladura, Oxford: The Clarendon Press, 1967.

Ubrurhe, John Oroshejide, Urohbo Traditional Medicine, Ibadan: Oputoru Books, 2001.

Van, Dalen, Understanding Educational Research, New York: Mac-Graw-Hill, 1979.

Van-Dolson, Leo R and R. Spangler, eds., Health, Happy, Holy, Washington, DC: Review and Herald Publishing Association, 1975.

Venden, M. I. Faith That Works, Washington DC: Review and Herald Publishing Association, 1980.

Warner, Richard, Morality in Medicine: An Introduction to Medical Ethics, California: Alfred Publishers Co., Inc., 1984.

White, Ellen G. A Call to Medical Evangelism and Health Education, Tennessee: Southern Publishing Association, 1954.

_____ Counsels on Health, Ontario: Pacific Press Publishing Association, 1954.

_____ Evangelism, Washington DC: Review and Herald Publishing Association, 1974.

_____ Healthful Living, California: Northwestern Publishing Association, 1982.

_____ Manuscript Releases, Vol. 1-21, Washington, DC: Review and Herald Publishing Association, 1981.

_____ Medical Ministry, Ontario: Pacific Press Publishing Association, 1992.

_____ Messages to Young People, Washington, DC: Review and Herald Publishing Association, 1958.

_____ Selected Messages, Book 2. Washington DC: Review and Herald Publishing Association, 1958.

_____ Temperance, Mountain View, California: 1949.

_____ Testimonies on Sexual Behaviour, Adultery, and Divorce, Maryland: The Ellen White Estate: Pacific Press Publishing Association, 1989.

_____ Testimonies for the Church, vols. 1-9, Ontario: Pacific Press Publishing Association, 1942.

_____ The Desire of Ages, Ontario: Pacific Press Publishing Association, 1993.

_____ The Ministry of Healing, Ontario: Pacific Press Publishing Association, 1942.

_____ The Story of Prophets and Kings, Ontario: Pacific Press Publishing Association. 1993.

_____ The Story of Patriarchs and Prophets, Ontario: Pacific Press Publishing Association, 1993.

_____ True Education, Idaho: Pacific Press Publishing Association, 2000.

Wills, Richard J. B., A-Z of Health, Liconshire: The Stanborough Press, 2003.

_____ The Kellogg Imperative, Linconshire: The Stanborough Press, 2000.

Wotogho-Weneka, Wellington O., ed., Religion and Spirituality, Port Harcourt: Emhai Printing and Publishing Company, 2001.

Woodhead, Linda, Religion in Modern World, London: Routledge, 2002.

Yandell, Keith E., Philosophy of Religion. A Contemporary Introduction, London: Routledge, 1999.

B. JOURNAL ARTICLES

Agbedahunsi, J. M. "Plant Utilization in Indigenous Medical System" in Africana Marburgensia, XXVI, 1+2 1993.

Agbaje, Bode. "Incantations as a Means of Healing in Yorubaland" in Africana Marburgensia, XXVI, 1+2 1993.

Akpan, Enomfon J. "Current Trends in Natural Pathy" in Traditional Medicine in Nigeria, Ibadan: Toyin Okebunmi Printers, 1998.

Alvares, Claude. "Genetically Modified Crops-Greed on Need?" Footsteps, Middlesex: Tearfund, 2001

Anamed, Schafweide. "Natural Remedies" in Footsteps, Middlesex: Tearfund, 2001.

Babalola, Elisha O. "The Persistence of African Traditional Medicine in Contemporary Nigerian Society" in Africana Marburgensia XXVI, 1+2 1993.

_____ Medical Dialogue Between Orthodox and Traditional Healers: The Complete Solution to Basic Medical Problems in the Nigerian Community" being a research proposal submitted to the National Universities Commission, Abuja, 2003.

_____ "The Concept of (Ofo) Incantation As An Aspect of Traditional Medicine in Yorubaland" Department of Religious Studies, Obafemi Awolowo University, Ile-Ife, Nigeria, 2002.

_____ "African Traditional Medicine as an Important Factor of Social Integration in Yorubaland" a paper presented at the 23rd Annual NASR Conference held at Benue State University, Markurdi, Nigeria, October 14-18, 2002.

_____ "The Scientific Basis of African Traditional Medicine: The Yoruba Example" Department of Religious Studies, Obafemi Awolowo University, Ile-Ife, November, 2002.

_____ "The Relevance of Herbal Medicine to the Practice of African Traditional Religion, Islam and Christianity in Yorubaland" Department of Religious Studies, Obafemi Awolowo University, 2002.

_____ "Clinical Management of Coronary Heart Disease with the use of Herbal Medicine and Food Therapy: A Contemporary Analysis" Department of Religious Studies, Obafemi Awolowo Universities, Ile-Ife, Nigeria, 2003.

Baldwin Martha B. "Toads and Plague: The Amulet Controversy in Seventh- century Medicine" in <u>Bulletin of the History of Medicine</u>. The American Association for the History of Medicine, Grieger GErt & Jerome J. Bylebyl, eds., Maryland: The Johns Hopkins University Press, 1993.

Carter Isabel. "Production of Traditional Medicine", Footsteps", Middlesex: Tearfund Press, 2001.

Dickson Trudi. "Improving Biochemistry at Local Level" in Footsteps, Middlesex: Tearfund, 2001.

Dopamu, P. Ade, "Scientific Basis of African Magic and Medicine: The Yoruba Experience" in Workshop Reader on African Culture, Modern Science and Religious Thought held at the University of Ilorin, Nigeria in collaboration with the Center for Theology and Natural Sciences, Bekeley, California, USA, October 19-24, 2001.

_____ "Yoruba Magic and Medicine and Their Relevance for Today" in <u>RELIGIONS</u>: Journal of the Nigerian Association for the Study of Religions, vol. 4, 1979.

_____ "Religion and Health Among the Traditional Yoruba" in <u>ORITA:</u> Ibadan: Journal of Religious Studies, vol. XXIV/1-2, June & December, 1992.

_____ "Health and Healing Within the Traditional African Religious Context" in "<u>ORITA</u>" Ibadan: Journal of Religious Studies, Vol. XVII/2, December 1985.

Elujoba, A. A. Laxative Activity of Africana Carsia Species with Reference to Senna in <u>Traditional Medicine in Nigeria</u>, Ibadan: Toyin Okebunmi Printers, 1998.

Hall, Avice, "Farmers' Question About Bio-diversity and GM Crops" in Footsteps. Middlesex: Tearfund, 2001.

Hirt, D. M. & Keith Lindsay, (eds.), "Natural Medicine" in Footsteps. Middlesex: Tearfund, 2001.

Igwillo, C. I., "Traditional Medicine-Dosages and Norms. Belief Systems" in <u>Traditional Medicine in Nigeria</u>, Ibadan: Toyin Okebunmi Printers, 1998.

Ikenga-Metuh, E., "African Traditional Medicine and Healing: A Theological and Pastoral Appraisal" in <u>West African Association</u>

of Theological Institutions Proceedings of WAATI Conference in 1982 and 1983.

Kafaru, Elizabeth, "Application of Dosages and Norms in the Nigeria Traditional Healing Methods" Traditional Medicine in Nigeria, Ibadan: Toyin Okebunmi Printers, 1998.

Komolafe, Kolawole, "Curative Claims and Norms of Traditional Healers in Nigeria" in Traditional Medicine in Nigeria, Ibadan: Toyin Okebunmi Printers, 1998.

Lambo J. O. "Management of Hypertension in Traditional Medicine" in Antihyptertensive Agents from Natural Sources, Ile-Ife: University of Ife Press, 1975.

Lindsay, Keith and H. Hirt, eds., "Medicinal Gardens" in Footsteps. Middlesex: Tearfund, 2001.

Mabadeje, A. F. B. "The Scientific Basis of Traditional Medicine: What Hope for Standardization of Dosages in Nigeria", Traditional Medicine in Nigeria, Ibadan: Toyin Okebunmi Printers, 1998.

Marquis, V. O., "Experimental Pharmacology of some Antihypertensives from Nigerian Medicinal Plants" in Antihypetensive Agents from Natural Sources, Ile-Ife: University of Ife Press, 1975.

Mitchell, Harvey and Samuel S. Kottek, "An Eighteenth-Century Medical View of the Diseases of the Jews in Northeastern France: Medical Anthropology and the Politics of Jewish Emancipation" in Bulletin of the History of Religion—The American Association for the History of Medicine, Brieger, Gert & Jerome, J. Bylebyl, eds, Maryland: The John Hopkins University Press, 1993.

Muller, Markus and Innocent Balagiz, eds., "Traditional and Modern Medicine: The Need for Co-operation" in Footsteps. Middlesex: Tearfund, 2001.

Nasekwa, Mwakamubaya, "Promoting Public Health Among Displaced People" in Footsteps, Middlesex: Tearfund, 2001.

Nkwoka, A. O., "Healing: The Biblical Perspective" in Africana Marburgensia, XXVI, 1+2 1993.

Ogunkoya, L. and O. O. Olubajo, "Chemistry of Some Plants with Hypotensive Properties" in Antihypertensive Agents from Natural Sources, Ile-Ife: University of Ife Press, 1975.

Opefeyintimi, A., "Healing in Traditional Yoruba Religion" in Africana Marburgensia, XXVI,1+2, 1993.

Opeola, S. Modupeola, "Ifa Divination and Healing" in Africana Marburgensia, XXVI, 1+2, 1993.

Poole, Nigel. "Neem: Who Owns It?" Traditional Property Rights and Biopiracy" in Footsteps. Middlesex: Tearfund, 2001.

Prance, Ghillean, "Caring for Life on Earth" in Footsteps, Middlesex: Tearfund, 2001.

Shode, O. O., "Understanding Nigeria's Medicinal Plants as a Source of Nature's Medicine" in Traditional Medicine in Nigeria. Ibadan: Toyin Okebunmi Printers, 1998.

Simbard, Rene Gayuna, "Working with Traditional Medicines" in Footsteps. Middlesex: Tearfund, 2001.

Soung, B and Hang Sorya, "Traditional Practices in Childbirth" in Footsteps. Middlesex: Tearfund, 2001.

Wambebe, C. O., "Preliminary Evaluations of Local Herbal Medicinal Preparation. NIPRD 94/006/1-2) for the Management of HIV/AIDS" in Traditional Medicine in Nigeria, Ibadan: Toyin Okebunmi Printers, 1998

C. ENCYCLOPEDIA

Cayne Bernard S., ed., <u>The Encyclopedia Americana</u>, ed., Vols, 13 & 18, New York: Americana Corporation, 1977.

Don. F. Neufield, ed., <u>Seventh-day Adventist Encyclopedia</u>, vol. 10, Washington, DC: Review and Herald Publishing Association, 1976.

Halsy William D. & Bernard Johnston, eds., <u>Collier Encyclopedia</u>, vols. 11 & 15. London: Macmillan Educational Company, 1988.

Wuthnow Robert, ed.,<u>The Encyclopedia of Politics and Religion</u>, vols. 1 & 2. London: Routledge, 1998.

D. DICTIONARIES

Allen, Robert and Catherine Schwarz, eds., <u>The Chambers Dictionary</u>, Edinburgh: Chambers Harrap Publishers, 2002.

Don, F. Neufield, ed., <u>Seventh-day Adventist Bible Commentary</u>, Washington D.C: Review and Herald Publishing Association, 1979.

Metcalf, Jonathan, ed., <u>Illustrated Oxford Dictionary</u>, New York: Oxford University Press, 1998.

Mish, Fredrick C. ed., <u>Webster's Ninth New Collegiate Dictionary</u>, Ontario: Thomas Allen & Sons Limited, 1991.

E. COMMENTARIES

Clarke, Adams, Clarke's Commentary, Cincinnati: Applegate Pounds ford & Co., 1810.

Henry, Matthew, Matthew Henry's Commentary on the Whole Bible, Michigan: Zondervan Publishing House, 1961.

Nichol, Francis D., The Seventh-day Adventist Bible Commentary, Washington, DC: Review and Herald Publishing Association, 1978.

Spence, H. D.M. ed., The Pulpit Commentary, London: Funk & Wagnall Company, nd.

Torrance, David W. ed., Calvin's Commentary, Michigan: Wm. Eerdmans Publishing Company, 1959.

F. UNPUBLISHED MATERIALS

DISSERTATIONS

Babalola, David O. "The Seventh-day Adventist Church in Yorubaland-Nigeria (1914-1984)" P.hD Thesis, University of Ibadan, Nigeria, 1988.

Babalola, Elisha Oladele, "Abiku Concept Among The Owo (Yoruba) Community of Ondo State, Nigeria: A Socio-Religious Approach" P.hD Thesis, Department of Religious Studies, Obafemi Awolowo University, Ile-Ife, Nigeria, 1987.

Burt, Merlin D, "The Historical Background, Interconnected Development and Integration of the Doctrines of the Sanctuary, The Sabbath, and Ellen G. White's role in Sabbatarian Adventism from 1844 to 1849" P.hD Thesis, Andrews University, Michigan, United States of America, 2002.

Kuranga, Abraham Akanbi, "The Seventh-day Adventism in Western Nigeria, 1914-1981. A Study in the Relationship Between Christianity and African Culture from the Missionary Era to the Introduction of African Leadership" P.hD Thesis, The Graduate School, Miami University, United States of America, 1991.

Nyekwere, Dave M. "A Study of Medical Institutions of the Seventh-day Adventist Church in Southern Nigeria as an Instrument of Evangelization 1940-2000." Ph. D Dissertation, University of Port Harcourt, Nigeria, 2003

Olupona, Jacob Obafemi Kehinde, "A Phenomenological/ Anthropological Analysis of then Religion of the Ondo-Yoruba of Nigeria," P.hD Thesis, Graduate School, Boston University, United States of America, 1983.

Onibere, S. G. A., "The Concept of God Among the Isoko of Bendel State, Nigeria," P.hD. Thesis, University of Ife, 1982.

G. DAILIES

"65% of Nigerians Patronize Traditional Healers" Sunday Tribune, July 6, 2003.

"Alternative Remedies for Arthritis" The Guardian, January 13, 2000.

"Beneficial Effects of Sitz Baths" The Guardian, December 12, 1996.

"Combating Asthma Using Natural Remedies" The Guardian, November 4, 1999.

"Coping with Allergies", The Guardian, June 26.

"Ginger and Its Uses" The Guardian, July 25, 1996.

"Healing Properties of the Tropical Stinging Nettle" The Guardian, June 27, 1996.

"Many Uses of Carrot" The Guardian, March 28, 1996.

"Medicinal Values of Good Old Walnut and Garden Egg" The Guardian, August 19, 1999.

"Medicinal Values of Honey" The Guardian, January 6, 2000.

"Medicinal Values of Pal kernel Oil "The Guardian, September 9, 1999.

Nature's Answer to Kidney Diseases" The Guardian, March 26, 1998.

"The Different Uses of Medicinal Plants" The Guardian, July 11, 1996.

"The Different Uses of Garlic" The Guardian, January 16, 1997.

"The Healing Power of Vegetables (11)" The Guardian, October 17, 1996.

"The Many Uses of Onions" The Guardian, July 29, 1999.

"The Medicinal Uses of Cashew Tree" The Guardian, May 16, 1996.

"The Medicinal Values of Avocado Pear" The Guardian, May 23, 1996.

"Eat Right, Protect against breast Cancer" in the Guardian, Thursday, October 13, 2005.

"Eat beans, soy beans to beat lung cancer in the Guardian, Thursday October 6, 2005.

"How low calorie intake could affect life span premature birth" The Guardian, Tuesday, June 16, 2005.

"Natural tips to beat diabetes epidemic" The Guardian, June 2, 2005.

"African pear on Cure for skin, oral infection" The Guardian, Thursday, July 21, 2005.

The Guardian, August 11, 2005.

The Guardian, August 18, 2005

"Mango, pawpaw leaves effective against sleeping sickness" The Guardian, August 25, 2005.

"Bitter Kola Shows potential for managing glaucoma" The Guardian, September 8, 2005.

"Local herbal preparations maketh new conventional anti-malaria drugs" The Guardian, September 1, 2005.

"Restore sexual vitality, stabilizes nervous system, blood pressure with sesame" The Guardian, September 15, 2005.

"Crushed garlic, Aloe Vera show promise for severe gum disease" The Guardian, September 25, 2005.

"The Medicinal Values of Wild Lettuce" The Guardian, May 9, 1996.

"The Uses of Bitter Leaf" The Guardian, February 6, 1997.

"Understanding the Medicinal Values of Herbs" The Guardian, April 17, 1997.

"Unknown Medicinal Values of Little Ironwood", The Guardian, May 27, 1997.

"Urinary Tract Infection and the Treatment", Sunday Tribune, March 7, 2004.

H. INTERNET/WORLD WIDE WEB PAGES

http://www.infidels.org/library/modern/janet-brazill/religiondictates.html

http://nature.ac.uk/search.html?hub=biome&hublet=natural&steming=true&field . . .

http://www.anc.org.za/ancdoes/pubs/umrabul/umbrabula18/handbook.html

http://allafrica.com/stories/200311140802.html

http://www.mmegi.bw/2003/November/Wednesday19/344667161050.html

http://www.drgrotte.com/Africa%20Medicine.html

http://www.who.int/mediacentre/facetsheets/2003/fs134/cn/

http://www.who.int/inf-fs./cn/fact134.html

http://www.afro.who.int/press/2000/regionalcommittee/rc5005.html

http://www.llu.edu/inf/legacy/LegacyBhtml

http://www.aims-ministry.org/sge5.html

http://www.petspourri.com/herbs01.htm

http://www.coconut-connections.com/,

http://www.mercola.com/2001/mar/24/coconut-oil.htm

http://www.healthresearchforum.org.uk/sunlight.html

http://www.shirleys-wellness-café.com/sunabth.htm

http://www.gcrio.org/ozone/ozoneFAQs.html

http://www.laformechic.com/water.htm

http://www.bottledwaterblues.com/Better Drinking Habits.cfm

http://members.aol.com/SaveMoDoe2/importance.htm

http://www.hifit.co.uk/health-breaks/importance-exercise.htm

http://www.ihj.com/ihj/story.jhtml:sessionid=XBDTB5F1C224DQ
FIBQNSCZQ?storyid

http://www.laformechic.com/water.htm

http://www.bottledwaterblues.com/Better Drinking Habits.cfm

http://www.cpft.edu/ete/modules/waterq/wqwaterimport.html

http://www.pathlights.com/nr-encyclopedia/00print4c.htm

http://www.bcas.net/Env.Features/HumanHealth-
december2002/15%20to%2030.htm

http://www.rosary-center.org/1151n5.htm

http://www.hc-sc.gc.ca/hecs-sesc/air-quality/faq.htm

http://www.projectrestore.com/library/health/rest.htm

http://www.nisbett.com/egw/mol/Chapter28.html

http://www.bibleartistis.com/w-soap.htm

http://www.lff.net/about/issues/healingOT.htm

http://www.keymey.ca/htm20030221.htm

http://en.wikipedia.org/wiki/If%C3%A1

http://www.iyabo4senate.com/facts.html

APPENDICES

APPENDIX I

QUESTIONNAIRE ON AFRICAN TRADITIONAL MEDICINE AMONG SEVENTH-DAY ADVENTISTS

This is a research questionnaire designed to investigate the above topic. Your honest, precise and accurate response is highly solicited. You may avoid names or any elements that could lead to identification. All information in this questionnaire will be treated confidentially. Thanks

SECTION 1: DEMOGRAPHIC INFORMATION

(Tick ☐ the appropriate answer and complete the spaces provided below

1. Please indicate your gender   Male ☐   Female ☐

2. Age   (a) 10-19 years   ☐
         (b) 20-29 years   ☐
         (c) 30-39 years   ☐
         (d) above 40 years.   ☐

3. _____ Ethnic Group

4. _____ Nationality

5. Educational Status:
   (a) Primary ☐
   (b) Secondary ☐
   (c) Post Secondary ☐
   (d) Other ☐

6. Marital Status:
   (a) Single ☐
   (b) Married ☐
   (c) Widow ☐
   (d) Divorced/ Separated ☐
   (e) Other ☐

7. What was your religious affiliation before you become a Seventh-day Adventist member:
   (a) Christian ☐
   (b) Muslim ☐
   (c) African Religion ☐
   (d) Another Religion (Specify) ☐

8. How long have you been a Seventh-day Adventist adherent?
   (a) 0-12 months ☐
   (b) 1-10 years ☐
   (c) 11-20 years ☐
   (d) Above 20 years ☐

SECTION II. IMPACT OF TRADITIONAL MEDICINE ON SDAs

9. Apart from orthodox medication, have you ever received healing from any alternative traditional method for any sickness in the past?
   (a) Yes ☐
   (b) No ☐

10. Where did you get that medication when you were sick?
    (a) Chemist's shop ☐
    (b) Herbal/ Traditional Medicine Dealer ☐
    (c) Self Help ☐
    (d) Another Method (Specify) ☐

11. If your answer to No. 10 question above is "b", why did you seek for Herbal or Traditional Medicine when you were sick?
    (a) It is affordable ☐
    (b) It is available ☐
    (c) It is more effective ☐
    (d) Another reason ☐

12. What motivated you to go for Herbal/ Traditional Medication?
    (a) My sickness defied orthodox medication ☐
    (b) Someone persuaded me to try traditional medicine ☐
    (c) My family member usually get cured with herbal medicine ☐
    (d) Another Reason (specify)_____ ☐

13. In what part of your body did you have the ill-health that led you to the traditional healer
    (a) Head ☐
    (b) Limbs ☐
    (c) Visceral organs ☐
    (d) Others (specify)_____ ☐

14. In what form did you receive your traditional medicine?
    (Tick as many as are applicable
    (a) Liquid ☐   (b) Gaseous ☐
    (c) Powder ☐   (d) Solid ☐
    (e) Poultice ☐   (f) Roots ☐
    (g) Rhizomes ☐   (h) Bark ☐
    (i) Leaves ☐

15. How long have you used traditional medicine?
    (a) 1-12 months ☐
    (b) 1-10 years ☐
    (c) 11-20 years ☐
    (d) 21 years and above ☐

16. How often do you use traditional medicine?
    (a) Daily ☐
    (b) Weekly ☐
    (c) Monthly ☐
    (d) As the need arises ☐

17. What is the nature of the sickness/ ill-health?
    (a) Child bearing/ pregnancy ☐
    (b) Accident induced ☐
    (c) Bone Setting ☐
    (d) Hypertension ☐
    (e) Jaundice ☐
    (f) Mystic ☐
    (g) Swelling ☐
    (h) Headache ☐
    (i) Blood related ☐
    (j) Psychological ☐
    (k) Others ☐

18. In your own opinion, what do you consider to be a better way of treating diseases that tend to defy orthodox medication
    (a) By praying and fasting in a religious environment ☐
    (b) By applying traditional medication ☐
    (c) Combing orthodox and traditional medicines ☐
    (d) Any other (specify)_____ ☐

19. Does the Seventh-day Adventist Church support the use of traditional medicine as a way of healing its members?
    (a) Yes ☐
    (b) No ☐
    (c) I Do not Know ☐

20. If your answer to No. 19 above is "yes", indicate three ways by which the Seventh-day Adventist Church does this?
    (a) Natural Therapy ☐
    (b) Herbs/ Leaves ☐
    (c) Feeding Habits ☐
    (d) Economic ☐

21. If your answer in No 19 above is "No", why do you think the SDA Church does not encourage her members to embrace traditional medical practice?
    (a) Idolatrous practice ☐
    (b) Mystic ☐
    (c) Unrefined ☐
    (d) Incantations ☐
    (e) Alcohol Mixture ☐
    (f) Sacrifice ☐
    (g) Any other ☐

22. In your opinion, is herbal or traditional medicine practice biblical?
    (a) Yes ☐
    (b) No ☐
    (c) I do not know ☐

23. If your answer to question No. 22 above is yes, could you supply some examples from the Bible?
    (a) _____
    (b) _____
    (c) _____

24. Who introduced you to the use of traditional medicine?
    (a) Your Spouse ☐
    (b) Your Friend ☐
    (c) Fellow Church Member ☐
    (d) Medical Personnel (by referral) ☐
    (e) A Co-worker ☐
    (f) Co-resident ☐
    (g) Divine Inspiration ☐
    (h) others _____

25. Do you know of any case or cases where orthodox medicine could not help someone to recover from a particular sickness whereas traditional medicine was used to save/heal such a person?
    (a) Yes ☐
    (b) No ☐

26. If your answer to question No. 25 above is "Yes" briefly identify the nature of the sickness that led to the use of traditional medicine
    (a) Leprosy ☐
    (b) Diabetes ☐
    (c) Child Bearing ☐
    (d) Hypertension ☐
    (e) Bone Setting ☐
    (f) Mystic ☐
    (g) Oedema ☐
    (h) Jaundice ☐
    (i) Cancer ☐
    (j) Osteoporosis ☐

27. What time of the day do you normally go for your traditional medication or treatment?
    (a) Before dawn ☐
    (b) Before nightfall ☐
    (c) Anytime of the day ☐
    (d) At night ☐
    (e) Others ☐
    (f) Do not Know ☐

28. What are your reasons for going at the time specified in No. 27 above to collect your traditional medicine or treatment?
    _____
    _____

29. Do other church members know you were taking traditional medicine?
    (a) Yes ☐
    (b) No ☐
    (c) Do not Know ☐

30. What was the attitude of the Church members when they discovered?
    (a) They were surprised ☐
    (b) They were apprehensive ☐
    (c) They made negative comments ☐
    (d) They were indifferent ☐
    (e) Do not Know ☐
    (f) Another ☐

31. What was the attitude of your pastor when he learnt you were taking traditional medication?
    (a) He was surprised ☐
    (b) He was apprehensive ☐
    (c) He made negative comments ☐
    (d) He was indifferent ☐
    (e) Do not Know ☐
    (f) Another ☐

32. Has there been any education by the Church leadership on the importance of traditional medicine in your local congregation?
    (a) Yes ☐
    (b) No ☐
    (c) Do not Know ☐

33. Has the Seventh-day Adventist Church ever disciplined any member of your congregation as a result of using traditional medicine?
    (a) Yes ☐
    (b) No ☐
    (c) Do not Know ☐

34. Has the practice of traditional medicine made any impact in your life?
    (a) Yes ☐
    (b) No ☐

35. Mention some of the impacts which traditional medical practice has made in your life?
    (a) _____
    (b) _____
    (c) _____

36. What notable impacts have traditional medical practice made on your family?
    (a) _____
    (b) _____
    (c) _____

37. List some impacts which the practice of traditional medicine have made on the members of your church?
    (a) _____
    (b) _____
    (c) _____

38. To what extent do you think one can go in the use of traditional medicine?
    _____
    _____
    _____

39. Are there some evils/ dangers in the use of traditional medicine?
    (a) Yes ☐
    (b) No   ☐
    (c) Do not Know ☐

40. If your answer to 39 above is "Yes" mention two of such dangers?
    (a) Unbiblical ☐
    (b) No Dosage ☐
    (c) Ignorance ☐
    (d) No Expiry date ☐
    (e) Idolatrous ☐
    (f) Unhygienic ☐

41. What are the reasons some of your Seventh-day Adventist friends (if there are any) do not like to practice traditional medicine?
    _____
    _____
    _____

NOTE: Questions without responses are adjudged "Do not Know"

APPENDIX II

INTERVIEW QUESTIONS

SECTION A:

Please Sir/Madam, may I know:

1. Your name _____
2. Your address_____
3. Your occupation_____
4. Length of time at present occupation_____
5. Your age _____ Gender _____
6. Your denomination_____
7. Duties performed in the Church_____

SECTION B:

1. What do you understand by African traditional medicine?
2. What materials are used in this type of medical practice?
3. Who introduced you to African traditional medicine?
4. Are there some benefits one can derive from the use of African traditional medicine?
5. Are there some dangers that you have discovered in the practice and use of this medicine?

6. Mention some of such dangers
7. Comparing the traditional with the modern ways of medication, which is a better way of treating diseases that affect humanity?
8. Have you ever referred any patient to a traditional medical healer? (Question for modern medical workers)
9. Has any patient been referred to you from any modern medical worker or hospital? (Question for traditional healers)
10. What was the nature of the sickness referred to you?
11. What is your opinion on the combination of African traditional medicine and modern ways of healing to achieve complete health for man?

APPENDIX III

LETTER OF PERMISSION TO DISTRIBUTE RESEARCH QUESTIONNAIRES

January 13, 2003

The Executive Committee,
South West Nigeria Conference of Seventh-day Adventists,
Akure,
Ondo State.

My Dear God's People,

REQUEST FOR PERMISSION TO DISTRIBUTE RESEARCH QUESTIONNAIRES AMONG SEVENTH-DAY ADVENTIST CHURCH MEMBERSHIP IN REMOLAND

Greetings in the name of the LORD.

I write to request for permission to distribute my research questionnaires among all Seventh-day Adventists in Remoland of Ogun State. I am currently carrying out a research titled: AFRICAN TRADITIONAL MEDICINE AMONG SEVENTH-DAY

ADVENTISTS. The information collected would be used for academic purposes only.

Please, kindly communicate your response to me by the end of April, 2003.

Thanks and God bless you abundantly.

Sincerely Yours

Philemon O. Amanze

APPENDIX IV

A LETTER REQUESTING FOR CHURCH MEMBERSHIP IN REMOLAND

January 13, 2003

The Executive Committee,
South West Nigeria Conference of Seventh-day Adventists,
Akure,
Ondo State.

My Dear God's People,

REQUEST FOR CHURCH MEMBERSHIP IN REMOLAND

Greetings in the name of the LORD.

I write to request that the membership of all Seventh-day Adventist Churches in Remoland of Ogun State be made available to me to facilitate the work I am currently doing titled: AFRICAN TRADITIONAL MEDICINE AMONG SEVENTH-DAY ADVENTISTS. Specifically, I will need the membership of the following:

A. Baptized membership in Remoland
B. Sabbath School membership in Remoland
C. Membership for the Adventist Youth, Men and Women's Ministries Departments.

Please, kindly make this information available to me by the end of April, 2003.

Thanks and God bless you abundantly.

Sincerely Yours

Philemon O. Amanze

FIG. LXIV MAP OF NIGERIA SHOWING YORUBA SPEAKING AREA

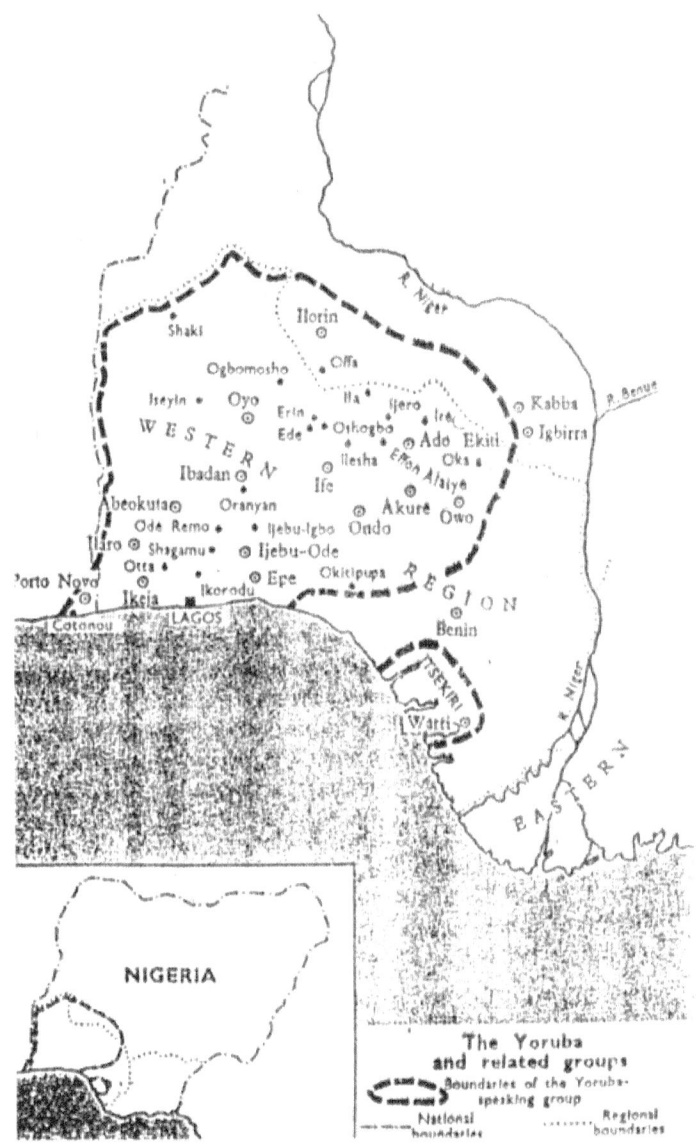

FIG. LXV MAP OF NIGERIA SHOWING ALL THE STATES INCLUDING OGUN WHERE THE STUDY WAS MADE

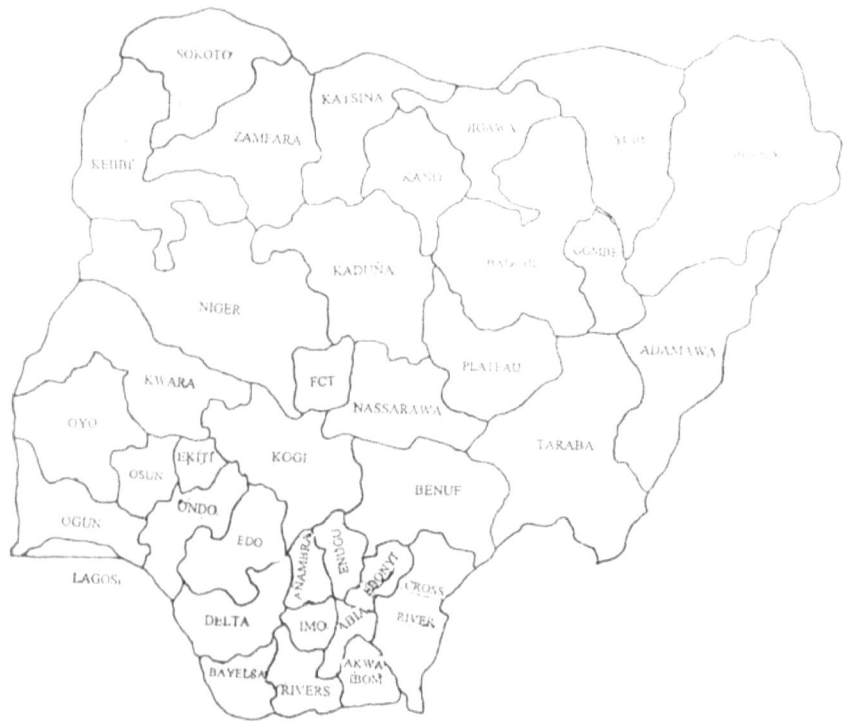

FIG. LXVI MAP OF OGUN STATE SHOWING DIFFERENT SECTIONS OF REMOLAND

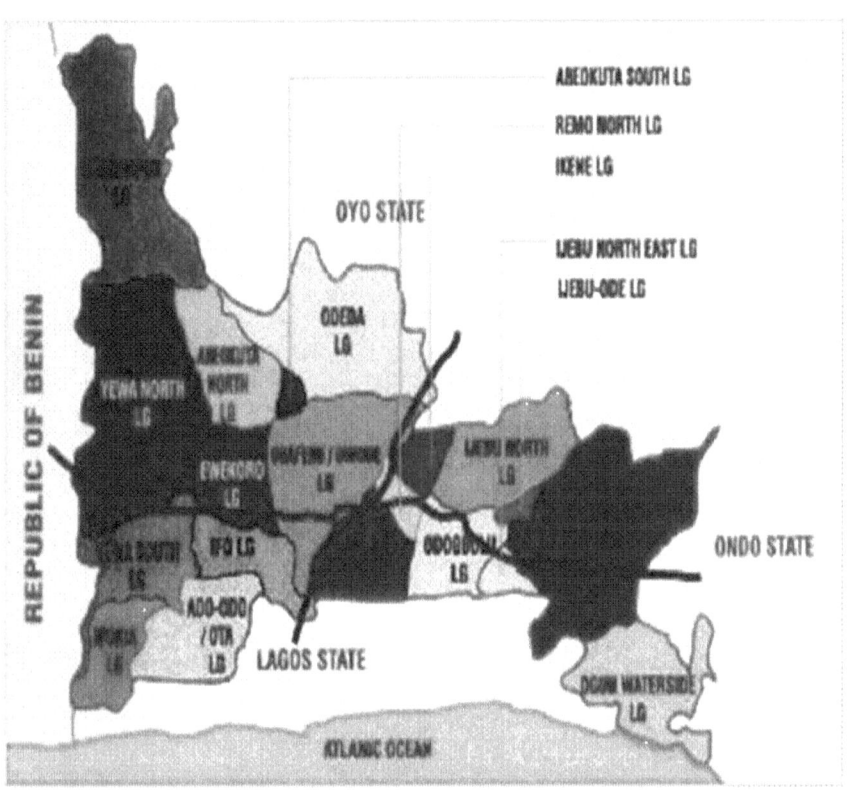

Source: http://www.iyabo4senate.com/facts.html

www.ingramcontent.com/pod-product-compliance
Lightning Source LLC
Chambersburg PA
CBHW031813170526
45157CB00001B/46